Updates in Hypertension and Cardiovascular Protection

Series Editors
Giuseppe Mancia, Milan, Italy
Enrico Agabiti-Rosei, Brescia, Italy

The aim of this series is to provide informative updates on both the knowledge and the clinical management of a disease that, if uncontrolled, can very seriously damage the human body and is still among the leading causes of death worldwide. Although hypertension is associated mainly with cardiovascular, endocrine, and renal disorders, it is highly relevant to a wide range of medical specialties and fields – from family medicine to physiology, genetics, and pharmacology. The topics addressed by volumes in the series *Updates in Hypertension and Cardiovascular Protection* have been selected for their broad significance and will be of interest to all who are involved with this disease, whether residents, fellows, practitioners, or researchers.

Pantelis Sarafidis • Roberto Pontremoli
Editors

Hypertension and Chronic Kidney Disease

Springer

Editors
Pantelis Sarafidis
1st Department of Nephrology
Aristotle University of Thessaloniki,
Hippokration Hospital
Thessaloniki, Greece

Roberto Pontremoli
University of Genoa Medical School and
Internal Medicine Unit
IRCCS Azienda Ospedaliera Metropolitana
Genova, Genova, Italy

ISSN 2366-4606 ISSN 2366-4614 (electronic)
Updates in Hypertension and Cardiovascular Protection
ISBN 978-3-032-29563-7 ISBN 978-3-032-29564-4 (eBook)
https://doi.org/10.1007/978-3-032-29564-4

This Springer imprint is published by the registered company Springer Nature Switzerland AG
The registered company address is: Gewerbestrasse 11, 6330 Cham, Switzerland

Contents

Hypertension in Chronic Kidney Disease: Epidemiology Basics (Prevalence, Association with TOD and Outcomes)

Lucia Del Vecchio, Stefania Comolli, Olga Balafa, and Leano Violo

Introduction

Hypertension is a common and clinically significant feature of chronic kidney disease (CKD), affecting the majority of patients across all stages of renal impairment.

In CKD, hypertension has also additional challenges, influencing outcome risk and treatment response. It is well known that non-dipping and nocturnal hypertension are highly prevalent in CKD. Moreover, a significant percentage of CKD patients meets the definition of resistant hypertension [1].

Prevalence of Hypertension in Chronic Kidney Disease

Hypertension prevalence in CKD ranges between 60% and 90%. In the Chronic Renal Insufficiency Cohort (CRIC), which included patients with an estimated glomerular filtration rate (eGFR) of 20–70 ml/min/1.73 m^2, approximately 90% had blood pressure >140/90 mmHg [2]. Similarly, data from the United States Renal Data System (USRDS) showed that hypertension affects a progressively greater percentage of patients with advancing CKD stages (23.3% in patients without CKD, 35.8% in stage 1, 48.1% in stage 2, 59.9% in stage 3, 84.1% in stages 4–5 CKD) [3].

L. Del Vecchio (✉) · L. Violo
Department of Nephrology and Dialysis, Sant'Anna Hospital, ASST Lariana, Como, Italy
e-mail: lucia.delvecchio@asst-lariana.it; Leano.violo@asst-lariana.it

S. Comolli
Department of Nephrology and Dialysis, ASST Sette Laghi, Varese, Italy
e-mail: Stefania.comolli@asst-settelaghi.it

O. Balafa
Department of Nephrology, General Hospital "G. Hatzikosta", Ioannina, Greece
e-mail: olgabalafa@gmail.com

P. Sarafidis, R. Pontremoli (eds.), *Hypertension and Chronic Kidney Disease*, Updates in Hypertension and Cardiovascular Protection,
https://doi.org/10.1007/978-3-032-29564-4_1

As expected, the prevalence of hypertension among individuals with CKD increases with advancing age. The Irish Longitudinal Study on Ageing (TILDA) showed that hypertension was present in over 80% of adults with CKD older than 50 years old compared to 60% in those without the disease, with an age gradient with increasing prevalence for older age (87.1% among those aged 75 years and older) [4].

The etiology of CKD influences the prevalence of hypertension. According to data from the Global Burden of Disease (GBD) study, the global prevalence of CKD attributed to hypertension, in 2021, was more than 24 million subjects. In a study of 1921 patients with various renal diseases, the prevalence of hypertension was also high among those with polycystic kidney disease (74%), diabetic nephropathy (87%), and renovascular disease (93%) [5]. In the same study, the prevalence of hypertension was 54% in chronic glomerulonephritis and 62% in chronic pyelonephritis. Across all nephropathies studied, hypertension prevalence was higher in patients with renal insufficiency.

In a cohort of 288 patients with primary chronic glomerulonephritis, 23.3% had hypertension compared to 12.8% in a control group from the same study area. However, among patients with glomerulonephritis and preserved renal function, hypertension prevalence was similar to controls (12.7%). Hypertension was more common in patients with membranous glomerulonephritis (26%) and focal segmental glomerulosclerosis (30%) [6].

With reference to the grade renal impairment, the CRIC study showed that prevalence of hypertension progressively increases with the worsening of renal function: prevalence was 67% in the group with eGFR ≥60 ml/min, 88% in patients with eGFR 40–49 ml/min, and 92% with eGFR 30 ml/min/m^2 [7].

Hypertension prevalence among CKD patients varies significantly across racial and ethnic groups. The Modification of Diet in Renal Disease (MDRD) study showed a higher prevalence rate in Afro-Americans than in Caucasians (93% vs. 81%) [8]. Similarly, the CRIC study showed a higher prevalence of hypertension in Afro-Americans than in Caucasians (93% vs. 80%). Hispanic and South Asian populations show intermediate risk, whereas prevalence of hypertension in CKD among White and East Asian individuals is relatively lower but increasing, paralleling global demographic aging and urbanization.

Sex Disparities

There are limited data about sex disparities in hypertension in CKD. The mean office BP levels do not consistently differ between sexes and seem not to modify CKD progression [9, 10]. Interestingly, more women have adequate controlled BP in screening programs compared to men [11], but this can be attributed to social deprivation or gender inequities. Ambulatory BP measurements in CKD patients reveal a higher prevalence of masked and sustained hypertension, which is more strongly associated with CKD progression, cardiovascular events, and mortality compared to office BP [12, 13]. Regarding sex disparities in CKD, a Spanish study demonstrated that male sex was an independent factor for higher systolic BP variability [14]. A prospective Italian study [15] further highlighted sex differences in BP phenotypes with men presenting higher 24-h, daytime and nighttime BP compared to women. Although men showed higher risks of both end-stage kidney failure (ESKF) and death, these differences became statistically insignificant after adjustment for ambulatory BP control, implying that protective effects associated with controlled ambulatory BP do not differ between sexes in CKD. Finally in dialysis and transplantation, small studies show that ambulatory BP levels are higher in male than females [16, 17], while office BP levels are similar. So far, we have no data exploring the biological mechanisms, social factors, or clinical impacts of these differences.

Associations with Type 2 Diabetes, Obesity and Metabolic Syndrome

Type 2 diabetes mellitus (T2DM) and hypertension are major, frequently coexisting risk factors for CKD development and progression. These conditions act synergistically to accelerate renal damage and worsen cardiovascular outcomes. Hypertension is highly prevalent among patients with T2DM, while diabetes promotes hypertension through endothelial dysfunction, insulin resistance, and enhanced sympathetic nervous system activity. In the United States, 50–80% of individuals with T2DM have hypertension. This percentage markedly increases in the presence of CKD [18, 19]. As expected, the burden of hypertension increases as CKD progresses. Data coming from the United States Renal Data System (USRDS) show that the prevalence of hypertension in patients with T2DM increases from ~36% in CKD stage 1 to ~84% in more advanced CKD stages 4 and 5. Oppositely, epidemiological studies have shown that the coexistence of T2DM and hypertension markedly increases the risk of CKD itself [20, 21].

Obesity is highly represented in the CKD population, either with or without T2DM, especially in high-income countries [22]. It induces hypertension through increased renal sodium reabsorption mediated by kidney compression from adipose tissue, elevated sympathetic nerve activity, renin-angiotensin-aldosterone system activation, and leptin-driven neurohormonal dysregulation [23]. Commonly, obesity-induced hypertension occurs prior to CKD development and contributes to more rapid CKD progression.

Recently, a new definition of the strict intertwining between metabolic risk factors has been made, called cardiovascular-kidney-metabolic syndrome (CKM) [24]. This new entity recognizes the interconnected nature of cardiovascular disease, CKD, and metabolic disorders (such as diabetes, obesity, and metabolic syndrome), emphasizing how these conditions influence each other and share common risk factors and pathophysiological mechanisms. According to a recent prospective observational study, up to 40% of adults with essential hypertension have CKM at any stage, and 15% having CKM at the more advanced stages (3 and 4) [25]. As expected, patients with CKM stage 4 had significantly higher creatinine values

(2.51 ± 1.13 mg/dl) compared with the other stages. Although clinic BP measurements showed no differences, 24-h ambulatory BP monitoring (ABPM) revealed significantly higher SBP in CKM 4 patients (134.75 ± 21.7 mmHg) compared to CKM 1–3 groups (129.5–132.4 mmHg; $p < 0.05$). Additionally, CKM 4 patients had lower hypertension control rates than CKM 1 patients (19.2% vs. 33.3%; $p < 0.05$).

Hypertension and Target Organ Damage

Left Ventricular Hypertrophy and Heart Failure

Long-term hypertension can lead to anatomical and functional changes in the cardiovascular system such as left ventricular hypertrophy (LVH), left atrial dilation, left ventricular diastolic dysfunction, and mitral valve regurgitation.

LVH has been shown to be strictly associated with albuminuria [26, 27]. The two are independent and additive predictors of heart failure. This was confirmed by a secondary analysis of the SPRINT (systolic blood pressure intervention trial) [28]. Among 8511 participants followed for a median of 3.2 years, concurrent albuminuria and LVH conferred greater risk of acute decompensated heart failure (HR 4.95, 95% CI 3.22–7.62) than either condition alone (HR 2.04, 95% CI 1.39–3.00; HR 1.47, 95% CI 0.93–2.32) with significant additive interaction ($p = 0.01$).

The maladaptive changes occurring with LVH predispose to the development of arrhythmias and increase the risk by 3.4-fold for supraventricular arrhythmias and 2.8-fold for ventricular arrhythmias as reported by Chatterjee et al. [29]. These changes also increase the risk of sudden cardiac death by six to eight times in men and three times in women [30].

LVH is observed in 48–84% of pre-dialysis patients and up to 90% of hemodialysis patients [31–34].

Cerebrovascular System

Hypertension is an important risk factor for acute cerebrovascular events such as ischemic stroke, intracranial hemorrhage, and transient ischemic attack, but also for chronic brain damage that can lead to dementia [35]. It induces significant structural changes in the wall of cerebral microvessels that damage the structure, architecture, and function of the microvascular network and contribute to the genesis of cerebral microhemorrhages and lacunar infarcts [36]. In addition, hypertension can also cause lesions in the white matter with an increased risk of stroke and cognitive decline.

In severe cases of uncontrolled hypertension, brain involvement may manifest as hypertensive encephalopathy, observed in approximately 10% of patients with associated retinal abnormalities. Even in the absence of overt neurologic symptoms, magnetic resonance imaging may reveal posterior reversible encephalopathy syndrome (PRES) [37]. This condition often presents with altered consciousness, including delirium or slowed mental activity, and may progress to loss of consciousness. The most serious complications are cerebral hemorrhage and intracranial herniation.

CKD is an independent risk factor for the development of cerebrovascular events. As the glomerular filtration rate (GFR) decreases, the risk of stroke increases by three to seven times going from stage III to stage V of CKD. Albuminuria is also a risk factor for the development of stroke [38].

In patients with CKD, cerebrovascular events are attributed to a combination of traditional and non-traditional mechanisms. Among traditional factors, hypertension has an important role, together with diabetes, atrial fibrillation, heart failure, obesity, dyslipidemia, and carotid disease. Non-traditional factors related to CKD can also increase the risk of cerebrovascular events. The hemodialysis population has additional risk factors, including cerebral hypoperfusion, increased arterial stiffness, and heightened BP variability. Additionally, CKD is strongly associated with cerebral small vessel disease, characterized by white matter lesions, silent cerebral hemorrhages, enlarged perivascular spaces, and cerebral microbleeds.

Renal Damage

In the last 30 years, there has been a substantial increase of the number of incident cases of hypertension-induced CKD globally. This also applies to adolescents and young adults [39]. NHANES data from 1988 to 1994 demonstrated that hypertensive individuals had an eight-fold increased prevalence of elevated serum creatinine (9.1%) compared to normotensive participants [40]. According to USRDS, hypertension accounted for approximately 25% of CKD cases [41].

Hypertension is also an important mediator of CKD progression, with a clear association between higher BP values and faster progression rate [42]. Notably, the worsening in renal function correlated with BP even within the normotensive range [43]. The negative effect of high BP values is more evident for SBP than for diastolic BP (DBP) [44]. The Multiple Risk Factor Intervention Trial (MRFIT) gave important epidemiological insights into the relationship between BP and CKD progression [45]. The decline in renal function was significantly greater in individuals with elevated SBP and DBP, with patients having DBP ≥95 mmHg experiencing a progressive decline. More recently, the FROM-J (Frontier of Renal Outcome Modifications in Japan) showed that among DBP categories, only values ≥90 mmHg correlated with significantly worse renal outcomes. Another study of 2939 patients with advanced CKD (stages G3b-G5) from two international cohorts demonstrated a strong dose-dependent relationship between BP and kidney disease progression over a median follow-up of 4.7 years [46]. The decline of eGFR accelerated with increasing SBP, ranging from −1.20 ml/min/1.73 m^2/year in the lowest category to −2.48 ml/min/1.73 m^2/year in the highest. DBP demonstrated comparable associations with CKD progression.

Proteinuria is an indicator of early renal damage, and the degree of proteinuria correlates with disease progression. Each 1 mmHg increase in SBP was associated with a 3% increased risk of having microalbuminuria in hypertensive patients ($p = 0.04$) [47]. This means that a 10 mmHg increase in SBP roughly corresponds to a 30% higher odds of microalbuminuria. No relationship was found for DBP. Another large observational study found that higher SBP was associated with a 50% increased odds of albuminuria per 20 mmHg increment among patients with hypertension (OR 1.50, 95% CI 1.42–1.60) [48].

Retinal and Microvascular Damage

One of the most significant complications of microcirculatory damage in hypertension is hypertensive retinopathy, characterized by endothelial dysfunction and smooth muscle cell remodeling within retinal arterioles [49]. Although hypertensive retinopathy is often asymptomatic in its early stages, the progressive nature of retinal damage can lead to significant visual impairment. In advanced stages, complications such as retinal ischemia, hard exudates, and, in severe cases, damage to the optic nerve may occur, potentially resulting in irreversible vision loss.

The Keith-Wagner-Barker classification is based on fundoscopy and allow to distinguish four grades of hypertensive retinopathy [50]. Different studies found a correlation between the degree of hypertensive retinopathy and the worsening of GFR in CKD [51, 52]. In hemodialysis patients, hypertensive retinal changes are often overlooked. However, the presence of arteriosclerotic retinopathy may be associated with increased arterial stiffness and history of CVD [53].

Hypertension and Outcomes in Chronic Kidney Disease

Mortality Risk

As for the general population, in CKD high BP correlates strongly with increased all-cause mortality. Mortality attributable to hypertensive kidney disease has risen by 48% in the United States over the past quarter-century, with men and ethnic minorities facing disproportionately higher risks [54]. GBD analyses also identify hypertension as a primary driver of CKD mortality worldwide, particularly in geographic areas with elevated SBP prevalence [55].

Large epidemiological cohort studies show a strong, independent, and graded relationship between BP levels and mortality risk. A Spanish primary care cohort of CKD patients followed for more than 43,000 person-years revealed elevated mortality rates among individuals with hypertension, T2DM, or both conditions [20]. Patients with coexisting hypertension and T2DM exhibited the greatest mortality risk, indicating a synergistic effect. The CDC WONDER (Wide-ranging Online Data for Epidemiologic Research) database demonstrated a 48% rise in age-adjusted mortality rates attributed to hypertensive kidney disease from 1999 to 2023.

All-cause mortality risk increased in patients with SBP either <100 mmHg or >120 mmHg, with the strongest associations observed in those treated with antihypertensive medications. A 5-year retrospective analysis of older CKD patients demonstrated that SBP ≤130 mmHg significantly increased mortality risk (HR 1.22), while elevated SBP (≥160 mmHg) paradoxically showed minimal impact on survival (HR 1.06) [56]. This U-shaped or J-shaped mortality pattern, where both hypotension and severe hypertension increase risk, appears particularly pronounced in elderly CKD populations and those on antihypertensive therapy. In a large retrospective study of 651,749 CKD patients, the lowest mortality occurred with BP readings between 130–149 and 70–89 mmHg [57]. Conversely, extreme BP values (either very high or very low combinations) were associated with increased mortality risk.

Notably, patients with more advanced CKD demonstrate more pronounced J-curve relationships, particularly with BP <110/70 mmHg being a marker of higher mortality in older individuals.

Cardiovascular Outcomes

In a large prospective cohort involving 12,523 Chinese CKD patients, BP levels of ≥130/90 mmHg significantly predicted increased CV events [58]. SBP showed a direct linear relationship with cardiovascular events down to 90 mmHg. DBP exhibited a J-shaped cardiovascular risk pattern, except in individuals <60 years where the relationship was linear (p for interaction <0.001). CV risk increased significantly at BP ≥130/90 mmHg vs. 90–119/50–69 mmHg.

Older CKD patients (eGFR ≤60 ml/min/1.73 m^2) demonstrated increased CV hospitalization at both SBP extremes (≤130 mmHg: HR 1.10; ≥160 mmHg: HR 1.26). While SBP maintained linear associations with events to 90 mmHg, DBP patterns varied by age (J-shaped in elderly, linear in <60 years). Stroke risk followed a CKD-specific J-curve, with optimal outcomes at SBP < 125 mmHg.

A similar J-curve was observed between SBP levels and the risk of stroke in another cohort of elderly individuals with CKD [59]. Those with SBP below 125 mmHg demonstrated significantly better stroke-free survival compared to the 125–139 mmHg group, while stroke survival rates declined progressively at SBP levels exceeding 140 mmHg. This J-shaped relationship was not found in patients without CKD.

Another analysis of nearly 340,000 patients with newly diagnosed CKD confirmed age-dependent relationships between BP and clinical outcomes [60]. Systolic hypertension (>140 mmHg) significantly increased all major cardiovascular adverse events, and death. However, this relationship progressively weakened with advancing age. Furthermore, while SBP below 110 mmHg reduced cardiovascular and cerebrovascular events, it increased overall mortality, highlighting the complexity of the J-curve phenomenon in CKD. Isolated diastolic hypotension (<70 mmHg) proved to be a selective mortality predictor, showing no relationship with other cardiovascular endpoints.

Recent data also showed the importance not only of a single point measurement of BP but rather the SBP time-in-target range. According to a Korean nation-wide study of 193,289 patients with CKD who underwent at least two health checkups between 2012 and 2015, for those not taking antihypertensive medications, a lower time-in-target range of SBP within 110–130 mmHg was associated with a higher risk of CVD events [61].

End-Stage Kidney Failure

Hypertensive kidney disease is the second most frequent cause of dialysis worldwide. Large epidemiological data demonstrate a clear relationship between elevated BP and progression to ESKF. Back in the 90 s, the MRFIT documented a 22-fold increased risk of ESKF in patients with stage 4 hypertension compared to those with BP <120/80 mmHg, independent of baseline renal function, proteinuria, demographics, and comorbidities [62]. Analysis of Kaiser Permanente members without baseline CKD confirmed progressively increasing ESKF risk beginning at prehypertensive levels (120–129/80–84 mmHg), with relative risks ranging from 1.6 at high-normal values to over 4.0 at severely elevated pressures [63]. For the same BP values, the risk for ESKF was much higher for African Americans than for Caucasians, and for those with T2DM.

Recently, a meta-analysis collected data from six cohorts, including 2,382,712 individuals and 6856 incident CKD events, and 833 ESKF events [64]. Interestingly, the relative risk for incident CKD or ESKF associated with SBP ≥140 mmHg vs. SBP < 120 mmHg was lower in women than in men.

The relation between elevated BP and increased risk of ESKF is confirmed also in the presence of established CKD, as shown by a study of 2939 patients with advanced CKD (stages G3b–G5) from two international cohorts [46]. Compared to SBP <120 mmHg, progressively higher BP categories (120–129, 130–139, and ≥140 mmHg) were associated with incrementally greater risk of the composite outcome (≥50% eGFR decline or kidney replacement therapy initiation), with HR of 1.33, 1.48, and 1.82, respectively.

Conclusions

Hypertension affects the majority of CKD patients and accelerates kidney disease progression while increasing CV and cerebrovascular complications. The relationship between elevated BP and declining renal function varies by age, ethnicity, sex, and comorbidity status. In older and more advanced CKD populations, mortality risk demonstrates a J-shaped curve, with both very low and very high BP associated with increased mortality. These findings indicate that BP management in CKD requires consideration of individual patient characteristics and baseline kidney function.

References

1. Noubiap JJ, Nansseu JR, Nyaga UF, Sime PS, Francis I, Bigna JJ. Global prevalence of resistant hypertension: a meta-analysis of data from 3.2 million patients. Heart. 2019;105(2):98–105.
2. Lash JP, Go AS, Appel LJ, He J, Ojo A, Rahman M, Townsend RR, Xie D, Cifelli D, Cohan J, Fink JC, Fischer MJ, Gadegbeku C, Hamm LL, Kusek JW, Landis JR, Narva A, Robinson N, Teal V, Feldman HI, Chronic Renal Insufficiency Cohort (CRIC) Study Group. Chronic renal insufficiency cohort (CRIC) study: baseline characteristics and associations with kidney function. Clin J Am Soc Nephrol. 2009;4:1302–11.
3. United States Renal Data System. US Renal Data System 2010 Annual Data Report. Am J Kidney Dis. 2011;57(1 Suppl 1):A8, e1–e526. https://doi.org/10.1053/j.ajkd.2010.10.007. pubmed.ncbi.nlm.nih+2.
4. Browne LD, Alamin MY, Miri HH, Hall R, Tandan M, Sexton D, Stack AG. Prevalence, awareness, treatment, and control of hypertension in community-dwelling older adults with chronic kidney disease: the Irish longitudinal study on ageing. Clin Kidney J. 2024;8:sfae184. https://doi.org/10.1093/ckj/sfae184.
5. Ridao N, Luño J, García de Vinuesa S, Gómez F, Tejedor A, Valderrábano F. Prevalence of hypertension in renal disease. Nephrol Dial Transplant. 2001;16(Suppl 1):70–3.
6. Orofino L, Quereda C, Lamas S, Orte L, Gonzalo A, Mampaso F, Ortuño J. Hypertension in primary chronic glomerulonephritis: analysis of 288 biopsied patients. Nephron. 1987;45:22–6.
7. Muntner P, Anderson A, Charleston J, Chen Z, Ford V, Makos G, O'Connor A, Perumal K, Rahman M, Steigerwalt S, Teal V, Townsend R, Weir M, Wright JT Jr, Chronic Renal Insufficiency Cohort (CRIC) Study Investigators. Hypertension awareness, treatment, and control in adults with CKD: results from the Chronic Renal Insufficiency Cohort (CRIC) study. Am J Kidney Dis. 2010;55(3):441–51.
8. Buckalew VM Jr, Berg RL, Wang SR, Porush JG, Rauch S, Schulman G. Prevalence of hypertension in 1795 subjects with chronic renal disease: the modification of diet in renal disease study baseline cohort. Modification of diet in renal disease study group. Am J Kidney Dis. 1996;28(6):811–21.
9. Minutolo R, Garofalo C, Borrelli S, Chiodini P, Provenzano M, Locatelli F, Conte G, De Nicola L. Sex differences in the progression of CKD among older patients: pooled analysis of 4 cohort studies. Am J Kidney Dis. 2020;75(1):30–8.
10. Ricardo AC, Yang W, Sha D, Appel LJ, Chen J, Krousel-Wood M, Manoharan A, Steigerwalt S, Wright J, Rahman M, Roy JA, Lash JP, CRIC Study Investigators. Sex-related disparities in CKD progression. J Am Soc Nephrol. 2019;30(1):137–46.
11. Duru OK, Li S, Jurkovitz C, Bakris G, Brown W, Chen SC, Collins A, Klag M, McCullough PA, McGill J, Norris K, Whaley-Connell A, Vassalotti J, KEEP Investigators. Race and sex differences in hypertension control in CKD: results from the Kidney Early Evaluation Program (KEEP). Am J Kidney Dis. 2008;51(2):192–8.
12. Minutolo R, Agarwal R, Borrelli S, Chiodini P, Bellizzi V, Nappi F, Cianciaruso B, Zamboli P, Conte G, Gabbai FB, De Nicola L. Prognostic role of ambulatory blood pressure measurement in patients with nondialysis chronic kidney disease. Arch Intern Med. 2011;171(12):1090–8.
13. Mallamaci F, Minutolo R, Leonardis D, D'Arrigo G, Tripepi G, Rapisarda F, Cicchetti T, Maimone I, Enia G, Postorino M, Santoro D, Fuiano G, De Nicola L, Conte G, Zoccali C. Blood pressure variability, mortality, and cardiovascular outcomes in CKD patients. Clin J Am Soc Nephrol. 2019;14(2):233–40.
14. Sarafidis PA, Ruilope LM, Loutradis C, Gorostidi M, de la Sierra A, de la Cruz JJ, Vinyoles E, Divisón-Garrote JA, Segura J, Banegas JR. Blood pressure variability increases with advancing chronic kidney disease stage: a cross-sectional analysis of 16 546 hypertensive patients. J Hypertens. 2018;36(5):1076–85.
15. Minutolo R, Borrelli S, Mallamaci F, Tripepi G, Fuiano L, Garofalo C, Provenzano M, Morrone LF, Santoro D, Postorino M, De Nicola L, Zoccali C, Conte G. Sex difference in

ambulatory blood pressure control associates with risk of ESKD and death in CKD patients receiving stable nephrology care. Nephrol Dial Transplant. 2021;36(11):2000–7.
16. Theodorakopoulou MP, Dipla K, Boutou AK, Papadopoulos CE, Zafeiridis A, Faitatzidou D, Koutroumpas K, Alexandrou ME, Sarafidis PA. Sex differences in ambulatory blood pressure levels, control and phenotypes of hypertension in hemodialysis patients. J Hypertens. 2022;40(9):1735–43.
17. Korogiannou M, Xagas E, Marinaki S, Sarafidis P, Kanakakis I, Liakopoulos V, Boletis JN. Sex differences in ambulatory blood pressure levels, control, and phenotypes of hypertension in kidney transplant recipients. J Hypertens. 2022;40(2):356–63.
18. Verma A, Vyas S, Agarwal A, Abbas S, Agarwal DP, Kumar R. Diabetic kidney disease and hypertension: a true love story. J Clin Diagn Res. 2016;10(3):OC11-3.
19. Collins AJ, Vassalotti JA, Wang C, Li S, Gilbertson DT, Liu J, Foley RN, Chen SC, Arneson TJ. Who should be targeted for CKD screening? Impact of diabetes, hypertension, and cardiovascular disease. Am J Kidney Dis. 2009;53(3 Suppl 3):S71–7.
20. Cunillera-Puértolas O, Vizcaya D, Cobo-Guerrero S, Romano-Sánchez J, Bundó-Luque D, Arbiol-Roca A, Salvador-González B. Chronic kidney disease progression in patients with previous type 2 diabetes and/or hypertension: a population-based cohort study from primary care in Spain. BMJ Open. 2025;15(1):e086919.
21. Shi W, Wang H, Zhou Y, Sun Y, Chen Y. Synergistic interaction of hypertension and diabetes on chronic kidney disease: insights from the National Health and Nutrition Examination Survey 1999–2006. J Diabetes Complicat. 2020;34(2):107447.
22. Friedman AN, Kaplan LM, le Roux CW, Schauer PR. Management of obesity in adults with CKD. J Am Soc Nephrol. 2021;32:777–90.
23. Hall JE, do Carmo JM, da Silva AA, Wang Z, Hall ME. Obesity, kidney dysfunction and hypertension: mechanistic links. Nat Rev Nephrol. 2019;15:367–85.
24. Ndumele CE, Rangaswami J, Chow SL, Neeland IJ, Tuttle KR, Khan SS, Coresh J, Mathew RO, Baker-Smith CM, Carnethon MR, Despres JP, Ho JE, Joseph JJ, Kernan WN, Khera A, Kosiborod MN, Lekavich CL, Lewis EF, Lo KB, Ozkan B, Palaniappan LP, Patel SS, Pencina MJ, Powell-Wiley TM, Sperling LS, Virani SS, Wright JT, Rajgopal Singh R, Elkind MSV, American Heart Association. Cardiovascular-kidney-metabolic health: a presidential advisory from the American Heart Association. Circulation. 2023;148(20):1606–35.
25. Petramala L, Gigante A, Sarlo F, Servello A, Circosta F, Marino L, Ciccarelli A, Cavallaro G, Letizia C. Relevance of obesity-related organ damage and metabolic syndrome classification in cardiovascular and renal risk stratification in patients with essential hypertension. Front Cardiovasc Med. 2024;11:1369090.
26. Wu N, Zhao W, Ye K, Li Y, He M, Lu B, Hu R. Albuminuria is associated with left ventricular hypertrophy in patients with early diabetic kidney disease. Int J Endocrinol. 2014;2014:351945.
27. Leoncini G, Viazzi F, Conti N, Baratto E, Tomolillo C, Bezante GP, Deferrari G, Pontremoli R. Renal and cardiac abnormalities in primary hypertension. J Hypertens. 2009;27(5):1064–73.
28. Ahmad MI, Kazibwe R, Soliman MZ, Singh S, Chen LY, Soliman EZ. Joint Association of Albuminuria and Left Ventricular Hypertrophy with incident heart failure in high-risk adults with hypertension: a SPRINT substudy. Am J Cardiol. 2023;208:75–82.
29. Chatterjee S, Bavishi C, Sardar P, Agarwal V, Krishnamoorthy P, Grodzicki T, Messerli FH. Meta-analysis of left ventricular hypertrophy and sustained arrhythmias. Am J Cardiol. 2014;114:1049–52.
30. Cunningham KS, Spears DA, Care M. Evaluation of cardiac hypertrophy in the setting of sudden cardiac death. Forensic Sci Res. 2019;4:223–40.
31. Park M, Hsu CY, Li Y, Mishra RK, Keane M, Rosas SE, Dries D, Xie D, Chen J, He J, Anderson A, Go AS, Shlipak MG, Chronic Renal Insufficiency Cohort (CRIC) Study Group. Associations between kidney function and subclinical cardiac abnormalities in CKD. J Am Soc Nephrol. 2012;23:1725–34.
32. Levin A, Singer J, Thompson CR, Ross H, Lewis M. Prevalent left ventricular hypertrophy in the predialysis population: identifying opportunities for intervention. Am J Kidney Dis. 1996;27:347–54.

33. Paoletti E, Bellino D, Cassottana P, Rolla D, Cannella G. Left ventricular hypertrophy in nondiabetic predialysis CKD. Am J Kidney Dis. 2005;46:320–7.
34. London GM, Pannier B, Guerin AP, Blacher J, Marchais SJ, Darne B, Metivier F, Adda H, Safar ME. Alterations of left ventricular hypertrophy in and survival of patients receiving hemodialysis: follow-up of an interventional study. J Am Soc Nephrol. 2001;12:2759–67.
35. Ungvari Z, Toth P, Tarantini S, Prodan CI, Sorond F, Merkely B, Csiszar A. Hypertension-induced cognitive impairment: from pathophysiology to public health. Nat Rev Nephrol. 2021;17:639–54.
36. Vermeer SE, Longstreth WT Jr, Koudstaal PJ. Silent brain infarcts: a systematic review. Lancet Neurol. 2007;6:611–9.
37. Potter T, Agarwal A, Schaefer TJ. Hypertensive encephalopathy. In: StatPearls [Internet]. Treasure Island: StatPearls Publishing; 2024. https://www.ncbi.nlm.nih.gov/books/NBK554499/. Accessed 2 Feb 2024.
38. Kelly DM, Ademi Z, Doehner W, Lip GYH, Mark P, Toyoda K, Wong CX, Sarnak M, Cheung M, Herzog CA, Johansen KL, Reinecke H, Sood MM. Chronic kidney disease and cerebrovascular disease: consensus and guidance from a KDIGO controversies conference. Stroke. 2021;52(7):e328–46.
39. Wang T, Pan R, Li C, Qin Y, Song C. A epidemiological trend of chronic kidney disease due to hypertension among adolescents and young adults: global burden and future 2035 projections. Front Public Health. 2025;13:1618416.
40. Klag MJ, Whelton PK, Randall BL, Neaton JD, Brancati FL, Stamler J, Pan W, Ford CE. Blood pressure and end-stage renal disease in men. N Engl J Med. 1996;334(1):13–8.
41. USRDS. 2013 Annual Data Report: Atlas of chronic kidney disease and end-stage renal disease in the United States. Bethesda: United States Renal Data System, National Institutes of Health, National Institute of Diabetes and Digestive and Kidney Diseases; 2013.
42. Brazy PC, Stead WW, Fitzwilliam JF. Progression of renal insufficiency: role of blood pressure. Kidney Int. 1989;35:670–4.
43. Tiernay WM, McDonald CJ, Luft FC. Renal disease in hypertensive adults: effect of race and type II diabetes mellitus. Am J Kidney Dis. 1989;13:485–93.
44. Perry HM, Miller JP, Fornoff JR, Baty JD, Sambhi MP, Rutan G, Moskowitz DW, Carmody SE. Early predictors of 15-year end-stage renal disease in hypertensive patients. Hypertension. 1995;25:587–94.
45. Walker WG, Neaton JD, Cutler JA, Neuwirth R, Cohen JD. Renal function change in hypertensive members of the multiple risk factor intervention trial. Racial and treatment effects. The MRFIT research group. JAMA. 1992;268(21):3085–91.
46. Park CH, Kim HW, Park JT, Chang TI, Yoo TH, Oh KH, Anderson AH, Yang W, Cohen JB, Rahman M, Kang SW, Han SH, on the behalf of CRIC Study and KNOW-CKD Investigators. BP and kidney disease progression in advanced CKD: findings from the chronic renal insufficiency cohort and KoreaN cohort study for outcome in patients with CKD studies. Clin J Am Soc Nephrol. 2025;20(9):1179–89.
47. Coşkun Ş, Cordan J, Mehmetoğlu E, Sağ S, Yeşilbursa D, Serdar OA. Association between microalbuminuria and pulse pressure among patients with isolated systolic and diastolic hypertension. J Updates Cardiovasc Med. 2021;9(1):39–48.
48. Shin JI, Chang AR, Grams ME, Coresh J, Ballew SH, Surapaneni A, Matsushita K, Bilo HJG, Carrero JJ, Chodick G, Daratha KB, Jassal SK, Nadkarni GN, Nelson RG, Nowak C, Stempniewicz N, Sumida K, Traynor JP, Woodward M, Sang Y, Gansevoort RT, CKD Prognosis Consortium. Albuminuria testing in hypertension and diabetes: an individual-participant data meta-analysis in a global consortium. Hypertension. 2021;78(4):1042–52.
49. Breslin DJ, Gifford RW Jr, Fairbairn JF 2nd, Kearns TP. Prognostic importance of ophthalmoscopic findings in essential hypertension. JAMA. 1966;195:335–8.
50. Modi P, Arsiwalla T. Hypertensive retinopathy. In: StatPearls [Internet]. Treasure Island: StatPearls Publishing; 2023.
51. Adappa K, Channabasappa S, Vinutha J, Chandana S, Mohan S. A study to correlate hypertensive retinopathy with chronic kidney disease. Int J Med Ophthalmol. 2024;6(2):35–9.

52. Dahyabhai RK, Mer BG. Hypertensive retinopathy changes in chronic kidney disease: observational study. Int J Acad Med Pharm. 2025;7(2):436–9.
53. Nokiba H, Takei T, Suto C, Nitta K. Association between ophthalmological changes and cardiovascular diseases in patients with chronic kidney disease undergoing hemodialysis. J Atheroscler Thromb. 2015;22(12):1248–54.
54. American Heart Association. Deaths from high blood pressure-related kidney disease up nearly 50% in the past 25 years. American Heart Association; 2024. https://newsroom.heart.org/news/deaths-from-high-blood-pressure-related-kidney-disease-up-nearly-50-in-the-past-25-years. Accessed 7 Oct 2025.
55. Lai Y, Long H, Liang Z, Wu C, Wu L, Liu C, Meng X. Global burden and risk factors of chronic kidney disease due to hypertension in adults aged 20 plus years, 1990–2021. Front Public Health. 2025;13:1503837.
56. Weiss JW, Johnson ES, Petrik A, Smith DH, Yang X, Thorp ML. Systolic blood pressure and mortality among older community-dwelling adults with CKD. Am J Kidney Dis. 2010;56:1062–71.
57. Kovesdy CP, Bleyer AJ, Molnar MZ, Ma JZ, Sim JJ, Cushman WC, Quarles LD, Kalantar-Zadeh K. Blood pressure and mortality in U.S. veterans with chronic kidney disease: a cohort study. Ann Intern Med. 2013;159:233–42.
58. Wu S, Li M, Lu J, Tang X, Wang G, Zheng R, Niu J, Chen L, Huo Y, Xu M, Wang T, Zhao Z, Wang S, Lin H, Qin G, Yan L, Wan Q, Chen L, Shi L, Hu R, Su Q, Yu X, Qin Y, Chen G, Gao Z, Shen F, Luo Z, Chen Y, Zhang Y, Liu C, Wang Y, Wu S, Yang T, Li Q, Mu Y, Zhao J, Ning G, Bi Y, Wang W, Xu Y, China Cardiometabolic Disease and Cancer Cohort (4C) Study Group. Blood pressure levels, cardiovascular events, and renal outcomes in chronic kidney disease without antihypertensive therapy: a Nationwide population-based cohort study. Hypertension. 2023;80(3):640–9.
59. Fu C, Zhang D, Chen H, Zhang H. Timed-averaged blood pressure showed a J-curve association with stroke in elderly chronic kidney disease patients. Ren Fail. 2022;44(1):1677–86.
60. Kovesdy CP, Alrifai A, Gosmanova EO, Lu JL, Canada RB, Wall BM, Alagiakrishnan K, Fyfe B, Nuti R, Sumida K, Streja E, Molnar MZ, Kalantar-Zadeh K. Age and outcomes associated with BP in patients with incident CKD. Clin J Am Soc Nephrol. 2016;11:821–31.
61. Yoon SY, Jeong SJ, Kim JS, Hwang HS, Jeong K. Time in target range of systolic blood pressure and cardiovascular disease in patients with chronic kidney disease: a Korean Nationwide cohort study. Am J Nephrol. 2025;57:30–41.
62. Klag MJ, Whelton PK, Randall BL, Neaton JD, Brancati FL, Ford CE, Shulman NB, Stamler J. Blood pressure and end-stage renal disease in men. N Engl J Med. 1996;334(1):13–8.
63. Hsu C, McCulloch CE, Darbinian J, Go AS, Iribarren C. Elevated blood pressure and risk of end-stage renal disease in subjects without baseline kidney disease. Arch Intern Med. 2005;165(8):923–8.
64. Weldegiorgis M, Woodward M. The impact of hypertension on chronic kidney disease and end-stage renal disease is greater in men than women: a systematic review and meta-analysis. BMC Nephrol. 2020;21(1):506.

Pathophysiology of Hypertension in Chronic Kidney Disease: Role of the Renin-Angiotensin System

Panagiota Anyfanti

Introduction

As early as in 1898, Tigerstedt and Bergman published their research on a substance isolated from kidney extracts, specifically the renal cortex, which was named "renin" and elicited consistent blood pressure (BP) rising effects [1]. Although the role of renin-angiotensin system (RAS) was not fully understood for decades, it is established to date as a powerful hormonal system modulating hypertension and cardio-renal disease. Classically, the main effector peptide of the RAS is angiotensin II (Ang II), which is produced through a cascade of enzymatic reactions involving two biologically important enzymes: renin and angiotensin-converting enzyme (ACE) (Fig. 1).

P. Anyfanti (✉)
Third Department of Internal Medicine, Papageorgiou Hospital, Aristotle University of Thessaloniki, Thessaloniki, Greece

P. Sarafidis, R. Pontremoli (eds.), *Hypertension and Chronic Kidney Disease*, Updates in Hypertension and Cardiovascular Protection,
https://doi.org/10.1007/978-3-032-29564-4_2

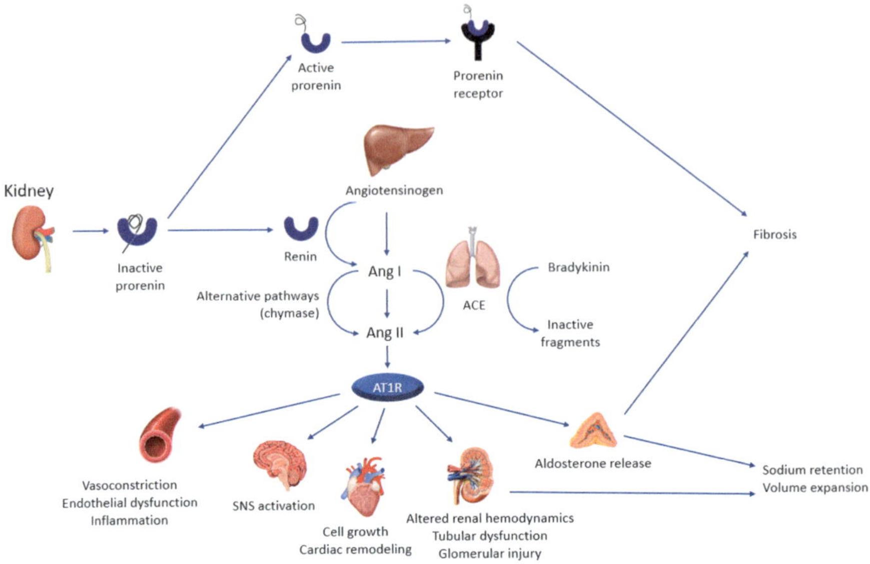

Fig. 1 The renin-angiotensin system. *ACE* angiotensin-converting enzyme, *Ang I* angiotensin I, *Ang II* angiotensin II, *AT1R* type 1 angiotensin receptor

Physiological Role of RAS Components

Renin is secreted by exocytosis from the cells of the renal juxtaglomerular apparatus. Major stimuli for increased renin synthesis include glomerular hypoperfusion, reduced sodium (and chloride) concentration at macula densa area, and increased activity of the sympathetic nervous system. Prorenin was long regarded as the inactive precursor of renin, processed in the endoplasmic reticulum and packaged into secretory granules of the renal juxtaglomerular cells. This view has long changed following the discovery of the prorenin receptor in the kidneys and the heart, whose binding to prorenin leads to its non-enzymatic activation [2]. Under normal circumstances, circulating prorenin levels exceed circulating renin levels by 10 times and reportedly, although not consistently, increase even further in disease states such as diabetes, implying a potential biological role [3, 4]. Both renin and prorenin are now considered to exert direct renal and cardiac toxic effects through receptor binding [5]. However, the main substrate for renin is angiotensinogen, a serpentine polypeptide synthesized mainly in the liver. In the classic systemic RAS, circulating renin cleaves angiotensinogen to produce angiotensin I (Ang I), an inactive decapeptide, which is then converted by angiotensin-converting enzyme (ACE) to Ang II, the major active component of RAS. ACE is abundantly present in the pulmonary endothelial cells, but is also expressed in various tissues including the kidney. ACE plays a role both in RAS and the kallikrein-kinin system by breaking down bradykinin, a potent vasodilator [6]. Chymase, a serine protease, offers an alternative route of Ang I to Ang II conversion in the heart and arteries [7].

Ang II is a vasoactive peptide with multiple functions produced systemically and locally within the vascular wall. It exerts its physiological effects primarily through binding to two distinct types of G-protein coupled angiotensin receptors. Activation of angiotensin receptor type 1 (AT1) results in potent vasoconstriction and BP elevation, sodium retention, and vascular cell production of reactive oxygen species (ROS) via redox-sensitive processes. It further acts as a pro-inflammatory, pro-fibrotic molecule and stimulates vascular cell hypertrophy and hyperplasia, which are important in vascular injury and remodeling in cardiovascular diseases. In contrast, activation of AT2 receptors induces antiproliferative, proapoptotic, and vasodilatory effects, but while these counteracting effects are important in the fetus, in adults they are largely outweighed by AT1 receptor-mediated functions [8]. Differential downstream effects of each receptor activation are further presented in Table 1.

Ang II stimulates aldosterone secretion from the adrenal cortex. Aldosterone promotes sodium reabsorption, water retention, and potassium excretion in its primary sites of action, which include the principal cells of the collecting tubules. Aldosterone binds to intranuclear mineralocorticoid receptors and exerts its genomic effects through activation of gene transcription, resulting in synthesis or activation of the Na^+-K^+-ATPase pump on the basolateral epithelial membrane and stimulation of the amiloride-sensitive sodium channels on the luminal side of the epithelial membrane. Under physiological conditions, the effects of aldosterone on pressure-natriuresis resemble those observed for Ang II; low sodium intake acts as a trigger to aldosterone to promote sodium retention, whereas during high sodium intake, suppression of aldosterone attenuates sodium retention and increases in BP [9]. Circulating aldosterone perpetuates the Ang II-induced vascular inflammation and fibrosis through stimulation of mineralocorticoid receptors expressed in both epithelial tissues like the kidney and colon, and nonepithelial tissues such as the heart and brainstem circumventricular organs, as well as through non-genomic effects mediated by other pathways [10].

Table 1 Diverse downstream effects triggered by angiotensin II binding to each receptor subtype (AT1 or AT2)

AT1R	AT2R
↑ Vasoconstriction	↑ Vasodilation
↑ Aldosterone, endothelin, and vasopressin	↑ Nitric oxide
↑ Tubular sodium reabsorption	↑ Natriuresis
↑ Cell proliferation and hypertrophy	↓ Cell growth
↑ Inflammation	↓ Inflammation
↑ Fibrosis	↑ Apoptosis
↑ Thrombosis	↓ Angiogenesis
↑ ROS generation	↓ Renin secretion
↑ SNS activation	

AT1R type 1 angiotensin receptor, *AT2R* type 2 angiotensin receptor, *ROS* reactive oxygen species, *SNS* sympathetic nervous system

The Role of RAS Activation in Hypertension of Chronic Kidney Disease

Several experimental and clinical studies have overtly demonstrated a trilateral association between RAS, hypertension, and chronic kidney disease (CKD). Ang II exerts both indirect effects on the kidney, though systemic BP increase, and direct effects, by triggering inflammation and fibrosis within the renal tissue and vascular wall. Kidney injury is closely linked to hypertension and each condition exacerbates the other in a vicious circle perpetuated by RAS overactivation.

Mutations in the genes encoding components of the RAS including renin, angiotensinogen, ACE, and AT1 receptor have been associated with renal tubular dysgenesis and susceptibility to arterial hypertension [11, 12]. In experimental models, renin overexpression in the collecting ducts caused spontaneous hypertension, whereas renin deletion in the collecting ducts was protective against Ang II-induced hypertension [13, 14]. In patients with CKD, a direct relationship of plasma renin activity with BP levels is often observed [15]. While "inappropriately normal" renin levels may be detected in these patients using conventional measurements methods, increased renin is secreted in areas of poor perfusion, such as cysts or scars, in areas of tubulo-interstitial inflammation, or in response to microangiopathic injury, resulting in a state of relatively high renin levels for a patient with hypertension, sodium retention, and volume overload [16].

The increase in sympathetic nervous system activity typically observed in CKD contributes, among other factors, to an increase in renin secretion via an increased sympathetic input into the juxtaglomerular apparatus through the β_1-adrenoreceptor [17]. At the same time, increased levels of Ang II in CKD act centrally within the brain neuroanatomical regions responsible for sympathetic activation, and further augment sympathetic outflow to organs such as the heart, the kidney, and the vasculature resulting in BP elevation.

The Role of the Intrarenal RAS

Apart from the well-described systemic RAS that requires interaction of multiple organs via circulation, multiple independently functioning tissue RASs exist, the most important of which is the intrarenal RAS. The intrarenal RAS is regulated in an autocrine/paracrine manner that is independent of systemic RAS and is characterized by an excessive amount of Ang II produced by kidney cells and detected in the proximal tubular fluid; this may exceed the circulating Ang II by as much as 1000 times [18]. Aside from the classic RAS pathways, prorenin receptors and chymase are also implicated in local Ang II formation in the kidney [19, 20]. Experimental studies have demonstrated that enhanced intrarenal RAS activity is more directly involved in kidney injury than systemic RAS [21, 22].

In concordance with the above, recent evidence from a large prospective CKD cohort supports that intrarenal RAS activity modifies the association between BP and adverse kidney outcomes, and that the clinical significance of BP control with respect to CKD progression may be diluted in patients with elevated intrarenal RAS activity [23]. Regardless of its origin, Ang II can affect both renal hemodynamics and tubular function, and RAS overactivation has been described a major factor contributing to glomerular hypertension.

Ang II-Mediated Renal Hemodynamic and Glomerular Effects Promoting Hypertension in CKD

In CKD secondary to vascular disease, diabetes, or polycystic kidney disease, increased formation of local and intrarenal Ang II in areas of renal injury or ischemia has been associated with exacerbation of systemic hypertension [16]. Physiologically, the powerful vasoconstrictive action of Ang II is mainly exerted to the postglomerular efferent arterioles rather than the preglomerular vessels, which are selectively protected by autacoid mechanisms such as prostaglandins or endothelial-derived nitric oxide. Increases in BP are counterbalanced by the Ang II-induced proportionate vasoconstriction of the preglomerular vasculature in order to relieve the pressure load transmitted from the systemic circulation to the glomerular capillary network. Thus, a relatively constant glomerular hydrostatic pressure regardless of systemic BP fluctuations is pertained in the normal kidney. In CKD, this auto-control response is blunted, particularly in patients where the afferent autoregulation is impaired, such as those with obesity and diabetes commonly presenting with afferent vasodilation; thus, glomerular hydrostatic pressure is increased, resulting in renal microvascular injury, hyperfiltration, and proteinuria, further contributing to the progression of CKD. Regardless of hemodynamic changes, locally produced Ang II directly induces podocyte impairment, promotes cellular hypertrophy, and induces oxidative stress through activation of AT1 receptor [24]. Hemodynamic actions of Ang II on glomerular microcirculation in normal conditions and in CKD are further presented in Fig. 2.

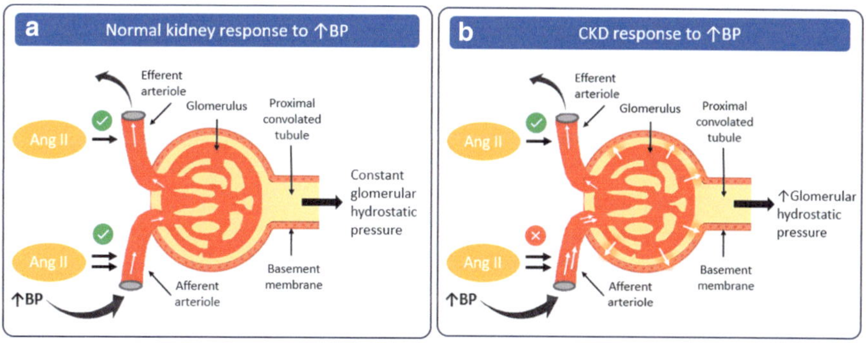

Fig. 2 Hemodynamic actions of Ang II on glomerular microcirculation in normal conditions (**a**) and in CKD (**b**). Abolishment of the auto-control response in CKD results in increased hydrostatic pressure within the glomerulus, which promotes renal microvascular injury, hyperfiltration, and proteinuria. *Ang II* angiotensin II, *BP* blood pressure, *CKD* chronic kidney disease

Renal glomerular or interstitial fibrosis characterizes virtually all progressive human kidney diseases [25]. Apart from its hemodynamic effects, Ang II possesses strong proinflammatory and profibrotic actions. Ang II plays a key role in glomerulosclerosis by stimulating mesangial cell synthesis of matrix proteins, increasing matrix protein receptors, and altering protease/protease-inhibitor balance, thereby inhibiting matrix degradation. These effects are mediated by Ang II directly through AT1 receptor activation, and indirectly through increased expression of profibrotic molecules such as transforming growth factor β (TGF-β), fibronectin, and collagen type I [26]. Although generally considered as renoprotective, activation of AT2 receptors plays a redundant role in the progression of kidney damage and subsequently hypertension, through an increase in apoptosis of glomerular and tubular cells that has been observed following renal injury in CKD [27]. In addition to renal fibrosis, Ang II produced in excess amounts in CKD promotes generation of ROS and proinflammatory cytokines, such as tumor necrosis factor α, and upregulates transcription factors such as nuclear factor kappa B [28]. Altogether, these profibrotic, pro-inflammatory effects of Ang II in the kidney mediate structural alterations that are critical to the exacerbation of hypertension in kidney disease.

Renal Tubular Effects of Ang II in Hypertension in CKD: A Cause for Salt-Sensitivity

Ang II effects on tubular function are largely mediated by increased Ang II-stimulated aldosterone release resulting in sodium and water retention, which typically characterizes patients with CKD. Aldosterone is a major contributor to hypertension in CKD as it upregulates sodium reabsorption both through epithelial sodium transporter channels and in the sodium chloride channels (the thiazide-sensitive channels) of the distal tubule. At the same time, other aldosterone-mediated actions include inhibition of nitric oxide action, hyperfiltration and proteinuria, inflammation and glomerular hypertrophy, generation of ROS and podocyte injury, all of which promote kidney damage and hypertension [29, 30]. Notwithstandingly, ineffective suppression of RAS in the presence of sodium loading has been implicated as a key mechanism in the pathogenesis of hypertension associated with CKD. Normally, increased dietary sodium intake results in suppressed renin activity and reduced production of Ang II, in order to prevent BP elevation through a prompt, precise, and effective sodium excretion from the kidneys, but this physiological counterbalancing mechanism is abolished in CKD resulting in impaired pressure natriuresis (Fig. 3). The salt-sensitivity of BP in CKD is exacerbated by impaired renal function that directly or indirectly increases sodium reabsorption and decreases glomerular capillary filtration coefficient. On the other hand, volume expansion in CKD patients perpetuates RAS activation and promotes its vasoactive effects resulting in the establishment and progression of hypertension in CKD [31].

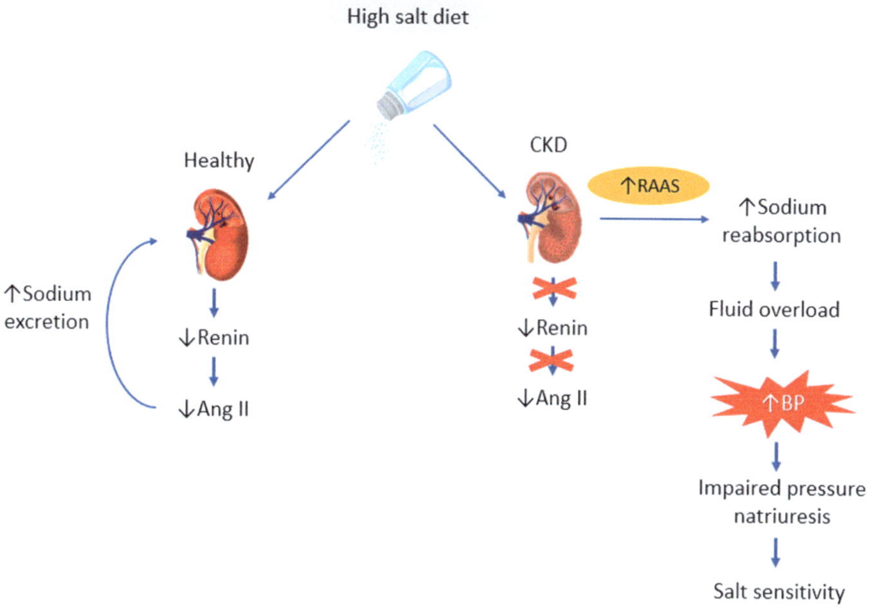

Fig. 3 Absence of Ang II suppression in CKD is an impaired counter-regulatory mechanism resulting in impaired pressure natriuresis and sustained BP increases. *Ang II* angiotensin II, *BP* blood pressure, *CKD* chronic kidney disease, *RAAS* renin-angiotensin aldosterone system

Conclusion

RAS is a major enzymatic cascade regulating BP and fluid balance in humans. RAS overactivation is critically involved in the pathogenesis of hypertension in CKD, considering its multifaceted modulation of vascular, neuronal, pro-inflammatory, and pro-fibrotic pathways impacting renovascular control of BP. Augmented Ang II, the main biologically active peptide of the RAS, is mutually reinforcing hypertension and CKD progression in a positive feedback loop. The catalytic role of RAS is most evident when considering the effectiveness of RAS inhibitors in controlling BP in CKD that provides, at the same time, a route of renoprotection beyond BP control. Expanding pathophysiological knowledge of the role of the core as well as non-classical RAS components has the potential of providing novel therapeutical approaches for hypertension in CKD.

References

1. Phillips MI, Schmidt-Ott KM. The discovery of renin 100 years ago. News Physiol Sci. 1999;14:271–4.
2. Nguyen G, Delarue F, Burcklé C, Bouzhir L, Giller T, Sraer JD. Pivotal role of the renin/prorenin receptor in angiotensin II production and cellular responses to renin. J Clin Invest. 2002;109(11):1417–27.
3. Senbonmatsu T. Prorenin: what are its functions? Hypertens Res. 2022;45(12):2021–3.
4. Mercure C, Prescott G, Lacombe MJ, Silversides DW, Reudelhuber TL. Chronic increases in circulating prorenin are not associated with renal or cardiac pathologies. Hypertension. 2009;53(6):1062–9.
5. Laragh JH. Abstract, closing summary, and table of contents for Laragh's 25 lessons in pathophysiology and 12 clinical pearls for treating hypertension. Am J Hypertens. 2001;14(12):1173–7.
6. Berkenboom G. Bradykinin and the therapeutic actions of angiotensin-converting enzyme inhibitors. Am J Cardiol. 1998;82(10A):11S–3S.
7. Miyazaki M, Takai S. Tissue angiotensin II generating system by angiotensin-converting enzyme and chymase. J Pharmacol Sci. 2006;100(5):391–7.
8. Nguyen Dinh Cat A, Montezano AC, Burger D, Touyz RM. Angiotensin II, NADPH oxidase, and redox signaling in the vasculature. Antioxid Redox Signal. 2013;19(10):1110–20.
9. Fuller PJ, Young MJ. Mechanisms of mineralocorticoid action. Hypertens. 2005;46(6):1227–35.
10. Briet M, Schiffrin EL. Vascular actions of aldosterone. J Vasc Res. 2013;50(2):89–99.
11. Gribouval O, Gonzales M, Neuhaus T, Aziza J, Bieth E, Laurent N, et al. Mutations in genes in the renin-angiotensin system are associated with autosomal recessive renal tubular dysgenesis. Nat Genet. 2005;37(9):964–8.
12. Wang L, Hou L, Li H, Chen J, Kelly TN, Jaquish CE, et al. Genetic variants in the renin-angiotensin system and blood pressure reactions to the cold pressor test. J Hypertens. 2010;28(12):2422–8.
13. Ramkumar N, Ying J, Stuart D, Kohan DE. Overexpression of renin in the collecting duct causes elevated blood pressure. Am J Hypertens. 2013;26(8):965–72.
14. Ramkumar N, Stuart D, Rees S, Van HA, Sigmund CD, Kohan DE. Collecting duct-specific knockout of renin attenuates angiotensin II-induced hypertension. Am J Physiol Renal Physiol. 2014;307(8):F931–8.
15. Boer P, Dorhout Mees EJ, Roos JC, Koomans HA, Geyskes GG. Renin and body fluid volumes in chronic renal disease. Relations between arterial pressure, plasma renin activity, blood volume, and extracellular volume in chronic renal disease, as compared with essential hypertension. Acta Med Scand. 1981;210(3):207–12.
16. Rosenberg ME, Smith LJ, Correa-Rotter R, Hostetter TH. The paradox of the renin-angiotensin system in chronic renal disease. Kidney Int. 1994;45(2):403–10.
17. Kaur J, Young BE, Fadel PJ. Sympathetic overactivity in chronic kidney disease: consequences and mechanisms. Int J Mol Sci. 2017;18(8):1682.
18. Carey RM. The intrarenal renin-angiotensin system in hypertension. Adv Chronic Kidney Dis. 2015;22(3):204–10.
19. Wei CC, Tian B, Perry G, Meng QC, Chen YF, Oparil S, et al. Differential ANG II generation in plasma and tissue of mice with decreased expression of the ACE gene. Am J Physiol Heart Circ Physiol. 2002;282(6):H2254–8.
20. Ichihara A, Kaneshiro Y, Takemitsu T, Sakoda M, Nakagawa T, Nishiyama A, et al. Contribution of nonproteolytically activated prorenin in glomeruli to hypertensive renal damage. J Am Soc Nephrol. 2006;17(9):2495–503.
21. Graciano ML, Cavaglieri R d C, Dellê H, Dominguez WV, Casarini DE, Malheiros DMAC, et al. Intrarenal renin-angiotensin system is upregulated in experimental model of progressive renal disease induced by chronic inhibition of nitric oxide synthesis. J Am Soc Nephrol. 2004;15(7):1805–15.

22. Yamamoto T, Nakagawa T, Suzuki H, Ohashi N, Fukasawa H, Fujigaki Y, et al. Urinary angiotensinogen as a marker of intrarenal angiotensin II activity associated with deterioration of renal function in patients with chronic kidney disease. J Am Soc Nephrol. 2007;18(5):1558–65.
23. Park CH, Kim HW, Park JT, Chang TI, Yoo TH, Lee J, et al. Intrarenal renin-angiotensin system activation alters relationship between systolic blood pressure and progression of chronic kidney disease. Hypertens. 2023;80(5):1024–34.
24. Santos PCJL, Krieger JE, Pereira AC. Renin-angiotensin system, hypertension, and chronic kidney disease: pharmacogenetic implications. J Pharmacol Sci. 2012;120(2):77–88.
25. Boor P, Ostendorf T, Floege J. Renal fibrosis: novel insights into mechanisms and therapeutic targets. Nat Rev Nephrol. 2010;6(11):643–56.
26. Iglarz M, Touyz RM, Viel EC, Amiri F, Schiffrin EL. Involvement of oxidative stress in the profibrotic action of aldosterone. Am J Hypertens. 2004;17(7):597–603.
27. Ding G, Reddy K, Kapasi AA, Franki N, Gibbons N, Kasinath BS, et al. Angiotensin II induces apoptosis in rat glomerular epithelial cells. Am J Physiol Renal Physiol. 2002;283(1):F173–80.
28. Ameer OZ. Hypertension in chronic kidney disease: what lies behind the scene. Front Pharmacol. 2022;13:949260.
29. Martín-Fernández B, Rubio-Navarro A, Cortegano I, Ballesteros S, Alía M, Cannata-Ortiz P, et al. Aldosterone induces renal fibrosis and inflammatory M1-macrophage subtype via mineralocorticoid receptor in rats. PLoS One. 2016;11(1):e0145946.
30. Rozansky DJ, Cornwall T, Subramanya AR, Rogers S, Yang YF, David LL, et al. Aldosterone mediates activation of the thiazide-sensitive Na-Cl cotransporter through an SGK1 and WNK4 signaling pathway. J Clin Invest. 2009;119(9):2601–12.
31. Hall JE. Renal dysfunction, rather than nonrenal vascular dysfunction, mediates salt-induced hypertension. Circulation. 2016;133(9):894–906.

Pathophysiology of Hypertension in Chronic Kidney Disease: Role of Dietary Sodium Consumption and Sodium Sensitivity

Artemios G. Karagiannidis and Pantelis Sarafidis

Introduction

Sodium has occupied a prominent place in history for millennia, long before its vital physiological roles were scientifically understood. From being used as food preservative, purifier in several religious rituals, natural remedy, and even currency in ancient times, salt has invaded every aspect of human civilization. This deep-rooted reverence contributed to the widespread belief in its health benefits. It was not until the latter half of the twentieth century that the important role of excessive sodium intake in the development of hypertension and cardiovascular diseases was recognized [1].

Chronic kidney disease (CKD) is a growing health issue worldwide, accounting for 1.5% of global deaths [2]. Major cardiovascular events represent the leading cause of death in CKD and their incidence progressively increases with advancing CKD stages [3]. This is attributed to the synergistic effects of traditional and nontraditional risk factors [4, 5]; among the traditional risk factors, hypertension is by far the most common, and its prevalence is gradually increased with advancing CKD stages, reaching ~95% of patients with CKD G4 and G5 [6]. In these patients, hypertension is independently associated with cardiovascular morbidity and mortality [6] and progression of kidney damage [7].

In the context of CKD, dietary sodium intake plays a central role in the pathogenesis of hypertension. The phenotype of sodium sensitivity, i.e., the exaggerated response of blood pressure (BP) to sodium load, is highly prevalent among CKD patients. This chapter delves into the role of sodium in the pathogenesis of hypertension in CKD, providing an overview of the role of high dietary sodium intake, the

A. G. Karagiannidis (✉) · P. Sarafidis
1st Department of Nephrology, Aristotle University of Thessaloniki, Hippokration Hospital, Thessaloniki, Greece

P. Sarafidis, R. Pontremoli (eds.), *Hypertension and Chronic Kidney Disease*, Updates in Hypertension and Cardiovascular Protection,
https://doi.org/10.1007/978-3-032-29564-4_3

phenomenon of sodium sensitivity and its entailed mechanisms, with a focus on the recently described role of uromodulin in sodium sensitivity. Additionally, the role of kidneys in BP regulation and the development of hypertension is also discussed.

Dietary Sodium Intake and Hypertension

The central role of increased sodium intake in the pathogenesis of hypertension is supported by a plethora of preclinical, epidemiological, and clinical studies published over many decades [8]. Based on these data, it is clear that strict sodium restriction (40–50 mmol/day) leads to a significant drop in BP in both hypertensive and normotensive individuals [9]; however, some researchers have raised serious doubts about the benefits of reducing dietary sodium intake to such low levels, given the potential risks [10]. Nonetheless, given that the average daily dietary sodium intake in the Western world far exceeds the above levels, and acknowledging the undeniable value of dietary sodium restriction, international guidelines systematically recommend dietary sodium restriction is proposed as a basic lifestyle change for all hypertensive patients and one of the most cost-effective public health measures to prevent cardiovascular disease at the general population [11]. According to several health organizations, sodium intake should be limited to no more than 2.3 g/day of sodium corresponding to 5.8 g (or 100 mmol) of salt [11–14].

The evidence supporting the central role of high sodium intake in the development of hypertension can be grouped into three major categories: (a) preclinical studies, (b) observational human studies, and (c) interventional human studies. A detailed description of all relevant evidence is beyond the scope of this chapter, but the main points are summarized below.

Preclinical Studies

Numerous preclinical studies support that increased dietary sodium intake is linked to the development of hypertension. As early as the 1960s, Dahl et al. showed that high salt intake leads to an increase in BP of mice, which in two-third of cases ultimately progresses to permanent hypertension, even after high salt intake is discontinued later in the experiment [15]. The same researchers also showed that the increase in BP in response to a high-sodium diet is much more pronounced in genetically predisposed mice [16], a finding that laid the foundations for the description of the phenomenon of sodium sensitivity and the role of renal sodium retention in the development of hypertension.

In the years that followed, various research groups verified the relationship between high sodium intake and the development of hypertension in several animal models. The most striking evidence, however, is derived from the studies of Denton et al. in free-living chimpanzees. In a preliminary study of this group, 26 chimpanzees were divided into two groups; the first group continued their habitual low-sodium diet of fruits and vegetables, whereas the other one received progressively increasing amounts of sodium up to 15 g/day (equivalent to our contermporary high-salt diet) [17]. Over a period of 20 months, BP in the second group rose an average of 33/10 mmHg, returning to baseline after the excess sodium was removed from the diet. Consistent with interindividual differences in sodium sensitivity, BP did not increase in all members of the second group, a fact highlighting the need for genetic predisposition for developing hypertension under high sodium intake.

In more recent studies by the same group, approximately 130 free-living chimpanzees were fed a diet with varying sodium content (from 35 to 250 mmol/day, roughly corresponding to 1–6 g of sodium per day) for extended periods. After long-term follow-up, a linear relationship between sodium intake and increased BP was observed (an average increase of 10/5 mmHg per 100 mmol/day of sodium). These experiments performed in higher mammals phylogenetically closer to *Homo sapiens* than any other species constitute some of the best experimental evidence for the relationship between dietary sodium intake and increased BP and underscore the importance of modern diet in the development of hypertension.

Observational Human Studies

The evidence from population-based studies supporting the relationship between sodium intake and the development of hypertension is overwhelming.

A significant association between dietary sodium intake and BP levels or hypertension incidence has been demonstrated by a large number of studies in various large populations [18–21]. The strongest evidence is derived from the INTERSALT study, which measured 24-h urine electrolytes and BP in over 10,000 men and women aged 20–60 years from 52 population samples worldwide. For all 52 centers, there was a positive correlation between 24-h urine sodium excretion and both systolic and diastolic BP, but an even stronger association between sodium excretion and the slope (increase) of BP with age (Fig. 1). Based on these data, it was estimated that an increase in habitual population sodium intake by 100 mmol/day is associated with an increase in BP by 3–6/0–3 mmHg [19]. Many additional studies have explored the relationship between sodium intake and BP, with one of the most recent being the NHANES-2014 examination, which confirmed a strong direct relationship between sodium intake (based on 24-h urine collection), BP, and prevalence of hypertension [22].

Additionally, it has long been recognized that indigenous populations, isolated in various parts of the planet, who consume a low-sodium diet (<1 g/day), resembling the diet followed by primitive humans, do not develop hypertension and their BP does not rise with age [23, 24]. In the INTERSALT study, only four out of 52 populations had a sodium intake close to 50 mmol/day; notably, these populations did not exhibit hypertension nor an increase in BP with age [25, 26]. When individuals from such populations migrate to Western countries and adopt Western dietary lifestyles, they experience an increase in BP and the occurrence of hypertension becomes similar to that of the native population [27, 28].

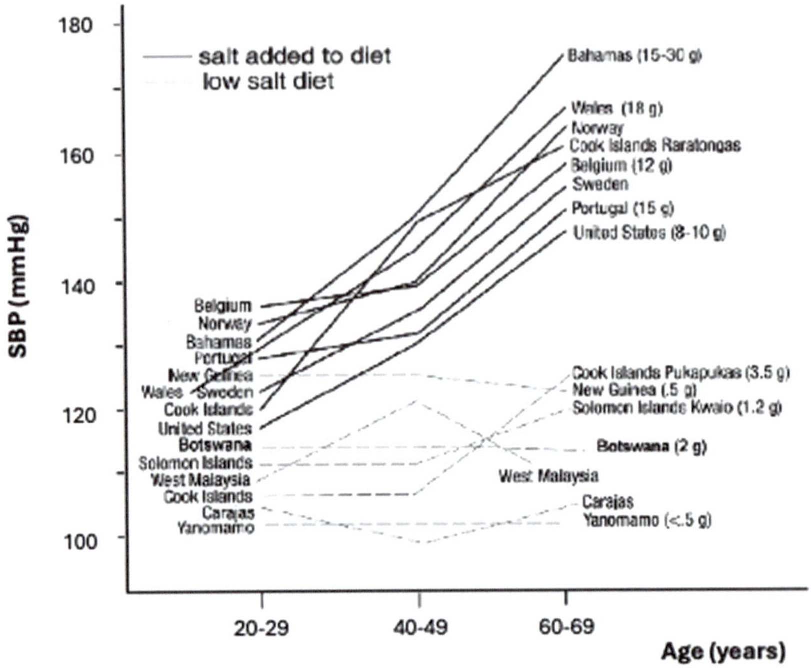

Fig. 1 Diagram of the mean increase in systolic blood pressure (SBP) over 40 years (from the age group of 20–29 to that of 60–69) based on the dietary salt intake in the various Western and isolated populations studied in the INTERSALT study

The aforementioned data have shaped the hypothesis that the development of hypertension is largely due to the mismatch between human evolutionary physiology, which has a tendency toward consuming salt, and the modern high-salt diet [24]. Our herbivorous ancestors probably consumed less than 10 mmol of sodium per day, whereas our carnivorous ancestors might have eaten around 30 mmol/day [29]. Prehistoric humans were forced to cross great continental distances to secure food, with salt being scarcely available; thus, their preference for salt was a physiological adaptation that facilitated salt intake at every opportunity. In parallel, our kidneys evolved efficient transport mechanisms to retain filtered sodium, an adaptation that enhanced survival during salt and water deprivation [24]. However, the diet of prehistoric humans, which mainly included fruits and vegetables, was high in potassium and low in sodium.

In contrast, in modern developed societies, the total sodium intake is much higher (100–250 mmol/day) [25], while the potassium intake is much lower. Importantly, more than 75% of sodium is thought to be added during the processing and preparation of food products [30], and our current preference for salty foods is not innate but rather an acquired taste, developing early in childhood [31]. Accumulating evidence suggests that there is a population "threshold" (i.e., 50–100 mmol/day) below which the human body can handle dietary sodium without increasing BP (depending largely on individual predisposition, as described below) [24, 32]. Unfortunately, modern Western societies have a much higher average dietary sodium intake than this level. Thus, the phylogenetic "adaptive" preference of the human species for salt is now considered "maladaptive" and a primary contributor to the development of hypertension.

Interventional Human Studies

Numerous clinical studies have unequivocally demonstrated the beneficial effects of sodium restriction on BP levels. This was already known since the beginning of the last century [33]. Strict restriction of dietary sodium has proven highly effective in reducing BP and has been systematically applied in clinical practice since the 1950s, when the need to treat hypertension became clear and therapeutic options were limited [34].

In recent decades, a large number of randomized clinical trials (RCTs) applying mild dietary sodium restriction have been published. In a sub-study of the Dietary Approaches to Stop Hypertension (DASH) trial, participants receiving either the DASH diet (rich in fruits and vegetables) or the control diet were randomly assigned to sodium intakes of 145, 105, and 65 mmol/day. Both groups showed significant reductions in BP with the low-sodium phases of both diets (average difference in BP of −3.0/−1.6 and −6.7/−3.5 mmHg between the high-sodium and low-sodium phases of DASH diet and control diet, respectively) [35]. In the TONE study, which included 975 hypertensive patients aged 60–80 years, after 3 years of follow-up, significantly lower BP levels were seen in patients with sodium restriction alone or in combination with weight loss compared to the control group [36]. Based on data from several randomized studies, it appears that reducing sodium intake to <100 mmol/day in hypertensive patients leads to a reduction in BP by approximately 5/2.5 mmHg [37]. Accordingly, a series of studies in individuals with high-normal BP showed that mild sodium restriction reduces both BP and the incidence of hypertension in the long term [38].

Sodium Sensitivity—Definition and Diagnosis

The magnitude of the effects of dietary sodium on BP levels is heterogeneous and varies among populations with different characteristics. Although most adults have consumed a high-sodium diet since childhood, only a portion of them develop hypertension by the age of 55, suggesting a variable degree of BP sensitivity to sodium [39].

Sodium sensitivity is a physiological characteristic of rodents and mammals, including humans, in which BP changes in some individuals parallel changes in sodium intake [40]. As early as the 1960s, Dahl et al. observed that the degree of BP increase after sodium loading differs considerably between different populations of experimental animals (Sprague-Dawley rats). Through selective inbreeding, researchers developed two distinct populations, i.e., Dahl (or sodium)- sensitive and

Dahl (or sodium)-resistant rats. Sodium-sensitive animals experienced BP increase with acute sodium loading and a BP decrease with sodium depletion, whereas the sodium-resistant animals did not.

These findings have been also confirmed by corresponding clinical studies [41, 42]. In humans, the trait is normally distributed and the differentiation between sodium-sensitive and sodium-resistant individuals is made by selecting an arbitrary threshold for sodium-induced BP changes [1]. Weinberger et al. defined sodium sensitivity if at least a 10% increase in mean arterial pressure is found after a high-salt versus low-salt challenge; individuals exhibiting smaller increases were defined as sodium-resistant [43]. However, in general, there is no clear consensus on the definition of sodium sensitivity in clinical practice [44, 45]. Although the criteria and assessment methods for sodium sensitivity are not standardized, approximately 25% of normotensive and 30–50% of hypertensive patients are sodium-sensitive [1, 46]. In recent years, inverse sodium sensitivity, a new entity concerning 15% of the general population and defined as a paradoxical BP decrease in response to high sodium intake, has been identified as masquerading within the broad spectrum of sodium resistance [47, 48].

Genetic polymorphisms have been linked to sodium sensitivity, hypertension, and cardiovascular disease, with candidate genes including those that influence the expression of proteins involved in renal sodium transport [49]. Apart from hypertensive patients and genetic polymorphisms, sodium sensitivity is also increased with aging [50], in African-American individuals [51], and in patients with metabolic syndrome or obesity [52], diabetes [53], and CKD [54, 55]. What is also important is that sodium sensitivity in normotensive adults predicts future hypertension [50, 56].

Existing protocols for diagnosing sodium sensitivity are broadly divided into outpatient multiday dietary protocols (i.e., diets of specific low and high sodium content given sequentially for a given period, typically ~1 week each) and inpatient "acute" protocols (i.e., a 3-day protocol consisting of a rapid volume expansion with intravenous normal saline loading on the first day followed by sodium and volume depletion with dietary sodium restriction and diuretic administration upon the second day) [46]. All of these protocols are inherent to limitations, cannot be easily applied in everyday clinical settings, while BP responses to sodium challenge are poorly reproducible [57]. In parallel, dietary protocols lack standardization regarding sodium content of diets, order of administration, exposure duration, and subsequent washout periods between diets [58]. Moreover, given that subjects are classified as sodium-sensitive if the protocol achieves a BP change (either absolute or percentage) greater than an arbitrary, investigator-defined threshold, the cutoff levels for sodium-sensitive BP responses vary widely among studies [59]. Consequently, no consensus has been reached on which protocols should be universally used for diagnosing sodium sensitivity.

Mechanisms of Sodium Sensitivity

Based on the Guytonian model of pressure-natriuresis, any increase in BP increases renal perfusion pressure and renal interstitial hydrostatic pressure, decreases sodium reabsorption by the proximal tubules and increases natriuresis, thereby lowering systemic BP [60]. In response to high sodium intake, kidneys activate natriuretic systems [atrial natriuretic peptide (ANP), nitric oxide (NO)] and suppress anti-natriuretic systems [renin-angiotensin-aldosterone system (RAAS), sympathetic nervous system (SNS)] [61]. In sodium-sensitive individuals, pressure-natriuresis is impaired, with natriuretic and anti-natriuretic systems being ineffectively activated and suppressed, respectively. Therefore, the pressure-natriuresis curve shifts to the right and its slope declines, as higher BP is required to maintain sodium equilibrium. In contrast, in sodium-resistant individuals, the pressure-natriuresis curve shifts to the right without a change in slope (Fig. 2).

The putative pathophysiological defect leading to sodium sensitivity may involve several mechanisms, the common denominator of which is a natriuretic handicap [1]—i.e., a disruption of the kidney's ability to excrete excess sodium—essentially rendering sodium sensitivity the connecting link between increased sodium intake and kidneys in the development of hypertension. The existence of many plausible mechanisms reflects the lack of a major distinct cause of this phenomenon [43], and the possibility that different pathways are activated in different individuals. Regardless of the precise mechanisms, sodium sensitivity appears to be largely genetically predetermined, as shown by preclinical studies and the close

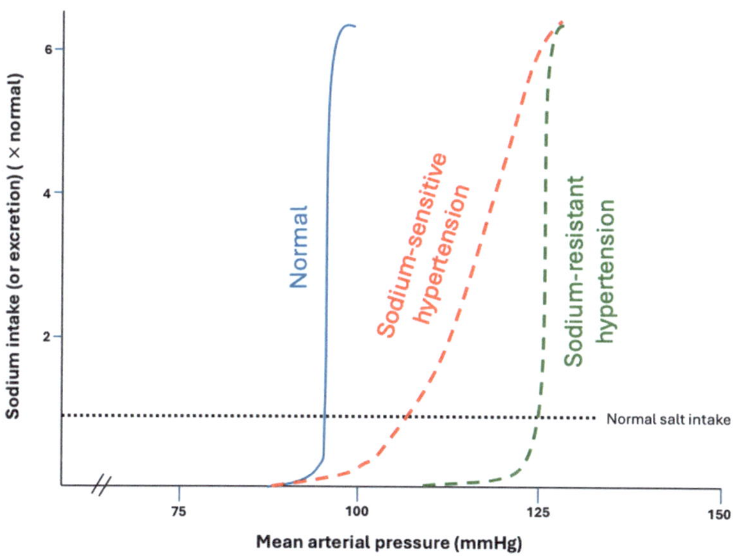

Fig. 2 Pressure-natriuresis curve. The relationship between mean arterial pressure (horizontal axis) and sodium intake (or excretion): (a) under normal conditions, (b) in patients with sodium-sensitive hypertension, and (c) in patients with sodium-resistant hypertension

resemblance in BP response to sodium restriction between normotensive mothers and healthy offsprings [62].

Several potential mechanisms have been proposed. Firstly, attenuated stimulation of RAAS by salt restriction [63, 64] and/or blunted suppression of renin in response to a salt load [65] have been manifested. Furthermore, impaired renal circulation (i.e., increased renal vasoconstriction and/or disrupted renal vasodilation), particularly in the renal medulla, results in an inability to excrete a chronic sodium load [66, 67]. Among other factors, decreased levels of endogenous NO [68], reduced renal kallikrein activity [69] and hyperuricemia [70] have been proposed as potential contributors. In parallel, overactivation of the sympathetic nervous system [71] is a common feature in sodium-sensitive subjects. Additionally, paradoxically reduced levels of ANP in response to a high-salt [72], oxidative stress [73, 74], hyperinsulinemia [75], and subclinical interstitial renal inflammation [76] also represent fundamental interrelated mechanisms. Our traditional view of sodium sensitivity as solely a manifestation of kidney malfunction has been lately challenged by recent seminal studies. It seems that non-osmotic sodium accumulation in the skin interstitium bound to negatively charged glycosaminoglycans [77] and endothelial dysfunction due to alterations in the endothelial surface layer characteristics [78] also play pivotal roles in sodium homeostasis and sodium sensitivity.

The Role of the Kidney in BP Regulation and the Development of Hypertension

Sodium-sensitive hypertension arises from an intrinsic renal defect in sodium excretion, although the kidney also contributes to hypertension in non-sodium-sensitive individuals. Many authors therefore regard hypertension as primarily a kidney disorder. Extensive research over recent decades has indicated several mechanistic pathways originating in the kidney that share a common feature: the inability of the kidneys to excrete excess sodium despite a normal glomerular filtration rate. While certain details remain unresolved, these mechanisms can be grouped into certain central "theories," outlined below. While these "theories" sometimes complement and sometimes contradict one another, they remain broadly consistent with the available experimental evidence.

Inherited Renal Defects in Sodium Excretion

The first theory in this field arose from Dahl's pioneering experiments and the development of animal models with sodium sensitivity and sodium resistance, which was attributed to a "genetic" defect of the kidney [16]. Dahl and colleagues extended their experiments to mice, showing that BP follows the kidney; when hypertensive mice received a kidney transplant from normotensive animals, BP returned to normal. Conversely, when normotensive animals received a kidney transplant from hypertensive ones, they developed hypertension [79]. It was therefore considered that hypertension is due to a genetically inherited disadvantage of the kidney that follows the kidney itself. Moreover, transplantation of a kidney from a hypertensive rat that had been briefly rendered normotensive with an angiotensin-converting enzyme inhibitor (ACEI) normalized BP in a hypertensive host.

This concept was partly confirmed by human transplant studies. In patients with renal failure due to hypertension, BP often normalized completely after receiving a kidney transplant from a normotensive donor [80]. Similarly, the development of hypertension in normotensive kidney recipients is more common when the graft comes from hypertensive donors [81].

At the time this theory was first formulated, it was not possible to identify the specific genetic defect of the kidney responsible for the long-term development of hypertension. Even after decades of research, no major single gene defect explaining most cases has been identified. However, rare monogenic forms of hypertension (e.g., Liddle's syndrome, Gordon's syndrome, etc.), in which a mutation of a single gene alters the function of a sodium renal transporter, demonstrate that such a mechanism is possible. Consequent research therefore focused on "mild" mutations of the corresponding genes that could produce subtler disturbances in these transporters and milder forms of hypertension in a large proportion of hypertensive patients [82]. Evidence supporting this possibility has begun to emerge in recent decades [83].

Heterogeneity of Nephrons and RAS Activation

This theory, formulated in the late 1980s by Laragh's group [84, 85], represents an evolution of Goldblatt's earlier views on renovascular hypertension [86]. Laragh and colleagues argued the existence of two distinct nephron populations [84, 85]. The first population consists of nephrons that are ischemic, either due to impaired autoregulation and vasoconstriction of the afferent arteriole or due to structural changes leading to glomerular ischemia. The second population, which constitutes the majority, undergoes compensatory hyperfunction and hyperfiltration, thereby maintaining a normal total glomerular filtration rate. The ischemic nephrons, however, exhibit increased renin release, which results in the production of angiotensin II and consequently enhanced sodium reabsorption in the proximal tubule of all nephrons (proportionally greater in the hyperfiltrating nephrons). Total plasma renin levels remain within normal limits, since the overproduction of renin by the ischemic nephrons is counterbalanced by renin suppression in the remaining nephrons. Thus, angiotensin II levels are slightly elevated compared to baseline but remain within the normal range. This modest elevation in angiotensin II is sufficient to increase sodium reabsorption in the hyperfunctioning nephrons, but not high enough to suppress renin release from ischemic nephrons (a process requiring a higher threshold). The net effect is a resetting of the pressure-natriuresis curve, such that BP is elevated for any given level of sodium excretion. In fact, hypertension is regarded as the "price" paid for ischemic nephrons to maintain their function independently of the remaining nephron population. Simultaneously, angiotensin II exerts trophic actions that, in combination with hyperfiltration, contribute to the development of kidney damage [84, 85].

This theory is consistent with a series of well-established observations: (i) total plasma renin levels in most hypertensive patients are within normal limits, yet remain "inappropriately high" for BP levels and are not fully suppressed, a finding that indicates impaired renal sodium excretion [87]; (ii) renin-angiotensin system blockers effectively reduce BP even when plasma renin levels are not elevated, possibly by interfering with renin derived from ischemic nephrons; and (iii) RAS blockers protect against progression of kidney damage in patients with proteinuric nephropathies or hyperfiltration [88].

Reduced Nephron Number

In the late 1980s, Brenner and coworkers advanced another influential theory regarding the renal origin of hypertension and progressive kidney disease [89]. Based on earlier observations that a nephron loss (e.g., surgical nephrectomy, renal diseases) accelerates hypertension and renal damage, they proposed that a reduced nephron number or filtration surface area limits sodium excretion, elevates BP, and forces sodium excretion at the cost of hypertension. This initiates a vicious cycle in which hypertension induces further renal injury and nephron loss [89, 90]. This model was subsequently used by the same authors to explain the vicious cycle of nephrosclerosis caused by nephron loss and hyperfunction of the remaining nephrons [90, 91].

Brenner and colleagues further hypothesized that congenital reduction in nephron number or filtration surface could account for differences in the prevalence of hypertension among populations (e.g., between Black and White patients). This concept was essentially incorporated into Barker's broader hypothesis of the fetal origin of adult disease [92, 93], which posits that neonates with low birth weight are at increased risk of cardiovascular disease later in adult life. A large number of epidemiological studies have since confirmed that neonates with low birth weight have higher risk for hypertension [94, 95], type 2 diabetes [96], and cardiovascular mortality [97]. One explanation supports that inadequate maternal nutrient supply during gestation forces the fetus to "prioritize" brain development at the expense of organs such as kidneys and pancreas (thrifty phenotype hypothesis) [98]. Another explanation, which has lately gained ground, is that the risk of adult disease is attributable less to low birth weight per se and more to the compensatory postnatal "catch-up growth" through overfeeding, which programs the infant for obesity, diabetes, hypertension, and cardiovascular disease in adult life [99].

With regard to the reduced nephron number, it has been demonstrated that the majority of nephrons are formed during the early weeks of the third trimester, and nephrogenesis ceases after 34–36 weeks of gestation [100]. A large body of studies have clearly shown that neonates with low birth weight have fewer nephrons (approximately 260,000 fewer per each kilogram decrease in birth weight) [101, 102] and that nephron number does not increase after birth, regardless of the quality of subsequent nutrition [100]. Thus, even if a neonate with low birth weight later attains normal body weight, it will still bear a higher functional "load" per nephron, necessitating hyperfiltration and initiating the vicious cycle leading to hypertension and renal injury. This theory was confirmed by an autopsy study of 10 hypertensive and 10 normotensive individuals (carefully matched for sex, age, and body size). Hypertensive patients had less than half the number of nephrons compared to normotensive individuals, and significantly larger nephron diameters, indicative of hyperfiltration. Moreover, hypertensive patients did not exhibit sclerotic glomeruli, suggesting that low nephron number was present from birth [103].

Natriuretic Factors

Another attractive theory linking a renal "defect" to the development of hypertension is that of the "natriuretic factors." This theory originating from Dahl's experiments has remained under investigation for more than 40 years. After the development of distinct strains of salt-sensitive and salt-resistant experimental animals, Dahl and colleagues observed in another experiment that chronic parabiosis of the two strains induced hypertension in animals previously salt-resistant. They hypothesized that a "humoral" factor was being transferred from one strain to the other [104]. Two years later, this factor was shown to act as a natriuretic hormone—initially paradoxically inducing both natriuresis and hypertension [105].

In the 1970s, this substance was found to inhibit the Na^+-K^+-ATPase pump [106] and increase intracellular calcium in vascular smooth muscle cells, elevating vascular resistance and BP [107]. These findings were further elaborated by de Wardener and McGregor, who proposed that the increase in natriuretic hormone represents a compensatory response to a renal "inability" to excrete sodium [108].

Over time, it became clear that this substance promotes renal sodium excretion by inhibiting of Na^+-K^+-ATPase located on the basolateral membrane of tubular epithelial cells, which constitutes the driving force for renal sodium reabsorption. However, this substance simultaneously inhibits Na^+-K^+-ATPase in the plasma membrane of all cells throughout the organism. Among others, in vascular smooth muscle cells, increased intracellular sodium raises intracellular calcium via the Na^+-Ca^{2+} exchanger. Thus, this substance was considered the missing link between natriuresis and BP elevation, as predicted by Guyton's original theory [108, 109].

The precise nature of this natriuretic hormone remains debated. The strongest candidate has been ouabain, shown to inhibit Na^+-K^+-ATPase by acting on the α_2-subunit of the enzyme, thereby increasing intracellular Ca^{2+} and raising BP in experimental animals [110–112]. However, the physiological relevance of endogenously produced ouabain is questioned, since it has not yet been conclusively demonstrated that it is synthesized in conditions and quantities sufficient to exert a physiological or pathophysiological role [113]. Instead, it has been argued that another peptide with similar properties, isolated from human plasma and possessing a bufadienolide structure, may represent the true natriuretic hormone [114]. Further research is warranted to clarify this intriguing issue.

Subclinical Renal Inflammation and Tubulointerstitial Injury

A more recent theory proposed by Johnson and colleagues focuses on subclinical renal inflammation [76, 115]. In models of sodium-sensitive hypertension, immune cell infiltrates and mild tubulointerstitial inflammation were identified; importantly, reducing this inflammation resulted in a decrease in BP levels. Detailed experiments led to the hypothesis that the infiltrating monocytes and macrophages produce angiotensin II and pro-inflammatory cytokines that interfere with tubular sodium excretion, promoting sodium-sensitive hypertension (Fig. 3) [115, 116]. The

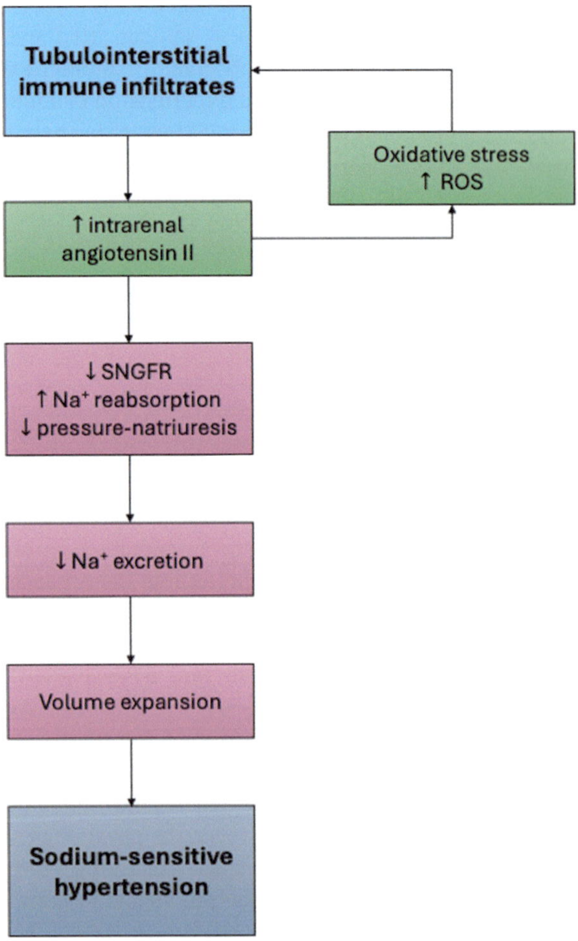

Fig. 3 Theory of subclinical renal inflammation and tubulointerstitial injury

researchers extended their observations and proposed that subclinical tubulointerstitial inflammation from various causes may trigger sodium retention and increase BP, and that chronic tubulointerstitial damage—resulting from hypertension, RAS activation, hyperuricemia, and other factors—may be the main cause of worsening BP control and the long-term transition of hypertension to a sodium-sensitive phenotype [117].

Dietary Sodium Intake in CKD

Sodium Loading

The role of dietary sodium intake in CKD has been extensively investigated, as it holds a central position in the pathogenesis of hypertension in these patients. Within the context of CKD, high salt intake is one of the most important modifiable factors for the development of resistant hypertension [118]. The main pathophysiological link lies in the fact that progressive renal impairment causes an increase in sodium sensitivity [54]. Notably, sodium sensitivity is not only limited to patients with advanced CKD stages, but seems to be present even before the onset of overt hypertension and severe renal dysfunction [119]. According to Guyton's pressure-natriuresis curve, sodium loading requires an increase in BP in order to excrete sodium. While sodium loading in healthy individuals and in patients with CKD leads in both cases to an increase in extracellular volume and fractional sodium excretion, it has different effects on BP, as a disproportionate increase is observed in patients with CKD [120]. This occurs because of the reduced ability to excrete sodium from the progressively declining number of functional nephrons [121]. Thus, in these patients, the expansion of extracellular volume restores external sodium balance, but at the cost of increased total body sodium and resistant hypertension [122, 123]. The extent of extracellular volume expansion is directly related to the degree of renal dysfunction and corresponds to approximately 5–10% of body weight, even in the absence of peripheral edema [122].

Higher sodium intake is consistently associated with adverse outcomes in patients with CKD. Sodium increases BP levels and the rate of appropriate BP control [124], worsens albuminuria [54, 125–127], limits the normal nocturnal BP dipping [128, 129], alters glomerular hemodynamics by inducing hyperfiltration [125, 127], attenuates the nephroprotective and antihypertensive effects of RAS blockers [130–133], and exerts a direct profibrotic effect on target organs (kidneys, heart, etc.) mediated by aldosterone due to sodium-dependent paradoxical activation of mineralocorticoid receptors [126, 134–136]. Regarding hard outcomes, in the CRIC (Chronic Renal Insufficiency Cohort) study, a large observational study with almost 4000 patients with CKD and ~7 years of follow-up, the group of patients with high sodium intake (i.e., urine sodium excretion >195 mmol/day) showed a higher risk for CKD progression [137]. Among participants, 804 composite cardiovascular events (575 heart failure, 305 myocardial infarctions, 148 strokes) occurred during the follow-up period, demonstrating a linear relationship between higher sodium intake and higher cardiovascular risk [138]. Additionally, a post hoc analysis of the first and second REIN (Ramipril Efficacy in Nephropathy) trials found a 1.61-fold higher risk of end-stage kidney disease for each 100-mEq/g increase in urine sodium-to-creatinine ratio [139].

Sodium Restriction

As extracellular volume overload is central to the pathogenesis of hypertension in CKD, sodium restriction is a key therapeutic strategy. Kempner was the first to recognize the benefits of limiting excess sodium intake in CKD patients, developing the strict "rice diet" a demanding dietary regimen restricting sodium intake to 0.15 g/day, and noting substantial reductions in oedema and other complications of fluid overload with this diet [140]. Since the 1960s, dietary sodium restriction has gained momentum for the prevention and treatment of cardiovascular and renal outcomes.

Several studies have examined the impact of sodium restriction in CKD. In 2021, McMahon et al. conducted an updated systematic review of 21 randomized controlled trials (RCTs) including 1197 participants, with a mean duration of 7 (1–36) weeks. Twelve studies enrolled patients in the earlier CKD stages (779 randomized participants), seven in dialysis (363 randomized participants), and two in post-transplant (55 randomized participants). Across studies, reducing sodium intake by 73.5 mmol/day consistently lowered BP by ~7/4 mmHg and reduced proteinuria in patients with earlier CKD stage (non-dialyzed, non-transplanted) by 34–36% [141]. Table 1 summarizes the main RCTs evaluating the impact of dietary sodium restriction on pre-dialysis CKD patients.

In light of the current evidence, guidelines for the management of CKD patients generally include recommendations on sodium intake [11, 142–144]. The 2024 KDIGO guidelines recommend targeting a sodium intake <2 g of sodium per day (or <90 mmol of sodium per day, or <5 g of sodium chloride per day) in CKD patients but suggests that this recommendation is based on weak evidence (2C grade) [142]. This cutoff is also suggested by 2023 ESH guidelines for all hypertensive patients [11], while the American Heart Association recommends <1.5 g of sodium per day (or <65 mmol of sodium per day, or <3.8 g of sodium chloride per day) for high-risk patients, including those with CKD [144].

However, sodium restriction remains one of the least successfully achieved targets in routine care of CKD patients [145, 146]. This is reflected in consistently high urinary sodium excretion in control groups of several studies. An analysis of the CRIC study showed a mean sodium intake of ~3.7 g/day, indicating that the vast majority of CKD patients do not comply with dietary sodium recommendations [138]. In fact, fewer than one in five CKD patients achieve the recommended target for dietary sodium restriction [146].

The most common barriers to effective dietary sodium restriction are practical (e.g., time, cost, limited availability of low-sodium foods, social constraints, lack of family support), perceptual (taste preferences, taste disorders), and educational

Table 1 Summary of main randomized controlled trials evaluating the effects of dietary sodium reduction on patients with pre-dialysis chronic kidney disease

Author, year	Country	Design	CKD stages	Number of patients	Intervention	Control	Modality of intervention	Intervention duration	Decrease in SBP/DBP
Konishi et al., 2001 [119]	Japan	Double-blind, cross-over RCT	N/A	38	*Target* Low sodium: 87 mmol/day *Mean 24-h urine sodium excretion* Low sodium: ~50 mmol/day	*Target* High sodium: 209 mmol/day *Mean 24-h urine sodium excretion* Low sodium: ~165 mmol/day	Provision of meals	1 week	−6.6/−4.0 mmHg
Vogt et al., 2008 [130]	The Netherlands	Double-blind, cross-over RCT	CKD stages 1–3	34	*Target* Low sodium: 50 mmol/day *Mean 24-h urine sodium excretion* Low sodium: ~90 mmol/day	*Target* High sodium: 200 mmol/day *Mean 24-h urine sodium excretion* High sodium: ~200 mmol/day	Individualized counselling by dietician	18 weeks	−6.0/−3.0 mmHg

(continued)

Table 1 (continued)

Author, year	Country	Design	CKD stages	Number of patients	Intervention	Control	Modality of intervention	Intervention duration	Decrease in SBP/DBP
Slagman et al., 2011 [174]	The Netherlands	Double-blind, cross-over RCT	CKD stages 1–3	52	*Target* Low sodium: 50 mmol/day *Mean 24-h urine sodium excretion* Low sodium: ~105 mmol/day	*Target* High sodium: 200 mmol/day *Mean 24-h urine sodium excretion* High sodium: ~185 mmol/day	Individualized counselling by dietician	6 weeks	−9.0/−7.0 mmHg
De Brito-Ashurst et al., 2013 [175]	United Kingdom (Bangladeshi origin patients)	Parallel, open-label RCT	CKD 3–4	*Intervention*, $n = 25$; *Control*, $n = 23$	*Mean 24-h urine sodium excretion* Low sodium: ~140 mmol/day	*Mean 24-h urine sodium excretion* High sodium: ~250 mmol/day	*Low sodium*: Individualized dietary education and cooking lessons; *High sodium*: Usual care (general low-salt advice sent with doctor's letter)	26 weeks	−8.0/−3.0 mmHg

McMahon et al., 2013 [176]	Australia	Double-blind, cross-over RCT	CKD stages 3–4	20	*Target* Low sodium: 60–80 mmol/day *Mean 24-h urine sodium excretion* Low sodium: ~75 mmol/day	*Target* High sodium: 180–200 mmol/day *Mean 24-h urine sodium excretion* High sodium: ~170 mmol/day	Dietary education from trained dietician	2 weeks	−9.70/−3.90 mmHg
Meuleman et al., 2017 [177]	The Netherlands	Open-label, parallel RCT	CKD stages 1–4	*Intervention*, $n = 67$; *Control*, $n = 71$	*Mean 24-h urine sodium excretion* Low sodium: ~150 mmol/day	*Mean 24-h urine sodium excretion* High sodium: ~175 mmol/day	*Low sodium*: Regular care plus self-management intervention comprising education, motivational interviewing, coaching, and self-monitoring of BP and 24-h urine sodium excretion; *high sodium*: Regular care	24 weeks	−2.0/−2.0 mmHg

(continued)

Table 1 (continued)

Author, year	Country	Design	CKD stages	Number of patients	Intervention	Control	Modality of intervention	Intervention duration	Decrease in SBP/DBP
Saran et al., 2017	USA	Open-label, cross-over RCT	CKD stages 3–4	58	*Target* Low sodium: <2000 mg/day *Mean 24-h urine sodium excretion* Low sodium: ~110 mmol/day	*Target* High sodium: (usual diet) *Mean 24-h urine sodium excretion* High sodium: ~170 mmol/day	Counselling by dietician	4 weeks	−10.80/−6.20 mmHg
Humalda et al., 2020 [178]	The Netherlands	Open-label, parallel RCT	CKD stages 1–4	*Intervention*, $n = 50$; *control*, $n = 40$	*Mean 24-h urine sodium excretion* Low sodium: *At 3 months*, ~148 mmol/day, *at 9 months*, ~160 mmol/day	*Mean 24-h urine sodium excretion* High sodium: *At 3 months*, ~174 mmol/day, *at 9 months*, ~154 mmol/day	*Low sodium*: Routine care and web-based self-management program, individual e-coaching and group meetings; *high sodium*: Routine care	12-week intervention period, 24-week maintenance period	*At 3 months*: −4.7/−1/8 mmHg; *at 9 months*: −4.3/−1.5 mmHg

Trakarnvanich et al., 2024 [179]	Thailand	Open-label, parallel RCT	CKD stages 1–3	*Intervention*, $n = 99$; *control*, $n = 95$	*Target* Low sodium: ~65 mmol/day *Mean 24-h urine sodium excretion* Low sodium: ~125 mmol/day	*Target* High sodium: (usual diet) *Mean 24-h urine sodium excretion* High sodium: ~135 mmol/day	Provision of meals	12 weeks	−6.6/−4.3 mmHg

(limited awareness of benefit or difficulty identifying low-sodium foods) reasons [147]. Patients with CKD often experience salt taste disorders due to reduced sensitivity (increased threshold) of the taste buds due to various causes, such as zinc deficiency, hypovolemic dry mouth, peripheral neuropathy, uremia, or as an adverse effect of medications [148]. In fact, a positive correlation has been demonstrated between taste dysfunction and sodium intake in patients with pre-dialysis CKD. However, only 1 week of low-sodium diet increases the taste sensitivity of these patients to salt [149]. Consequently, even short-term sodium restriction per se may improve compliance by removing taste restriction. On the other hand, the majority of consumed sodium derives mostly from hidden sources (preservatives, canned products, condiments, sweets, deli meats, cured meats, baked products, cheeses, and other processed food items) and restaurant food, and only ~15% from added table salt or home cooking [150]; therefore, sodium overconsumption could be significantly reduced by simply checking food labels. At the same time, regular measurement of 24-h urinary sodium excretion and provision of feedback by treating physicians are also effective strategies to improve patient adherence to dietary instructions and to identify errors in food selection or fatigue with dietary efforts.

The Role of Uromodulin in Sodium Sensitivity: Rediscovery of an Old Molecule

Uromodulin, also known as Tamm-Horsfall protein, is a kidney-specific glycoprotein which is exclusively produced by the epithelial cells lining the thick ascending limb (TAL) (85–90%) and early distal convoluted tubule (DCT) (10–15%) and shows a bilateral secretion (apical and basolateral). This results in several uromodulin forms, i.e., intracellular, urinary (uUMOD), interstitial, and serum uromodulin (sUMOD), each of which possesses a discrete biological role [151]. Although uromodulin was firstly discovered in 1950, its role remained unclear for many years. During the past two decades, uromodulin gained extensive scientific interest and was recognized as a multifaceted player in various physiological and pathological processes. Among them, uromodulin has been widely recognized as a pivotal factor accounting for sodium homeostasis and thus is proposedly involved in sodium-sensitive hypertension.

The physiologic substrate lies in the tight functional connection of intracellular uromodulin with Na^+ tubular handling through modulation of Na^+ transporters' activity [152]. In particular, it increases the distal Na^+ reabsorption by activating the furosemide-sensitive Na^+-K^+-$2Cl^-$ cotransporter type 2 (NKCC2), located in the apical membrane of TAL cells [153]; additionally, uromodulin also activates the thiazide-sensitive, apical Na^+/Cl^- cotransporter (NCC) in DCT1 [154].

Preclinical studies have provided insights into the role of uromodulin in sodium sensitivity and hypertension. Uromodulin-deficient mice exhibit polyuria, salt wasting, reduced BP and eGFR, with impaired NKCC2/NCC activity leading to resistance to furosemide and metolazone but hyperresponsiveness to acetazolamide [155–158]. Their BP remains low compared to wild-type mice under basal salt conditions and resistant to dietary salt due to enhanced urinary sodium-wasting phenotype in response to salt loading. Similarly, hepsin-deficient mice, showing defective uromodulin processing, accumulate intracellular uromodulin, develop tubular damage and salt wasting, and do not display BP rises upon salt loading [159]. In contrast, *UMOD* risk variant transgenic mice overexpressing uromodulin display higher NKCC2 activity, hypertension, left ventricular hypertrophy, CKD-like changes, and enhanced furosemide responsiveness [160]; hypertension is *Umod* dosage-dependent and sodium-sensitive, as after an extremely salt-depleted diet BP is normalized in transgenic mice, while in normotensive wild-type mice no change on BP is evident under these conditions [160]. Consequently, uromodulin deficiency causes a leftward shift of pressure-natriuresis curve compared to wild-type mice when exposed to salt loading, a fact revealing that uromodulin deficiency results in the loss of the sodium sensitivity of BP [156]. Conversely, uromodulin excess causes a rightward shift of pressure-natriuresis curve compared to wild-type mice when exposed to salt restriction, indicating that uromodulin excess results in the acquisition of the sodium sensitivity of BP (Fig. 4) [151].

Genetic studies consistently link *UMOD* variants to sodium sensitivity and hypertension. *UMOD* promoter SNPs, such as rs13333226, rs4293393, and rs12917707, influence uromodulin expression and tubular sodium handling. A large

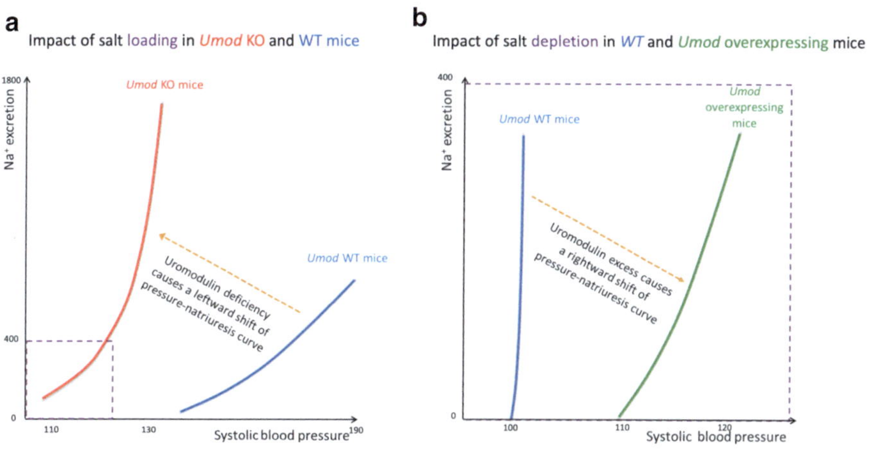

Fig. 4 Uromodulin and the pressure-natriuresis curve. (**a**) Uromodulin deficiency causes a leftward shift of pressure-natriuresis curve compared with wild-type (WT) mice, indicating that uromodulin deficiency results in the loss of the sodium sensitivity of blood pressure observed in WT mice: in the presence of uromodulin, higher sodium intake results in higher blood pressure values than in absence of uromodulin. (**b**) Uromodulin overexpression causes a rightward shift of pressure-natriuresis curve compared with WT mice when mice are salt-depleted (20-fold decrease in dietary NaCl), indicating that uromodulin excess results in the acquisition of the sodium sensitivity of blood pressure. On the contrary, in normotensive WT mice no effect on BP is evident under these experimental conditions. Na^+ excretion in μmol/24 h and systolic blood pressure (SBP) in mmHg. Inset in (**a**) displays the dimensions of panel (**b**). Notice that studies in panels (**a**) and (**b**) used different mouse strains and protocols. (Reproduced from Karagiannidis et al. [151], distributed under the terms of CC BY 4.0)

GWAS showed that the minor G allele of rs13333226 was associated with lower uUMOD, reduced BP, and decreased hypertension risk [161], while the rs4293393 T allele was associated with a stronger natriuretic and BP-lowering effect after furosemide [160]. Additionally, Mendelian randomization studies reinforce causality. Ponte et al. showed that genetically higher uUMOD levels were significantly associated with lower eGFR, higher odds for eGFR decline or CKD, and higher SBP or DBP, with the effect of uUMOD on BP being partially mediated by eGFR [162]. Further analyses in over a million individuals confirmed that *UMOD* variants driving higher uUMOD also raise hypertension incidence [163]. Finally, variants increasing uUMOD were associated with myocardial infarction, an effect largely explained by elevated BP [164].

Clinical studies have investigated the link between uromodulin, sodium sensitivity, and hypertension in diverse populations. In general population, individuals classified in the highest uUMOD strata (i.e., with 24-h uUMOD above the sex-specific median) showed a significant association of higher 24-h SBP and a non-significant trend of higher DBP levels in parallel with an increase in 24-h urinary Na^+ excretion [165]. Conversely, participants in the lowest uUMOD strata presented a significant association of lower 24-h ambulatory DBP levels and a non-significant trend for lower 24-h SBP in parallel to an increase in 24-h urinary Na^+ excretion [165]. These results were the first to reveal that uromodulin may have a differential impact on the development of either sodium sensitivity or inverse sodium sensitivity, depending on uUMOD levels. Newly diagnosed patients with mild hypertension exhibited higher uUMOD compared with controls, but without differences between sodium-sensitive and sodium-resistant patients [166, 167]. Furthermore, in a Croatian cohort of young untreated hypertensive patients, higher uUMOD was linked to higher SBP sleep-through surge levels and lower DBP dipping in prehypertensive subjects. This study was the first to show that uUMOD levels influence per se the circadian BP patterns and are linked to circadian BP alterations in prehypertensive subjects as a precursor of sustained hypertension [168]. Importantly, genotype-directed studies demonstrated that patients with *UMOD* risk alleles show greater BP reduction and enhanced natriuresis with loop diuretics, supporting genotype-guided therapy [160, 169]. Lastly, among children with CKD, higher uUMOD/Cr ratio was associated with lower BP in univariable but not multivariable analyses; in another pediatric study, a significant negative correlation between uUMOD/UCr and SBP (but not DBP) was reported [170]. However, these studies suffered from several limitations [171]. Moreover, in CKD and kidney transplant patients, lower uUMOD predicted reduced diuretic response to the furosemide stress, though associations weakened after adjusting for baseline eGFR and albuminuria [172]. Therefore, solid data on the link of uromodulin with sodium sensitivity in the setting of CKD are currently missing. The confirmation of such an association in the context of CKD is rather important, as these patients significantly differ from the ones studied so far (e.g., general population, hypertensive patients). CKD patients show decreasing uromodulin levels mirroring decreasing nephron and tubular mass with progression to ESKD [173], while eGFR seems to significantly mediate the effects of uromodulin on BP.

Conclusions

Sodium plays a central role in the development of hypertension, particularly in CKD patients, where impaired renal sodium excretion and elevated sodium sensitivity result in resistant hypertension, cardiovascular events, and CKD progression. Evidence from preclinical, observational, and clinical studies indicates that excessive sodium intake in Western societies coupled with defective renal sodium excretion is a principal mechanism that leads to development of hypertension, while dietary sodium restriction represents a cornerstone of effective antihypertensive treatment. The kidney is central to this process and possesses a dominant role in the development of sodium sensitivity. New scientific data elucidating mechanistic pathways involved in sodium sensitivity are being generated, expanding our current knowledge and providing novel therapeutic targets. Among them, uromodulin has been recently emerged as highly promising player in the development of sodium sensitivity. Further research into these interrelated and perplexed mechanisms may enable more precise, personalized strategies to prevent and treat hypertension, especially in CKD patients.

References

1. Kotchen TA, Cowley AW, Frohlich ED. Salt in health and disease—a delicate balance. N Engl J Med. 2013;368(13):1229–37. https://doi.org/10.1056/NEJMra1212606.
2. Webster AC, Nagler EV, Morton RL, Masson P. Chronic kidney disease. Lancet. 2017;389(10075):1238–52. https://doi.org/10.1016/S0140-6736(16)32064-5.
3. Go AS. Cardiovascular disease consequences of CKD. Semin Nephrol. 2016;36(4):293–304. https://doi.org/10.1016/j.semnephrol.2016.05.006.
4. Go AS, Chertow GM, Fan D, McCulloch CE, Hsu C, yuan. Chronic kidney disease and the risks of death, cardiovascular events, and hospitalization. N Engl J Med. 2004;351(13):1296–305. https://doi.org/10.1056/NEJMoa041031.
5. Shastri S, Sarnak MJ. Cardiovascular disease and CKD: core curriculum 2010. Am J Kidney Dis. 2010;56(2):399–417. https://doi.org/10.1053/j.ajkd.2010.03.019.
6. Johansen KL, Chertow GM, Gilbertson DT, et al. US renal data system 2021 annual data report: epidemiology of kidney disease in the United States. Am J Kidney Dis. 2022;79(4):A8–A12. https://doi.org/10.1053/j.ajkd.2022.02.001.
7. Tozawa M, Iseki K, Iseki C, Kinjo K, Ikemiya Y, Takishita S. Blood pressure predicts risk of developing end-stage renal disease in men and women. Hypertension. 2003;41(6):1341–5. https://doi.org/10.1161/01.HYP.0000069699.92349.8C.
8. Dahl LK. Role of dietary sodium in essential hypertension. J Am Diet Assoc. 1958;34(6):585–90.
9. Chobanian AV, Bakris GL, Black HR, et al. Seventh report of the joint National Committee on Prevention, Detection, Evaluation, and Treatment of High Blood Pressure. Hypertension. 2003;42(6):1206–52. https://doi.org/10.1161/01.HYP.0000107251.49515.c2.
10. Alderman MH. Salt, blood pressure, and human health. Hypertension. 2000;36(5):890–3. https://doi.org/10.1161/01.HYP.36.5.890.
11. Mancia G, Kreutz R, Brunström M, et al. 2023 ESH guidelines for the management of arterial hypertension the task force for the management of arterial hypertension of the European Society of Hypertension: endorsed by the International Society of Hypertension

(ISH) and the European renal association (ERA). J Hypertens. 2023;41(12):1874–2071. https://doi.org/10.1097/HJH.0000000000003480.
12. Whelton PK, Carey RM, Aronow WS, et al. 2017 ACC/AHA/AAPA/ABC/ACPM/AGS/APhA/ASH/ASPC/NMA/PCNA guideline for the prevention, detection, evaluation, and Management of High Blood Pressure in adults: a report of the American College of Cardiology/American Heart Association task force on clinical practice guidelines. Hypertension. 2018;71(6):e13–e115. https://doi.org/10.1161/HYP.0000000000000065.
13. World Health Organization. Guideline: sodium intake for adults and children. Geneva: World Health Organization; 2012. p. 1–46.
14. Health and Medicine Division, National Academies of Sciences, Engineering, and Medicine. Committee to review the dietary reference intakes for sodium and potassium, food and nutrition board. In: Stallings VA, Harrison M, Oria M, editors. Dietary reference intakes for sodium and potassium. Washington, DC: National Academies Press; 2019. p. 25353. https://doi.org/10.17226/25353.
15. Dahl LK. Effects of chronic excess salt feeding. Induction of self-sustaining hypertension in rats. J Exp Med. 1961;114(2):231–6. https://doi.org/10.1084/jem.114.2.231.
16. Dahl LK, Heine M, Tassinari L. Effects of chronia excess salt ingestion. Evidence that genetic factors play an important role in susceptibility to experimental hypertension. J Exp Med. 1962;115(6):1173–90. https://doi.org/10.1084/jem.115.6.1173.
17. Denton D, Weisinger R, Mundy NI, et al. The effect of increased salt intake on blood pressure of chimpanzees. Nat Med. 1995;1(10):1009–16. https://doi.org/10.1038/nm1095-1009.
18. Elliott P. Observational studies of salt and blood pressure. Hypertension. 1991;17(1_supplement):I3–8. https://doi.org/10.1161/01.HYP.17.1_Suppl.I3.
19. Stamler J. The INTERSALT study: background, methods, findings, and implications. Am J Clin Nutr. 1997;65(2):626S–42S. https://doi.org/10.1093/ajcn/65.2.626S.
20. Khaw KT, Bingham S, Welch A, et al. Blood pressure and urinary sodium in men and women: the Norfolk cohort of the European prospective investigation into cancer (EPIC-Norfolk). Am J Clin Nutr. 2004;80(5):1397–403. https://doi.org/10.1093/ajcn/80.5.1397.
21. Du Cailar G, Mimran A, Fesler P, Ribstein J, Blacher J, Safar ME. Dietary sodium and pulse pressure in normotensive and essential hypertensive subjects. J Hypertens. 2004;22(4):697–703. https://doi.org/10.1097/00004872-200404000-00011.
22. Jackson SL, Cogswell ME, Zhao L, et al. Association between urinary sodium and potassium excretion and blood pressure among adults in the United States: National Health and nutrition examination survey, 2014. Circulation. 2018;137(3):237–46. https://doi.org/10.1161/CIRCULATIONAHA.117.029193.
23. Oliver WJ, Cohen EL, Neel JV. Blood pressure, sodium intake, and sodium related hormones in the Yanomamo Indians, a "no-salt" culture. Circulation. 1975;52(1):146–51. https://doi.org/10.1161/01.CIR.52.1.146.
24. Denton D. Can hypertension be prevented? J Hum Hypertens. 1997;11(9):563–9. https://doi.org/10.1038/sj.jhh.1000489.
25. Elliott P, Stamler J, Nichols R, et al. Intersalt revisited: further analyses of 24 hour sodium excretion and blood pressure within and across populations. Intersalt Cooperative Research Group. BMJ. 1996;312(7041):1249–53. https://doi.org/10.1136/bmj.312.7041.1249.
26. Stamler J, Elliott P, Dyer AR, Stamler R, Kesteloot H, Marmot M. Commentary: Sodium and blood pressure in the Intersalt study and other studies—in reply to the Salt Institute. BMJ. 1996;312(7041):1285–7. https://doi.org/10.1136/bmj.312.7041.1285.
27. Poulter NR, Khaw KT, Hopwood BE, et al. The Kenyan Luo migration study: observations on the initiation of a rise in blood pressure. BMJ. 1990;300(6730):967–72. https://doi.org/10.1136/bmj.300.6730.967.
28. Klag MJ, He J, Coresh J, et al. The contribution of urinary cations to the blood pressure differences associated with migration. Am J Epidemiol. 1995;142(3):295–303. https://doi.org/10.1093/oxfordjournals.aje.a117635.

29. Eaton SB, Eaton SB, Konner MJ, Shostak M. An evolutionary perspective enhances understanding of human nutritional requirements. J Nutr. 1996;126(6):1732–40. https://doi.org/10.1093/jn/126.6.1732.
30. Mattes RD, Donnelly D. Relative contributions of dietary sodium sources. J Am Coll Nutr. 1991;10(4):383–93. https://doi.org/10.1080/07315724.1991.10718167.
31. Beauchamp GK, Engelman K. High salt intake. Sensory and behavioral factors. Hypertension. 1991;17(1 Suppl):I176–81. https://doi.org/10.1161/01.hyp.17.1_suppl.i176.
32. Kaplan NM, Victor RG. Primary hypertension: pathogenesis (with a special section on renal denervation and carotid baroreceptor pacing). In: Kaplan's clinical hypertension. 11th ed. Wolters Kluwer; 2015. p. 53–69.
33. Allen FM. Arterial hypertension. JAMA. 1920;74(10):652. https://doi.org/10.1001/jama.1920.02620100012005.
34. Kempner W. Treatment of hypertensive vascular disease with rice diet. Am J Med. 1948;4(4):545–77. https://doi.org/10.1016/0002-9343(48)90441-0.
35. Sacks FM, Svetkey LP, Vollmer WM, et al. Effects on blood pressure of reduced dietary sodium and the dietary approaches to stop hypertension (DASH) diet. N Engl J Med. 2001;344(1):3–10. https://doi.org/10.1056/NEJM200101043440101.
36. Whelton PK, Appel LJ, Espeland MA, et al. Sodium reduction and weight loss in the treatment of hypertension in older persons: a randomized controlled trial of non-pharmacologic interventions in the elderly (TONE). JAMA. 1998;279(11):839. https://doi.org/10.1001/jama.279.11.839.
37. Cutler J, Follmann D, Allender P. Randomized trials of sodium reduction: an overview. Am J Clin Nutr. 1997;65(2):643S–51S. https://doi.org/10.1093/ajcn/65.2.643S.
38. Effects of weight loss and sodium reduction intervention on blood pressure and hypertension incidence in overweight people with high-normal blood pressure. The Trials of Hypertension Prevention, phase II. The Trials of Hypertension Prevention Collaborative Research Group. Arch Intern Med. 1997;157(6):657–67.
39. Rodriguez-Iturbe B, Romero F, Johnson RJ. Pathophysiological mechanisms of salt-dependent hypertension. Am J Kidney Dis. 2007;50(4):655–72. https://doi.org/10.1053/j.ajkd.2007.05.025.
40. Elijovich F, Weinberger MH, Anderson CAM, et al. Salt sensitivity of blood pressure: a scientific statement from the American Heart Association. Hypertension. 2016;68(3):e7–e46. https://doi.org/10.1161/HYP.0000000000000047.
41. Luft FC, Grim CE, Higgins JT, Weinberger MH. Differences in response to sodium administration in normotensive white and black subjects. J Lab Clin Med. 1977;90(3):555–62.
42. Kawasaki T, Delea CS, Bartter FC, Smith H. The effect of high-sodium and low-sodium intakes on blood pressure and other related variables in human subjects with idiopathic hypertension. Am J Med. 1978;64(2):193–8. https://doi.org/10.1016/0002-9343(78)90045-1.
43. Weinberger MH. Salt sensitivity of blood pressure in humans. Hypertension. 1996;27(3 Pt 2):481–90. https://doi.org/10.1161/01.hyp.27.3.481.
44. Luzardo L, Noboa O, Boggia J. Mechanisms of salt-sensitive hypertension. Curr Hypertens Rev. 2015;11(1):14–21. https://doi.org/10.2174/1573402111666150530204136.
45. Rodriguez-Iturbe B, Vaziri ND. Salt-sensitive hypertension—update on novel findings. Nephrol Dial Transplant. 2007;22(4):992–5. https://doi.org/10.1093/ndt/gfl757.
46. Kurtz TW, DiCarlo SE, Pravenec M, Morris RC. An appraisal of methods recently recommended for testing salt sensitivity of blood pressure. J Am Heart Assoc. 2017;6(4):e005653. https://doi.org/10.1161/JAHA.117.005653.
47. Castiglioni P, Parati G, Lazzeroni D, et al. Hemodynamic and autonomic response to different salt intakes in normotensive individuals. J Am Heart Assoc. 2016;5(8):e003736. https://doi.org/10.1161/JAHA.116.003736.
48. Felder RA, Gildea JJ, Xu P, et al. Inverse salt sensitivity of blood pressure: mechanisms and potential relevance for prevention of cardiovascular disease. Curr Hypertens Rep. 2022;24(9):361–74. https://doi.org/10.1007/s11906-022-01201-9.

49. Armando I, Villar VA, Jose P. Genomics and pharmacogenomics of salt-sensitive hypertension. Curr Hypertens Rev. 2015;11(1):49–56. https://doi.org/10.2174/1573402111999150521102331.
50. Weinberger MH, Fineberg NS. Sodium and volume sensitivity of blood pressure. Age and pressure change over time. Hypertension. 1991;18(1):67–71. https://doi.org/10.1161/01.hyp.18.1.67.
51. Elijovich F, Kirabo A, Laffer CL. Salt sensitivity of blood pressure in Black people: the need to sort out ancestry versus epigenetic versus social determinants of its causation. Hypertension. 2024;81(3):456–67. https://doi.org/10.1161/HYPERTENSIONAHA.123.17951.
52. Chen J, Gu D, Huang J, et al. Metabolic syndrome and salt sensitivity of blood pressure in non-diabetic people in China: a dietary intervention study. Lancet. 2009;373(9666):829–35. https://doi.org/10.1016/S0140-6736(09)60144-6.
53. Strojek K, Grzeszczak W, Lacka B, Gorska J, Keller CK, Ritz E. Increased prevalence of salt sensitivity of blood pressure in IDDM with and without microalbuminuria. Diabetologia. 1995;38(12):1443–8. https://doi.org/10.1007/BF00400605.
54. Koomans HA, Roos JC, Boer P, Geyskes GG, Mees EJ. Salt sensitivity of blood pressure in chronic renal failure. Evidence for renal control of body fluid distribution in man. Hypertension. 1982;4(2):190–7. https://doi.org/10.1161/01.hyp.4.2.190.
55. Trepiccione F, Zacchia M, Capasso G. The role of the kidney in salt-sensitive hypertension. Clin Exp Nephrol. 2012;16(1):68–72. https://doi.org/10.1007/s10157-011-0489-y.
56. Sullivan JM. Salt sensitivity. Definition, conception, methodology, and long-term issues. Hypertension. 1991;17(1_supplement):I61–8. https://doi.org/10.1161/01.HYP.17.1_Suppl.I61.
57. Parksook WW, Williams GH. Challenges and approach to identifying individuals with salt sensitivity of blood pressure. Am J Nephrol. 2022;53(11–12):847–55. https://doi.org/10.1159/000529057.
58. Bailey MA, Dhaun N. Salt sensitivity: causes, consequences, and recent advances. Hypertension. 2024;81(3):476–89. https://doi.org/10.1161/HYPERTENSIONAHA.123.17959.
59. De Leeuw PW, Kroon AA. Salt and sensitivity. Hypertension. 2013;62(3):461–2. https://doi.org/10.1161/HYPERTENSIONAHA.113.01831.
60. Guyton AC. Renal function curve—a key to understanding the pathogenesis of hypertension. Hypertension. 1987;10(1):1–6. https://doi.org/10.1161/01.HYP.10.1.1.
61. Balafa O, Kalaitzidis RG. Salt sensitivity and hypertension. J Hum Hypertens. 2021;35(3):184–92. https://doi.org/10.1038/s41371-020-00407-1.
62. Miller JZ, Weinberger MH, Christian JC, Daugherty SA. Familial resemblance in the blood pressure response to sodium restriction. Am J Epidemiol. 1987;126(5):822–30. https://doi.org/10.1093/oxfordjournals.aje.a114719.
63. He FJ, Markandu ND, Sagnella GA, MacGregor GA. Importance of the renin system in determining blood pressure fall with salt restriction in black and white hypertensives. Hypertension. 1998;32(5):820–4. https://doi.org/10.1161/01.HYP.32.5.820.
64. He FJ, Markandu ND, MacGregor GA. Importance of the renin system for determining blood pressure fall with acute salt restriction in hypertensive and normotensive whites. Hypertension. 2001;38(3):321–5. https://doi.org/10.1161/01.HYP.38.3.321.
65. Yatabe MS, Yatabe J, Yoneda M, et al. Salt sensitivity is associated with insulin resistance, sympathetic overactivity, and decreased suppression of circulating renin activity in lean patients with essential hypertension. Am J Clin Nutr. 2010;92(1):77–82. https://doi.org/10.3945/ajcn.2009.29028.
66. Schmidlin O, Forman A, Tanaka M, Sebastian A, Morris RC. NaCl-induced renal vasoconstriction in salt-sensitive African Americans: antipressor and hemodynamic effects of potassium bicarbonate. Hypertension. 1999;33(2):633–9. https://doi.org/10.1161/01.HYP.33.2.633.
67. Bragulat E, Sierra ADL. Salt intake, endothelial dysfunction, and salt-sensitive hypertension. J Clin Hypertens. 2002;4(1):41–6. https://doi.org/10.1111/j.1524-6175.2002.00503.x.

68. Tolins JP, Shultz PJ. Endogenous nitric oxide synthesis determines sensitivity to the pressor effect of salt. Kidney Int. 1994;46(1):230–6. https://doi.org/10.1038/ki.1994.264.
69. Ferri C, Bellini C, Carlomagno A, Perrone A, Santucci A. Urinary kallikrein and salt sensitivity in essential hypertensive males. Kidney Int. 1994;46(3):780–8. https://doi.org/10.1038/ki.1994.333.
70. Johnson RJ, Segal MS, Srinivas T, et al. Essential hypertension, progressive renal disease, and uric acid: a pathogenetic link? J Am Soc Nephrol. 2005;16(7):1909–19. https://doi.org/10.1681/ASN.2005010063.
71. Campese VM, Romoff MS, Levitan D, Saglikes Y, Friedler RM, Massry SG. Abnormal relationship between sodium intake and sympathetic nervous system activity in salt-sensitive patients with essential hypertension. Kidney Int. 1982;21(2):371–8. https://doi.org/10.1038/ki.1982.32.
72. Campese VM, Tawadrous M, Bigazzi R, et al. Salt intake and plasma atrial natriuretic peptide and nitric oxide in hypertension. Hypertension. 1996;28(3):335–40. https://doi.org/10.1161/01.HYP.28.3.335.
73. Laffer CL, Bolterman RJ, Romero JC, Elijovich F. Effect of salt on isoprostanes in salt-sensitive essential hypertension. Hypertension. 2006;47(3):434–40. https://doi.org/10.1161/01.HYP.0000202480.06735.82.
74. Imanishi M, Okada N, Konishi Y, et al. Angiotensin II receptor blockade reduces salt sensitivity of blood pressure through restoration of renal nitric oxide synthesis in patients with diabetic nephropathy. J Renin-Angiotensin-Aldosterone Syst. 2013;14(1):67–73. https://doi.org/10.1177/1470320312454764.
75. Sarafidis PA, Bakris GL. The antinatriuretic effect of insulin: an unappreciated mechanism for hypertension associated with insulin resistance? Am J Nephrol. 2007;27(1):44–54. https://doi.org/10.1159/000098955.
76. Johnson RJ, Herrera-Acosta J, Schreiner GF, Rodríguez-Iturbe B. Subtle acquired renal injury as a mechanism of salt-sensitive hypertension. N Engl J Med. 2002;346(12):913–23. https://doi.org/10.1056/NEJMra011078.
77. Titze J, Shakibaei M, Schafflhuber M, et al. Glycosaminoglycan polymerization may enable osmotically inactive Na+ storage in the skin. Am J Physiol Heart Circ Physiol. 2004;287(1):H203–8. https://doi.org/10.1152/ajpheart.01237.2003.
78. Choi HY, Park HC, Ha SK. Salt sensitivity and hypertension: a paradigm shift from kidney malfunction to vascular endothelial dysfunction. Electrolyte Blood Press. 2015;13(1):7. https://doi.org/10.5049/EBP.2015.13.1.7.
79. Dahl LK, Heine M. Primary role of renal homografts in setting chronic blood pressure levels in rats. Circ Res. 1975;36(6):692–6. https://doi.org/10.1161/01.RES.36.6.692.
80. Curtis JJ, Luke RG, Dustan HP, et al. Remission of essential hypertension after renal transplantation. N Engl J Med. 1983;309(17):1009–15. https://doi.org/10.1056/NEJM198310273091702.
81. Guidi E, Menghetti D, Milani S, Montagnino G, Palazzi P, Bianchi G. Hypertension may be transplanted with the kidney in humans: a long-term historical prospective follow-up of recipients grafted with kidneys coming from donors with or without hypertension in their families. J Am Soc Nephrol. 1996;7(8):1131–8. https://doi.org/10.1681/ASN.V781131.
82. Luft FC. Monogenic hypertension: lessons from the genome. Kidney Int. 2001;60(1):381–90. https://doi.org/10.1046/j.1523-1755.2001.00810.x.
83. Tobin MD, Tomaszewski M, Braund PS, et al. Common variants in genes underlying monogenic hypertension and hypotension and blood pressure in the general population. Hypertension. 2008;51(6):1658–64. https://doi.org/10.1161/HYPERTENSIONAHA.108.112664.
84. Sealey JE, Blumenfeld JD, Bell GM, Pecker MS, Sommers SC, Laragh JH. On the renal basis for essential hypertension: nephron heterogeneity with discordant renin secretion and sodium excretion causing a hypertensive vasoconstriction-volume relationship. J Hypertens. 1988;6(11):763–77. https://doi.org/10.1097/00004872-198811000-00001.

85. Laragh J. Nephron heterogeneity: clue to the pathogenesis of essential hypertension and effectiveness of angiotensin-converting enzyme inhibitor treatment. Am J Med. 1989;87(6):S2–S14. https://doi.org/10.1016/0002-9343(89)90084-3.
86. Goldblatt H. Experimental renal hypertension: mechanism of production and maintenance. Circulation. 1958;17(4):642–7. https://doi.org/10.1161/01.CIR.17.4.642.
87. Harrap SB, Cumming AD, Davies DL, et al. Glomerular hyperfiltration, high renin, and low-extracellular volume in high blood pressure. Hypertension. 2000;35(4):952–7. https://doi.org/10.1161/01.HYP.35.4.952.
88. Sarafidis PA, Khosla N, Bakris GL. Antihypertensive therapy in the presence of proteinuria. Am J Kidney Dis. 2007;49(1):12–26. https://doi.org/10.1053/j.ajkd.2006.10.014.
89. Brenner BM, Garcia DL, Anderson S. Glomeruli and blood pressure: less of one, more the other? Am J Hypertens. 1988;1(4 Pt 1):335–47. https://doi.org/10.1093/ajh/1.4.335.
90. Brenner BM, Chertow GM. Congenital oligonephropathy: an inborn cause of adult hypertension and progressive renal injury? Curr Opin Nephrol Hypertens. 1993;2(5):691–5.
91. Brenner BM, Lawler EV, Mackenzie HS. The hyperfiltration theory: a paradigm shift in nephrology. Kidney Int. 1996;49(6):1774–7. https://doi.org/10.1038/ki.1996.265.
92. Barker DJ, Osmond C, Golding J, Kuh D, Wadsworth ME. Growth in utero, blood pressure in childhood and adult life, and mortality from cardiovascular disease. BMJ. 1989;298(6673):564–7. https://doi.org/10.1136/bmj.298.6673.564.
93. Barker D, Eriksson J, Forsén T, Osmond C. Fetal origins of adult disease: strength of effects and biological basis. Int J Epidemiol. 2002;31(6):1235–9. https://doi.org/10.1093/ije/31.6.1235.
94. Law CM, Shiell AW. Is blood pressure inversely related to birth weight? The strength of evidence from a systematic review of the literature. J Hypertens. 1996;14(8):935–41.
95. Irving RJ, Shore AC, Belton NR, Elton RA, Webb DJ, Walker BR. Low birth weight predicts higher blood pressure but not dermal capillary density in two populations. Hypertension. 2004;43(3):610–3. https://doi.org/10.1161/01.HYP.0000116029.85706.5f.
96. Johansson S, Iliadou A, Bergvall N, et al. The association between low birth weight and type 2 diabetes: contribution of genetic factors. Epidemiology. 2008;19(5):659–65. https://doi.org/10.1097/ede.0b013e31818131b9.
97. Barker DJP, Lackland DT. Prenatal influences on stroke mortality in England and Wales. Stroke. 2003;34(7):1598–602. https://doi.org/10.1161/01.STR.0000077257.27430.7E.
98. Hales CN, Barker DJ. The thrifty phenotype hypothesis. Br Med Bull. 2001;60:5–20. https://doi.org/10.1093/bmb/60.1.5.
99. Singhal A, Lucas A. Early origins of cardiovascular disease: is there a unifying hypothesis? Lancet. 2004;363(9421):1642–5. https://doi.org/10.1016/S0140-6736(04)16210-7.
100. Lucas A, Morley R. Does early nutrition in infants born before term programme later blood pressure? BMJ. 1994;309(6950):304–8. https://doi.org/10.1136/bmj.309.6950.304.
101. Mañalich R, Reyes L, Herrera M, Melendi C, Fundora I. Relationship between weight at birth and the number and size of renal glomeruli in humans: a histomorphometric study. Kidney Int. 2000;58(2):770–3. https://doi.org/10.1046/j.1523-1755.2000.00225.x.
102. Hughson M, Farris AB, Douglas-Denton R, Hoy WE, Bertram JF. Glomerular number and size in autopsy kidneys: the relationship to birth weight. Kidney Int. 2003;63(6):2113–22. https://doi.org/10.1046/j.1523-1755.2003.00018.x.
103. Keller G, Zimmer G, Mall G, Ritz E, Amann K. Nephron number in patients with primary hypertension. N Engl J Med. 2003;348(2):101–8. https://doi.org/10.1056/NEJMoa020549.
104. Dahl LK, Knudsen KD, Heine M, Leitl G. Effects of chronic excess salt ingestion. Genetic influence on the development of salt hypertension in parabiotic rats: evidence for a humoral factor. J Exp Med. 1967;126(4):687–99. https://doi.org/10.1084/jem.126.4.687.
105. Dahl LK, Knudsen KD, Iwai J. Humoral transmission of hypertension: evidence from parabiosis. Circ Res. 1969;24(5):21–33.

106. Overbeck HW, Pamnani MB, Akera T, Brody TM, Haddy FJ. Depressed function of a ouabain-sensitive sodium-potassium pump in blood vessels from renal hypertensive dogs. Circ Res. 1976;38(6 Suppl 2):48–52. https://doi.org/10.1161/01.res.38.6.48.
107. Blaustein MP. Sodium ions, calcium ions, blood pressure regulation, and hypertension: a reassessment and a hypothesis. Am J Phys. 1977;232(5):C165–73. https://doi.org/10.1152/ajpcell.1977.232.5.C165.
108. de Wardener HE. Franz Volhard lecture 1996. Sodium transport inhibitors and hypertension. J Hypertens Suppl. 1996;14(5):S9–18.
109. Blaustein MP. Endogenous ouabain: role in the pathogenesis of hypertension. Kidney Int. 1996;49(6):1748–53. https://doi.org/10.1038/ki.1996.260.
110. Iwamoto T, Kita S, Zhang J, et al. Salt-sensitive hypertension is triggered by Ca^{2+} entry via Na^+/Ca^{2+} exchanger type-1 in vascular smooth muscle. Nat Med. 2004;10(11):1193–9. https://doi.org/10.1038/nm1118.
111. Zhang J, Lee MY, Cavalli M, et al. Sodium pump alpha2 subunits control myogenic tone and blood pressure in mice. J Physiol. 2005;569(Pt 1):243–56. https://doi.org/10.1113/jphysiol.2005.091801.
112. Zhang J, Hamlyn JM, Karashima E, et al. Low-dose ouabain constricts small arteries from ouabain-hypertensive rats: implications for sustained elevation of vascular resistance. Am J Physiol Heart Circ Physiol. 2009;297(3):H1140–50. https://doi.org/10.1152/ajpheart.00436.2009.
113. Nicholls MG, Lewis LK, Yandle TG, Lord G, McKinnon W, Hilton PJ. Ouabain, a circulating hormone secreted by the adrenals, is pivotal in cardiovascular disease. Fact or fantasy? J Hypertens. 2009;27(1):3–8. https://doi.org/10.1097/HJH.0b013e32831101d1.
114. Hilton PJ, McKinnon W, Gravett EC, et al. Selective inhibition of the cellular sodium pump by emicymarin and 14β anhydroxy bufadienolides. Steroids. 2010;75(13–14):1137–45. https://doi.org/10.1016/j.steroids.2010.07.010.
115. Johnson RJ, Rodríguez-Iturbe B, Schreiner GF, Herrera-Acosta J. Hypertension: a microvascular and tubulointerstitial disease. J Hypertens Suppl. 2002;20(3):S1–7.
116. Rodríguez-Iturbe B, Quiroz Y, Herrera-Acosta J, Johnson RJ, Pons HA. The role of immune cells infiltrating the kidney in the pathogenesis of salt-sensitive hypertension. J Hypertens Suppl. 2002;20(3):S9–14.
117. Johnson RJ, Rodriguez-Iturbe B, Kang DH, Feig DI, Herrera-Acosta J. A unifying pathway for essential hypertension. Am J Hypertens. 2005;18(3):431–40. https://doi.org/10.1016/j.amjhyper.2004.08.035.
118. Sinnakirouchenan R, Kotchen TA. Role of sodium restriction and diuretic therapy for "resistant" hypertension in chronic kidney disease. Semin Nephrol. 2014;34(5):514–9. https://doi.org/10.1016/j.semnephrol.2014.08.005.
119. Konishi Y, Okada N, Okamura M, et al. Sodium sensitivity of blood pressure appearing before hypertension and related to histological damage in immunoglobulin a nephropathy. Hypertension. 2001;38(1):81–5. https://doi.org/10.1161/01.HYP.38.1.81.
120. Blythe WB. Natural history of hypertension in renal parenchymal disease. Am J Kidney Dis. 1985;5(4):A50–6. https://doi.org/10.1016/S0272-6386(85)80066-4.
121. Qian Q. Salt, water and nephron: mechanisms of action and link to hypertension and chronic kidney disease: salt, water and nephron. Nephrology. 2018;23:44–9. https://doi.org/10.1111/nep.13465.
122. De Nicola L, Minutolo R, Bellizzi V, et al. Achievement of target blood pressure levels in chronic kidney disease: a salty question? Am J Kidney Dis. 2004;43(5):782–95. https://doi.org/10.1053/j.ajkd.2004.01.009.
123. Vasavada N, Agarwal R. Role of excess volume in the pathophysiology of hypertension in chronic kidney disease. Kidney Int. 2003;64(5):1772–9. https://doi.org/10.1046/j.1523-1755.2003.00273.x.
124. Koo HS, Kim YC, Ahn SY, Oh SW, Kim S, Chin HJ. Analysis of correlation between 24-hour urinary sodium and the degree of blood pressure control in patients with chronic

kidney disease and non-chronic kidney disease. J Korean Med Sci. 2014;29(Suppl 2):S117. https://doi.org/10.3346/jkms.2014.29.S2.S117.
125. Weir MR, Dengel DR, Behrens MT, Goldberg AP. Salt-induced increases in systolic blood pressure affect renal hemodynamics and proteinuria. Hypertension. 1995;25(6):1339–44. https://doi.org/10.1161/01.HYP.25.6.1339.
126. Krikken JA, Laverman GD, Navis G. Benefits of dietary sodium restriction in the management of chronic kidney disease. Curr Opin Nephrol Hypertens. 2009;18(6):531–8. https://doi.org/10.1097/MNH.0b013e3283312fc8.
127. Bigazzi R, Bianchi S, Baldari D, Sgherri G, Baldari G, Campese VM. Microalbuminuria in salt-sensitive patients. A marker for renal and cardiovascular risk factors. Hypertension. 1994;23(2):195–9. https://doi.org/10.1161/01.HYP.23.2.195.
128. Fukuda M, Mizuno M, Kimura G. Nocturnal hypertension and chronic kidney disease. Curr Hypertens Rev. 2011;7(1):5–8. https://doi.org/10.2174/157340211795909025.
129. Fukuda M, Goto N, Kimura G. Hypothesis on renal mechanism of non-dipper pattern of circadian blood pressure rhythm. Med Hypotheses. 2006;67(4):802–6. https://doi.org/10.1016/j.mehy.2006.04.024.
130. Vogt L, Waanders F, Boomsma F, de Zeeuw D, Navis G. Effects of dietary sodium and hydrochlorothiazide on the antiproteinuric efficacy of losartan. J Am Soc Nephrol. 2008;19(5):999–1007. https://doi.org/10.1681/ASN.2007060693.
131. Buter H. The blunting of the antiproteinuric efficacy of ACE inhibition by high sodium intake can be restored by hydrochlorothiazide. Nephrol Dial Transplant. 1998;13(7):1682–5. https://doi.org/10.1093/ndt/13.7.1682.
132. Navis G, de Jong PE, Donker AJM, van der Hem GK, de Zeeuw D. Diuretic effects of angiotensin-converting enzyme inhibition: comparison of low and liberal sodium diet in hypertensive patients. J Cardiovasc Pharmacol. 1987;9(6):743–8. https://doi.org/10.1097/00005344-198706000-00016.
133. Esnault VLM, Ekhlas A, Delcroix C, Moutel MG, Nguyen JM. Diuretic and enhanced sodium restriction results in improved antiproteinuric response to RAS blocking agents. J Am Soc Nephrol. 2005;16(2):474–81. https://doi.org/10.1681/ASN.2004060505.
134. Blasi ER, Rocha R, Rudolph AE, Blomme EAG, Polly ML, McMahon EG. Aldosterone/salt induces renal inflammation and fibrosis in hypertensive rats. Kidney Int. 2003;63(5):1791–800. https://doi.org/10.1046/j.1523-1755.2003.00929.x.
135. Barrera-Chimal J, Girerd S, Jaisser F. Mineralocorticoid receptor antagonists and kidney diseases: pathophysiological basis. Kidney Int. 2019;96(2):302–19. https://doi.org/10.1016/j.kint.2019.02.030.
136. Nagase M, Matsui H, Shibata S, Gotoda T, Fujita T. Salt-induced nephropathy in obese spontaneously hypertensive rats via paradoxical activation of the mineralocorticoid receptor: role of oxidative stress. Hypertension. 2007;50(5):877–83. https://doi.org/10.1161/HYPERTENSIONAHA.107.091058.
137. He J, Mills KT, Appel LJ, et al. Urinary sodium and potassium excretion and CKD progression. J Am Soc Nephrol. 2016;27(4):1202–12. https://doi.org/10.1681/ASN.2015010022.
138. Mills KT, Chen J, Yang W, et al. Sodium excretion and the risk of cardiovascular disease in patients with chronic kidney disease. JAMA. 2016;315(20):2200. https://doi.org/10.1001/jama.2016.4447.
139. Vegter S, Perna A, Postma MJ, Navis G, Remuzzi G, Ruggenenti P. Sodium intake, ACE inhibition, and progression to ESRD. J Am Soc Nephrol. 2012;23(1):165–73. https://doi.org/10.1681/ASN.2011040430.
140. Kempner W. Some effects of the rice diet treatment of kidney disease and hypertension. Bull N Y Acad Med. 1946;22(7):358–70.
141. McMahon EJ, Campbell KL, Bauer JD, Mudge DW, Kelly JT. Altered dietary salt intake for people with chronic kidney disease. Cochrane Database Syst Rev. 2021;6(6):CD010070. https://doi.org/10.1002/14651858.CD010070.pub3.

142. Stevens PE, Ahmed SB, Carrero JJ, et al. KDIGO 2024 clinical practice guideline for the evaluation and management of chronic kidney disease. Kidney Int. 2024;105(4):S117–314. https://doi.org/10.1016/j.kint.2023.10.018.
143. NICE. Chronic kidney disease: assessment and management. London: National Institute for Health and Care Excellence (NICE); 2021. http://www.ncbi.nlm.nih.gov/books/NBK574714/. Accessed 27 Aug 2025.
144. Lloyd-Jones DM, Hong Y, Labarthe D, et al. Defining and setting National Goals for cardiovascular health promotion and disease reduction: the American Heart Association's strategic impact goal through 2020 and beyond. Circulation. 2010;121(4):586–613. https://doi.org/10.1161/CIRCULATIONAHA.109.192703.
145. De Nicola L, Minutolo R, Chiodini P, et al. Global approach to cardiovascular risk in chronic kidney disease: reality and opportunities for intervention. Kidney Int. 2006;69(3):538–45. https://doi.org/10.1038/sj.ki.5000085.
146. Van Zuilen AD, Wetzels JFM, Bots ML, Van Blankestijn PJ, MASTERPLAN Study Group. MASTERPLAN: study of the role of nurse practitioners in a multifactorial intervention to reduce cardiovascular risk in chronic kidney disease patients. J Nephrol. 2008;21(3):261–7.
147. McMahon EJ, Campbell KL, Mudge DW, Bauer JD. Achieving salt restriction in chronic kidney disease. Int J Nephrol. 2012;2012:1–10. https://doi.org/10.1155/2012/720429.
148. Tanaka M, Nishiwaki H, Kado H, et al. Impact of salt taste dysfunction on interdialytic weight gain for hemodialysis patients; a cross-sectional study. BMC Nephrol. 2019;20(1):121. https://doi.org/10.1186/s12882-019-1312-3.
149. Kusaba T, Mori Y, Masami O, et al. Sodium restriction improves the gustatory threshold for salty taste in patients with chronic kidney disease. Kidney Int. 2009;76(6):638–43. https://doi.org/10.1038/ki.2009.214.
150. Harnack LJ, Cogswell ME, Shikany JM, et al. Sources of sodium in US adults from 3 geographic regions. Circulation. 2017;135(19):1775–83. https://doi.org/10.1161/CIRCULATIONAHA.116.024446.
151. Karagiannidis AG, Theodorakopoulou MP, Pella E, Sarafidis PA, Ortiz A. Uromodulin biology. Nephrol Dial Transplant. 2024;39(7):1073–87. https://doi.org/10.1093/ndt/gfae008.
152. Karagiannidis AG, Theodorakopoulou MP, Iatridi F, Ortiz A, Sarafidis P. A salty symphony: unraveling the tale of uromodulin and sodium sensitivity. J Hum Hypertens. 2025;39(5):320–33. https://doi.org/10.1038/s41371-025-01013-9.
153. Boder P, Mary S, Mark PB, et al. Mechanistic interactions of uromodulin with the thick ascending limb: perspectives in physiology and hypertension. J Hypertens. 2021;39(8):1490–504. https://doi.org/10.1097/HJH.0000000000002861.
154. Tokonami N, Takata T, Beyeler J, et al. Uromodulin is expressed in the distal convoluted tubule, where it is critical for regulation of the sodium chloride cotransporter NCC. Kidney Int. 2018;94(4):701–15. https://doi.org/10.1016/j.kint.2018.04.021.
155. Bachmann S, Mutig K, Bates J, et al. Renal effects of Tamm-Horsfall protein (uromodulin) deficiency in mice. Am J Physiol Renal Physiol. 2005;288(3):F559–67. https://doi.org/10.1152/ajprenal.00143.2004.
156. Graham LA, Padmanabhan S, Fraser NJ, et al. Validation of uromodulin as a candidate gene for human essential hypertension. Hypertension. 2014;63(3):551–8. https://doi.org/10.1161/HYPERTENSIONAHA.113.01423.
157. Liu Y, Mo L, Goldfarb DS, et al. Progressive renal papillary calcification and ureteral stone formation in mice deficient for Tamm-Horsfall protein. Am J Physiol Renal Physiol. 2010;299(3):F469–78. https://doi.org/10.1152/ajprenal.00243.2010.
158. Liu Y, Goldfarb DS, El-Achkar TM, Lieske JC, Wu XR. Tamm-Horsfall protein/uromodulin deficiency elicits tubular compensatory responses leading to hypertension and hyperuricemia. Am J Physiol Renal Physiol. 2018;314(6):F1062–76. https://doi.org/10.1152/ajprenal.00233.2017.

159. Olinger E, Lake J, Sheehan S, et al. Hepsin-mediated processing of uromodulin is crucial for salt-sensitivity and thick ascending limb homeostasis. Sci Rep. 2019;9(1):12287. https://doi.org/10.1038/s41598-019-48300-3.
160. Trudu M, Janas S, Lanzani C, et al. Common noncoding UMOD gene variants induce salt-sensitive hypertension and kidney damage by increasing uromodulin expression. Nat Med. 2013;19(12):1655–60. https://doi.org/10.1038/nm.3384.
161. Padmanabhan S, Melander O, Johnson T, et al. Genome-Wide Association Study of blood pressure extremes identifies variant near UMOD Associated with Hypertension. PLoS Genet. 2010;6(10):e1001177. https://doi.org/10.1371/journal.pgen.1001177.
162. Ponte B, Sadler MC, Olinger E, et al. Mendelian randomization to assess causality between uromodulin, blood pressure and chronic kidney disease. Kidney Int. 2021;100(6):1282–91. https://doi.org/10.1016/j.kint.2021.08.032.
163. You R, Chen L, Xu L, et al. High level of uromodulin increases the risk of hypertension: a mendelian randomization study. Front Cardiovasc Med. 2021;8:736001. https://doi.org/10.3389/fcvm.2021.736001.
164. Jian Z, Yuan C, Ma Y. Blood pressure mediated the effects of urinary uromodulin levels on myocardial infarction: a mendelian randomization study. Hypertension. 2022;79(11):2430–8. https://doi.org/10.1161/HYPERTENSIONAHA.122.19670.
165. Ponte B, Pruijm M, Ackermann D, et al. Uromodulin, salt, and 24-hour blood pressure in the general population. Clin J Am Soc Nephrol. 2021;16(5):787–9. https://doi.org/10.2215/CJN.11230720.
166. Matafora V, Zagato L, Ferrandi M, et al. Quantitative proteomics reveals novel therapeutic and diagnostic markers in hypertension. BBA Clin. 2014;2:79–87. https://doi.org/10.1016/j.bbacli.2014.10.001.
167. Matafora V, Lanzani C, Zagato L, et al. Urinary proteomics reveals key markers of salt sensitivity in hypertensive patients during saline infusion. J Nephrol. 2021;34(3):739–51. https://doi.org/10.1007/s40620-020-00877-z.
168. Josipović J. Uromodulin—a link between sodium excretion and alteration in circadian blood pressure pattern in prehypertensives. Acta Clin Croat. 2023;62:313–22. https://doi.org/10.20471/acc.2023.62.02.09.
169. McCallum L, Lip S, McConnachie A, et al. UMOD genotype-blinded trial of ambulatory blood pressure response to Torasemide. Hypertension. 2024;81(10):2049–59. https://doi.org/10.1161/HYPERTENSIONAHA.124.23122.
170. Golob Jančič S, Močnik M, Filipič M, Homšak E, Svetej M, Marčun VN. Serum and urinary uromodulin concentration in children and young adults with chronic kidney disease. Pediatr Nephrol. 2025;40(5):1751–8. https://doi.org/10.1007/s00467-024-06630-z.
171. Karagiannidis AG, Baroutidou A, Iatridi F. Uromodulin in pediatric patients with chronic kidney disease: lessons unlearned regarding blood pressure. Pediatr Nephrol. 2025;40(9):3009–10. https://doi.org/10.1007/s00467-025-06781-7.
172. Bullen AL, Vaingankar S, Madero M, et al. Urine uromodulin, kidney tubulointerstitial fibrosis, and furosemide response. Nephron. 2024;148(7):443–7. https://doi.org/10.1159/000534578.
173. Pivin E, Ponte B, De Seigneux S, et al. Uromodulin and nephron mass. Clin J Am Soc Nephrol. 2018;13(10):1556–7. https://doi.org/10.2215/CJN.03600318.
174. Slagman MCJ, Waanders F, Hemmelder MH, et al. Moderate dietary sodium restriction added to angiotensin converting enzyme inhibition compared with dual blockade in lowering proteinuria and blood pressure: randomised controlled trial. BMJ. 2011;343:d4366. https://doi.org/10.1136/bmj.d4366.
175. de Brito-Ashurst I, Perry L, Sanders TAB, et al. The role of salt intake and salt sensitivity in the management of hypertension in south Asian people with chronic kidney disease: a randomised controlled trial. Heart. 2013;99(17):1256–60. https://doi.org/10.1136/heartjnl-2013-303688.

176. McMahon EJ, Bauer JD, Hawley CM, et al. A randomized trial of dietary sodium restriction in CKD. J Am Soc Nephrol. 2013;24(12):2096–103. https://doi.org/10.1681/ASN.2013030285.
177. Meuleman Y, Hoekstra T, Dekker FW, et al. Sodium restriction in patients with CKD: a randomized controlled trial of self-management support. Am J Kidney Dis. 2017;69(5):576–86. https://doi.org/10.1053/j.ajkd.2016.08.042.
178. Humalda JK, Klaassen G, de Vries H, et al. A self-management approach for dietary sodium restriction in patients with CKD: a randomized controlled trial. Am J Kidney Dis. 2020;75(6):847–56. https://doi.org/10.1053/j.ajkd.2019.10.012.
179. Trakarnvanich T, Chailimpamontree W, Kantachuvesiri S, et al. Effect of a low salt diet on the progression of chronic kidney disease: a prospective, open-label, randomized controlled trial. J Prim Care Community Health. 2024;15:21501319241297766. https://doi.org/10.1177/21501319241297766.

Pathophysiology of Hypertension in Chronic Kidney Disease: Role of the Sympathetic Nervous System Activation

Filippo Scalise, Evelina Toscano, Antonio Sorropago, Chiara Amman, and Guido Grassi

Introduction

The pathophysiology of hypertension in chronic kidney disease (CKD) is multifactorial, but the activation of the sympathetic nervous system (SNS) plays a central and well-established role.

Under normal conditions, the kidneys and the nervous system interact to maintain homeostasis. However, in chronic kidney disease (CKD), this balance is disrupted, leading to sustained overactivation of the sympathetic nervous system (SNS). In patients with chronic kidney failure, sympathetic nerve activity related to hypertension and cardiovascular events is significantly elevated [1, 2]. Evidence indicates that sympathetic overactivity, common in CKD, significantly raises cardiovascular risk [3]. It contributes to hypertension and organ damage progression in both CKD and hypertension [4]. Numerous studies have reported increased sympathetic nerve activity (SNA) in CKD [5, 6]. Studies have shown that plasma norepinephrine levels, the main neurotransmitter from sympathetic nerves, are significantly

F. Scalise (✉)
Department of Interventional Cardiology, Policlinico di Monza, Monza, Italy

ESH Excellence Center, Istituto Clinico Verano Brianza, Monza, Italy
e-mail: filippo.scalise@policlinicodimonza.it

E. Toscano · A. Sorropago
Department of Interventional Cardiology, Policlinico di Monza, Monza, Italy
e-mail: evelina.toscano@policlinicodimonza.it; antonio.sorropago@policlinicodimonza.it

C. Amman
School of Medicine, Università Vita e Salute San Raffaele, Milan, Italy
e-mail: chiara.amman@gmail.com

G. Grassi
Università degli Studi Milano Bicocca, Monza, Italy
e-mail: guido.grassi@unimib.it

P. Sarafidis, R. Pontremoli (eds.), *Hypertension and Chronic Kidney Disease*, Updates in Hypertension and Cardiovascular Protection,
https://doi.org/10.1007/978-3-032-29564-4_4

Table 1 Summary of clinical evidence

Evidence type	Key findings
MSNA (Microneurography)	Directly elevated SNS activity in CKD, increasing with disease progression
Plasma norepinephrine	Elevated in CKD and ESRD; associated with LVH and cardiovascular mortality
Baroreflex sensitivity tests	Blunted in CKD, allowing sustained SNS overactivity
Imaging (fMRI, PET)	Increased sympathetic centers activated in CKD patients
Drug trials (e.g., clonidine)	SNS inhibition lowers BP and improves outcomes
Renal denervation	Reduces BP and SNS activity in resistant hypertension (some CKD patients)

higher in renal failure patients [7]. CKD patients, especially those with ESRD, poor blood pressure control, left ventricular hypertrophy, or heart failure, often have elevated plasma norepinephrine levels. This finding reflects both increased central sympathetic outflow and reduced renal clearance of catecholamines. High norepinephrine levels are linked to cardiovascular risk, left ventricular mass, and mortality [8]. Microneurography, a technique that directly records postganglionic sympathetic nerve traffic through a microelectrode inserted into a peripheral nerve, has been widely used to assess muscle sympathetic nerve activity (MSNA). Studies [9] have found that MSNA is significantly elevated in CKD patients, even in early stages (Stage 2–3). As kidney function declines, MSNA progressively increases, demonstrating an inverse relationship between glomerular filtration rate (GFR) and sympathetic activity. Grassi et al. [5] studied mild-to-moderate CKD patients, dividing them into four groups based on their eGFR. Group I had the highest eGFR (95.4 ± 1.6 mL/min/1.73 m^2) while Group IV had the lowest (31.4 ± 1.8 mL/min/1.73 m^2). Resting MSNA significantly increased from the highest to the lowest eGFR quartile. Functional magnetic resonance imaging (fMRI) and positron emission tomography (PET) studies have demonstrated increased activation of brainstem regions involved in sympathetic regulation, particularly the rostral ventrolateral medulla. This may be due to altered brain autonomic regulation from kidney nerve signals or uremic toxins [10].

Further evidence of SNS activation is shown through Clinical Tests of Baroreflex Function. Baroreflex sensitivity, a key modulator of SNS activity, is reduced in CKD patients. This decreased response allows SNS overactivity when BP rises, especially in those with arterial stiffness or volume overload [11]. Recent studies on renal denervation in CKD patients with resistant hypertension show a high prevalence of uncontrolled BP due to persistent SNS activation [12]. This correlates with conditions like left ventricular hypertrophy, arrhythmias, and sudden cardiac death common in CKD and ESRD. Although still investigational, renal sympathetic denervation has shown to reduce BP in resistant hypertension patients (many with CKD), decrease muscle sympathetic nerve activity and norepinephrine spillover, but later-stage trials show mixed results due to patient variability and technical challenges (Table 1) [13].

Mechanisms of SNS Activation in CKD

The mechanisms of sympathetic nervous system (SNS) activation in chronic kidney disease (CKD) are intricate, yet they can be categorized into six primary pathways. Each pathway contributes to the overactivation of the SNS, which is pivotal in the progression of hypertension in CKD. Below is a comprehensive explanation:

1. Renal afferent nerve signaling
   The kidneys are innervated by chemoreceptors and baroreceptors that provide feedback to the brain to regulate sympathetic outflow and systemic blood pressure. Research from both animal and human studies suggests that neural signals originating from the kidney contribute to increased sympathetic outflow in chronic kidney disease (CKD) [14]. The brain's response is an increase in efferent sympathetic output, sending stronger signals to various organs. This results in systemic vasoconstriction, increased heart rate, and activation of the renin-angiotensin system.
2. Impaired clearance of sympathoexcitatory substances (uremic toxins)
   In chronic kidney disease (CKD), the renal system fails to sufficiently eliminate specific metabolites and toxins, such as guanidino compounds and indoxyl sulfate [15]. These substances accumulate in the bloodstream and activate sympathetic centers within the brain. The brain interprets this accumulation as a signal to elevate blood pressure, thereby increasing sympathetic output. This process contributes to the persistent elevation of sympathetic tone, particularly in advanced stages of CKD or end-stage renal disease.
3. Baroreceptor dysfunction
   Baroreceptors are pressure sensors located in the aortic arch and carotid sinus. They regulate blood pressure by sending feedback to the brain to modulate sympathetic activity. In chronic kidney disease (CKD), arterial stiffness, caused by hypertension or vascular calcification, and volume overload can impair these receptors. As a result, the baroreflex becomes less sensitive, preventing the brain from accurately detecting high blood pressure. This results in increased sympathetic activation, which contributes to hypertension [16].
4. Renin–angiotensin system
   The renin–angiotensin system is known to be activated in CKD. Renin from the kidney converts angiotensinogen to angiotensin I, which becomes angiotensin II (Ang II) via ACE. This activation raises Ang II levels in the blood, a common CKD feature. Ang II acts as a strong vasoconstrictor with various effects [17]. In summary, Ang II contributes to peripheral vasoconstriction and modulates peripheral sympathetic nerve activity (SNA) by enhancing norepinephrine release from sympathetic nerve terminals. Additionally, Ang II is involved in regulating sympathetic outflow from the brainstem. Although Ang II receptor blockers and ACE inhibitors are first-line treatments for patients with CKD, chronic administration of these medications only reduces MSNA without normalizing it [18]. In other words, MSNA remains elevated in CKD patients despite chronic treatment with Ang II receptor blockers and ACE inhibitors

when compared to healthy individuals. Consequently, it is clear that mechanisms beyond the renin–angiotensin system contribute to the sympathetic overactivity observed in CKD.

5. Nitric oxide pathway

   A potential mechanism for chronic sympathoexcitation in chronic kidney disease (CKD) is the reduction of nitric oxide (NO) bioavailability. Notably, systemic inhibition of NOS in healthy individuals leads to an immediate increase in arterial blood pressure due to the reduction of NO and endothelium-mediated vasodilation [19]. Evidence indicates that nitric oxide (NO) is a significant signaling molecule involved in regulating sympathetic outflow from the brainstem.

6. Oxidative stress

   CKD patients experience higher oxidative stress [20], potentially leading to chronic sympathoexcitation. Oxidative stress in the central nervous system plays a crucial role in controlling sympathetic outflow from the brainstem [21]. Reactive oxygen species (ROS), including superoxide ion, hydroxyl radical, and hydrogen peroxide, serve as crucial intracellular messengers. However, excessive production of ROS can be detrimental. Various animal studies have demonstrated that increased oxidative stress in the brain contributes to heightened central sympathetic outflow, either directly or through the scavenging of nitric oxide (NO) [22, 23]. Overall, the published studies suggest that oxidative stress is one of the mechanisms that increases sympathetic outflow from the brainstem and may be involved in elevated SNA in CKD.

Consequences of the Sympathetic Overactivity

Sympathetic overactivity is linked to several diseases and contributes to the advancement of cardiovascular, metabolic, and renal pathologies [24]. Hypertension, the most frequent adverse outcome of increased sympathetic nerve activity (SNA), affects 80% of patients with chronic kidney disease (CKD) [25, 26]. Hypertension results in structural and functional abnormalities such as left ventricular hypertrophy, increased vascular smooth muscle cell hyperplasia and hypertrophy, and endothelial dysfunction [27, 28]. The elevated SNS tone causes arteriolar constriction, increasing systemic vascular resistance, and blood pressure. SNS stimulates $\alpha 1$-adrenergic receptors on vascular smooth muscle, leading to vasoconstriction. This increases systemic vascular resistance (SVR) and elevates diastolic blood pressure. Chronic vasoconstriction also contributes to arterial stiffness and endothelial dysfunction. Chronic sympatho-excitation, independent of hypertension, has been associated with adverse effects. Research indicates that sub-hypertensive doses of norepinephrine can induce myocardial cell hypertrophy and left ventricular hypertrophy [29]. Additionally, elevated sympathetic nervous activity (SNA) has various harmful effects beyond increased blood pressure. These include, but are not limited to, pronounced coronary vasoconstriction [30], arrhythmogenicity [31], impaired renal function, glomerular podocyte injury [32], metabolic impairment [33], increased arterial stiffness [34], endothelial dysfunction [35], and the subsequent development of atherosclerosis, all contributing to an elevated risk of cardiovascular events. The overactivity of the sympathetic nervous system (SNS) in chronic kidney disease manifests both systemically—affecting the entire cardiovascular system—and specifically within the kidneys, directly impairing kidney function. This plays a crucial role in the pathogenesis of hypertension and the progression of renal decline.

Treatment Strategies

Overactivity of the sympathetic nervous system (SNS) is not merely a consequence of chronic kidney disease (CKD); it is also a therapeutic target (Table 2). Pharmacological interventions are a primary approach. Centrally Acting Sympatholytics like Clonidine, Moxonidine, and Methyldopa reduce central sympathetic outflow by targeting brainstem receptors [36] (e.g., α2-adrenergic or imidazoline receptors). This lowers blood pressure, improves baroreflex sensitivity, and decreases heart rate and plasma norepinephrine levels. Clonidine is used for resistant hypertension, including in dialysis patients, while Methyldopa is safe during pregnancy with CKD [37]. The use of beta-blockers, such as Atenolol, Bisoprolol, Carvedilol, and Nebivolol, can have a significant impact in these cases. They function by blocking β1-adrenergic receptors, leading to a reduction in heart rate, renin release, and cardiac output. This helps control blood pressure and sympathetic drive, reduce left ventricular hypertrophy, and lower the risk of sudden cardiac death [38]. The use of RAAS inhibitors (such as ACEIs, ARBs, and Direct Renin Inhibitors like Lisinopril, Losartan, and Aliskiren) can reduce vasoconstriction, sodium retention, and sympathetic tone. These mechanisms contribute to lowering blood pressure, reducing proteinuria, slowing CKD progression, and indirectly suppressing SNS activity by mitigating angiotensin II's central and peripheral effects. ACEIs and ARBs are recommended as first-line agents in proteinuric CKD, particularly in diabetes [39]. It is also important to mention the use of diuretics, specifically loop diuretics (furosemide) and thiazides, in managing volume overload, which is a key factor in stimulating sympathetic nervous system (SNS) overactivity. Loop diuretics are particularly crucial in cases of advanced chronic kidney disease (CKD)

Table 2 Treatment strategies

Therapy type	Examples	Effect on SNS overactivity
Centrally acting drugs	Clonidine, Moxonidine	↓ Central sympathetic tone
Beta-blockers	Bisoprolol, carvedilol	↓ Heart rate, ↓ renin, ↓ SNS output
RAAS inhibitors	ACEIs, ARBs, Aliskiren	↓ SNS indirectly via RAAS suppression
Diuretics	Furosemide, thiazides	↓ Volume → ↓ baroreflex stress → ↓ SNS
Renal denervation	RDN procedure	↓ Afferent and efferent renal nerve activity
Lifestyle/CPAP	Salt restriction, CPAP	↓ Sympathetic drive via improved systemic balance

Table 3 Benefits of RDN in CKD patients

Effect	Potential clinical benefit
Sympathetic activity	Slower progression of CKD, reduced LVH
Renin, Na^+ retention	Better BP and volume control
Systemic vascular resistance	Reduced cardiovascular workload
BP variability	Fewer hypertensive peaks → reduced end-organ damage
Improved patient compliance	Reduction in medication burden possible (in some responders)

(eGFR <30), where thiazides become less effective. Reducing volume can lower sympathetic tone and improve blood pressure control [40].

A second line of intervention involves device-based therapies such as Renal Sympathetic Denervation (RDN), which is a minimally invasive catheter-based procedure that ablates renal sympathetic nerves. This procedure targets both afferent (kidney to brain) and efferent (brain to kidney) sympathetic nervous system pathways. Clinical trials, including Symplicity HTN-3 and SPYRAL HTN-ON MED, indicate a blood pressure reduction in resistant hypertension and some improvement in renal function markers [41] However, it is still under investigation in chronic kidney disease (CKD) and is not yet considered routine therapy due to mixed results and the need for better patient selection (Table 3) [13].

Non-pharmacologic interventions, such as lifestyle modifications, are crucial. Sodium restriction helps reduce volume expansion and SNS activation. Weight loss and exercise improve insulin sensitivity and autonomic tone [42]. Smoking cessation decreases SNS stimulation and enhances vascular health [43]. Treating sleep apnea with CPAP is important since obstructive sleep apnea (OSA) is common in CKD and activates SNS. CPAP therapy reduces sympathetic outflow and improves BP control in CKD patients with OSA [44]. The fourth strategy involves dialysis techniques. Adequate dialysis is fundamental as it reduces uremic toxins that can activate the sympathetic nervous system (SNS) [45].

Conclusion

In chronic kidney disease (CKD), the activation of the sympathetic nervous system significantly contributes to hypertension through mechanisms such as renal afferent signaling, impaired baroreflexes, and increased renin release. This leads to widespread vasoconstriction, sodium retention, and further kidney damage, thereby perpetuating a detrimental cycle of escalating hypertension and progressive renal deterioration. Addressing sympathetic overactivity in chronic kidney disease (CKD) is crucial not only for managing hypertension, but also for mitigating kidney damage, lowering cardiovascular risk, and enhancing survival rates. An individualized, multimodal approach—which integrates pharmacologic, interventional, and lifestyle strategies—yields the most favorable outcomes.

References

1. Agarwal R. Systolic hypertension in hemodialysis patients. Semin Dial. 2003;16:208–13.
2. Masuo K, Lambert GW, Esler MD, Rakugi H, Ogihara T, Schlaich MP. The role of sympathetic nervous activity in renale injury and end-stage renal disease. Hypertens Res. 2010;33:521–8.
3. Zoccali C, Mallamaci F, Parlongo S, Cutrupi S, Benedetto FA, Tripepi G, Bonanno G, Rapisarda F, Fatuzzo P, Seminara G, et al. Plasma norepinephrine predicts survival and incident cardiovascular events in patients with end-stage renal disease. Circulation. 2002;105:1354–9.
4. Sousa F, Neves J, Ferreira R, et al. 1b.05: In hypertension the change from a non-dipper to a dipper pattern is associated with a better cardiovascular prognosis than the persistence within the non-dipper pattern. J Hypertens. 2015;33(Suppl. 1):e6.
5. Grassi G, Quarti-Trevano F, Seravalle G, Arenare F, Volpe M, Furiani S, Dell'Oro R, Mancia G. Early sympathetic activation in the initial clinical stages of chronic renal failure. Hypertension. 2011;57:846–51.
6. Grassi G, Seravalle G, Ghiadoni L, Tripepi G, Bruno RM, Mancia G, Zoccali C. Sympathetic nerve traffic and asymmetric dimethylarginine in chronic kidney disease. Clin J Am Soc Nephrol. 2011;6:2620–7.
7. Ligtenberg G, Blankestijn PJ, Oey PL, Klein IH, Dijkhorst-Oei LT, Boomsma F, Wieneke GH, van Huffelen AC, Koomans HA. Reduction of sympathetic hyperactivity by enalapril in patients with chronic renal failure. N Engl J Med. 1999;340:1321–8.
8. Grassi G, Fowler B, Scali B, Rossi F, Motto E, Pieruzzi F, Mancia G. Sympathetic activation and heart rate thresholds for cardiovascular risk in chronic kidney disease. J Hypertens. 2022;40(8):1530–6.
9. Grassi G, Biffi A, Seravalle G, Bertoli S, Airoldi F, Corrao G, Pisano A, Mallamaci F, Mancia G, Zoccali C. Sympathetic nerve traffic overactivity in chronic kidney disease: a systematic review and meta-analysis. J Hypertens. 2021;39(3):408–16.
10. Harrell W, Gipson DS, Belger A, Matsuda-Abedini M, Bjornson B, Hooper SR. Functional magnetic resonance imaging findings in children and adolescents with chronic kidney disease: preliminary findings. Semin Nephrol. 2021;41(5):462–75.
11. Kaur M, Chandran DS, Jaryal AK, Bhowmik D, Agarwal SK, Deepak KK. Baroreflex dysfunction in chronic kidney disease. World J Nephrol. 2016;5(1):53–65.
12. Schmieder RE. Renal denervation in patients with chronic kidney disease: current evidence and future perspectives. Nephrol Dial Transplant. 2023;38(5):1089–96.
13. Scalise F, Quarti-Trevano F, Toscano E, Sorropago A, Vanoli J, Grassi G. Renal denervation in end-stage renal disease: current evidence and perspectives. High Blood Press Cardiovasc Prev. 2024;31:7–13.
14. Ye S, Zhong H, Yanamadala V, Campese VM. Renal injury caused by intrarenal injection of phenol increases afferent and efferent renal sympathetic nerve activity. Am J Hypertens. 2002;15:717–24.
15. Marescau B, Nagels G, Possemiers I, De Broe ME, Becaus I, Billiouw JM, Lornoy W, De Deyn PP. Guanidino compounds in serum and urine of nondialyzed patients with chronic renal insufficiency. Metabolism. 1997;46(9):1024–31.
16. Lataro RM, Brognara F, Iturriaga R, Paton JFR. Inflammation of some visceral sensory systems and autonomic dysfunction in cardiovascular disease. Auton Neurosci. 2024;251:103–37.
17. Anguiano L, Riera M, Pascual J, Valdivielso JM, Barrios C, Betriu A, Clotet S, Mojal S, Fernandez E, Soler MJ. Circulating angiotensin converting enzyme 2 activity as a biomarker of silent atherosclerosis in patients with chronic kidney disease. Atherosclerosis. 2016;253:135–43.
18. Klein IH, Ligtenberg G, Oey PL, Koomans HA, Blankestijn PJ. Enalapril and losartan reduce sympathetic hyperactivity in patients with chronic renal failure. J Am Soc Nephrol. 2003;14:425–30.
19. Sakuma I, Togashi H, Yoshioka M, Saito H, Yanagida M, Tamura M, Kobayashi T, Yasuda H, Gross SS, Levi R. NG-methyl-L-arginine, an inhibitor of L-arginine-derived nitric oxide

synthesis, stimulates renal sympathetic nerve activity in vivo. A role for nitric oxide in the central regulation of sympathetic tone? Circ Res. 1992;70:607–11.
20. Dounousi E, Papavasiliou E, Makedou A, Ioannou K, Katopodis KP, Tselepis A, Siamopoulos KC, Tsakiris D. Oxidative stress is progressively enhanced with advancing stages of CKD. Am J Kidney Dis. 2006;48:752–60.
21. Hirooka Y, Kishi T, Sakai K, Takeshita A, Sunagawa K. Imbalance of central nitric oxide and reactive oxygen species in the regulation of sympathetic activity and neural mechanisms of hypertension. Am J Physiol Regul Integr Comp Physiol. 2011;300:R818–26.
22. Oliveira-Sales EB, Nishi EE, Carillo BA, Boim MA, Dolnikoff MS, Bergamaschi CT, Campos RR. Oxidative stress in the sympathetic premotor neurons contributes to sympathetic activation in renovascular hypertension. Am J Hypertens. 2009;22:484–92.
23. Campese VM, Ye S, Zhong H, Yanamadala V, Ye Z, Chiu J. Reactive oxygen species stimulate central and peripheral sympathetic nervous system activity. Am J Physiol Heart Circ Physiol. 2004;287:695–703.
24. Grassi G, Seravalle G, Dell'Oro R, Mancia G. Sympathetic mechanisms, organ damage, and antihypertensive treatment. Curr Hypertens Rep. 2011;13:303–8.
25. Smith PA, Graham LN, Mackintosh AF, Stoker JB, Mary DA. Relationship between central sympathetic activity and stages of human hypertension. Am J Hypertens. 2004;17:217–22.
26. Grassi G, Cattaneo BM, Seravalle G, Lanfranchi A, Mancia G. Baroreflex control of sympathetic nerve activity in essential and secondary hypertension. Hypertension. 1998;31:68–72.
27. Feihl F, Liaudet L, Levy BI, Waeber B. Hypertension and microvascular remodelling. Cardiovasc Res. 2008;78:274–85.
28. Folkow B. Physiological aspects of primary hypertension. Physiol Rev. 1982;62:347–504.
29. Simpson P. Norepinephrine-stimulated hypertrophy of cultured rat myocardial cells is an alpha 1 adrenergic response. J Clin Invest. 1983;72:732–8.
30. Coutsos M, Sala-Mercado JA, Ichinose M, Li Z, Dawe EJ, O'Leary DS. Muscle metaboreflex-induced coronary vasoconstriction limits ventricular contractility during dynamic exercise in heart failure. Am J Physiol Heart Circ Physiol. 2013;304:1029–37.
31. Volders PG. Novel insights into the role of the sympathetic nervous system in cardiac arrhythmogenesis. Heart Rhythm. 2010;7:1900–6.
32. Rafiq K, Noma T, Fujisawa Y, Ishihara Y, Arai Y, Nabi AH, Suzuki F, Nagai Y, Nakano D, Hitomi H, et al. Renal sympathetic denervation suppresses de novo podocyte injury and albuminuria in rats with aortic regurgitation. Circulation. 2012;125:1402–13.
33. Jamerson KA, Julius S, Gudbrandsson T, Andersson O, Brant DO. Reflex sympathetic activation induces acute insulin resistance in the human forearm. Hypertension. 1993;21:618–23.
34. Failla M, Grappiolo A, Emanuelli G, Vitale G, Fraschini N, Bigoni M, Grieco N, Denti M, Giannattasio C, Mancia G. Sympathetic tone restrains arterial distensibility of healthy and atherosclerotic subjects. J Hypertens. 1999;17:1117–23.
35. Hijmering ML, Stroes ES, Olijhoek J, Hutten BA, Blankestijn PJ, Rabelink TJ. Sympathetic activation markedly reduces endothelium-dependent, flow-mediated vasodilation. J Am Coll Cardiol. 2002;39:683–8.
36. Vongpatanasin W, Kario K, Atlas SA, Victor RG. Central sympatholytic drugs. J Clin Hypertens. 2011;13(9):658–61.
37. Wiles K, Chappell L, Clark K, Elman L, Hall M, Lightstone L, Mohamed G, Mukherjee D, Nelson-Piercy C, Webster P, Whybrow R, Bramham K. Clinical practice guideline on pregnancy and renal disease. BMC Nephrol. 2019;20(1):401.
38. Pepper GS, Lee RW. Sympathetic activation in heart failure and its treatment with β-blockade. Arch Intern Med. 1999;159(3):225–34.
39. Taler SJ, Agarwal R, Bakris GL, et al. KDOQI US commentary on the 2012 KDIGO clinical practice guideline for management of blood pressure in CKD. Am J Kidney Dis. 2013;62(2):201–13.
40. Joyner MJ, Charkoudian N, Wallin BG. Sympathetic nervous system and blood pressure in humans: individualized patterns of regulation and their implications. Hypertension. 2010;56(1):10–6.

41. Schmieder RE, Hettrick DA, Böhm M, et al. Novel approaches to define responders to interventional treatment in hypertension: insights from the SPYRAL HTN-OFF and HTN-ON MED trials. Hypertens Res. 2025;48:327–35.
42. Iaccarino G, Franco D, Sorriento D, et al. Modulation of insulin sensitivity by exercise training: implications for cardiovascular prevention. J Cardiovasc Transl Res. 2021;14:256–70.
43. Grassi G, Seravalle G, Calhoun DA, Bolla GB, Giannattasio C, Marabini M, Del Bo A, Mancia G. Mechanisms responsible for sympathetic activation by cigarette smoking in humans. Circulation. 1994;90(1):248–53.
44. Ruzicka M, Knoll G, Leenen FHH, Leech J, Aaron SD, Hiremath S. Effects of CPAP on blood pressure and sympathetic activity in patients with diabetes mellitus, chronic kidney disease, and resistant hypertension. CJC Open. 2020;2(4):258–64.
45. Cheng B-C, Lai Y-R, Huang C-C, Lu C-H. Improved cardiovascular autonomic function and decreased protein-bound uremic toxins in patients with end-stage renal disease after peritoneal dialysis. J Int Med Res. 2020;48(7):300060520933797.

Pathophysiology of Hypertension in Chronic Kidney Disease: The Complex Role of Arterial Stiffness

Christodoula Kourtidou and Panagiotis I. Georgianos

Introduction

Hypertension is the most frequent chronic disorder worldwide and represents an established risk factor for kidney injury progression and the second more frequent cause of chronic kidney disease (CKD) [1, 2]. Furthermore, the burden of CKD follows an increasing trend during the last two decades and is currently estimated to affect more than 10% of the adult population worldwide [3]. Among hypertensive patients with CKD, increased systolic BP (SBP), reduced diastolic BP (DBP), and elevation in pulse pressure (PP) are typical patterns of BP profile. This particular phenotype of isolated systolic hypertension reflects the arterial remodeling that occurs in CKD, which is characterized by early vascular aging and accelerated arterial stiffening [4–6]. Arterial stiffness is a long-term process of structural changes in the visco-elastic properties of the biomaterial constituting the media of the aortic wall. This remodeling begins from the early stages of CKD and progresses in parallel with kidney function decline, resulting in arterial enlargement, wall thickening, and hardening. Increased arterial rigidity is proposed as a main mechanistic mediator of left ventricular hypertrophy, subendocardial hypo-perfusion, and congestive heart failure [4, 5]. In this context, it should not come as a surprise the fact that several longitudinal studies have consistently shown that aortic pulse wave velocity (PWV), a direct marker of aortic stiffness, is a strong and independent predictor of adverse cardiovascular outcomes and all-cause death in several patient populations [7], including those with CKD [8].

Apart from the well-documented impact of arterial stiffness on the left ventricular work load, downstream transmission of pulsatile pressure to the level of microcirculation is a mechanism through which arterial stiffness induces injury to other

C. Kourtidou · P. I. Georgianos (✉)
2nd Department of Nephrology, AHEPA Hospital, School of Medicine, Aristotle University of Thessaloniki, Thessaloniki, Greece

P. Sarafidis, R. Pontremoli (eds.), *Hypertension and Chronic Kidney Disease*, Updates in Hypertension and Cardiovascular Protection,
https://doi.org/10.1007/978-3-032-29564-4_5

susceptible organs [9]. This may be of particular relevance for the progression of kidney damage, as unique features of renal microcirculation (i.e., continuous and passive renal perfusion, low input impedance of renal microvasculature, decreased wave reflections at the kidney level) make this organ particularly susceptible to the deleterious impact of excessive pulsatile energy transmission to the glomerulus [9, 10]. In this context, several cross-sectional studies showed an inverse relationship between aortic PWV and estimated-glomerular-filtration-rate (eGFR) in patients with or without established CKD [11, 12]. Accumulating evidence from prospective observational studies over the past few years suggests that increased arterial stiffness is strongly related to the annual rate of eGFR decline and is possibly an independent predictor of faster progression of CKD [13–16].

In this chapter, we explore the complex interrelation between arterial stiffness, CKD and hypertension. We provide an overview of earlier and more recent studies suggesting that arterial stiffness may not be simply the consequence of CKD, but a causal factor for new-onset CKD and more rapid eGFR decline in patients with preexisting CKD. Thus, in these patients arterial stiffness is not only a vascular mechanism of systolic BP elevation, but a promoter of BP increase through acceleration of kidney injury.

Pathophysiology: Cross-Talk Between Macrocirculation and Microcirculation in Primary Hypertension and in Patients with CKD

Microcirculation and macrocirculation are closely interconnected into a dangerous cross-link in hypertension. Microvascular damage involves functional (vasoconstriction, impaired vasodilatation) and structural abnormalities (mostly inward eutrophic remodeling). These abnormalities are major mediators of the increase in total peripheral resistance and mean BP in primary hypertension. In the long term, alterations in microcirculation promote the adverse remodeling of aorta and large central arteries leading to large arterial stiffening [17, 18]. In turn, stiffening of large central arteries elevates central systolic and pulse pressures, which are further augmented by the premature arrival of the reflected pulse wave in central aorta during the systolic instead of the diastolic phase of the cardiac cycle. The elevation in wave reflection from the peripheral segments of the arterial tree is largely attributable to structural alterations in small resistance arteries. Furthermore, transmission of high BP and flow pulsatility to small resistance arteries promotes the acceleration of functional and structural abnormalities, thus leading to further elevation in total peripheral resistance and mean BP [17, 18]. This cross-talk generates a dangerous vicious circle. Transmission of high pulsatile energy to microcirculation, in addition to higher mean BP, exaggerates end-organ damage and results in cardiovascular, cerebral, and renal complications.

In detail, healthy vascular aging is a measure to delay the progression of end-organ damage. In healthy persons, an impedance mismatch occurs in response to the stiffness gradient between the central elastic arteries and distal muscular-type arteries. This physiological phenomenon generates pressure wave reflection, limiting the transmission of pressure pulsatility to microcirculation. The largest part of the reflected pulsatile energy that propagates backward, toward the heart, travels at low velocity along the elastic arteries. As a result, the reflected pulse wave does not superimpose on the incident pressure wave. In this way, central BP remains normal. With aging or in clinical states of premature vascular aging, such as in patients with CKD, the stiffened central aorta loses its capacity to dampen the pulsatility of ventricular ejection. The microcirculation in the target organs is damaged by the hyperpulsatility. Because the stiffness of distal muscular-type arteries is not modified with aging, there is a decrease in the stiffness gradient between the central elastic arteries and peripheral muscular-type arteries. In this way, pressure pulsatility is transmitted to a larger extent toward small vessels of the target organs. The largest part of the reflected pulsatile energy that propagates backward, toward the heart, travels at high velocity along stiff arteries. Therefore, the reflected pulse wave returns early and it superimposes on the incident pressure wave during systole rather than diastole, leading to an augmented central aortic systolic BP and pulse pressure [17, 18]. This is a typical mechanism of CKD leading through several pathways to increased arterial stiffness, which, in turn would lead to increased systolic BP.

With respect to the microvascular damage at the kidney level, the perfusion of this organ is characterized by a high-flow, low-impedance microcirculation [19, 20]. These particular features of renal perfusion make the kidney vulnerable to high pressure pulsatility that can penetrate deeply into the microvascular bed. In the renal microcirculation, myogenic tone primarily mediates the autoregulatory response, a compensatory mechanism that protects the kidney mircovessels from hypertensive injury. When renal autoregulatory capacity is impaired, even modest increments in systemic BP can be transmitted to the glomerular capillaries [21–23]. Therefore, the impaired myogenic tone of the renal microcirculation, such as that identified in vessels from hypertensive patients with type 2 diabetes (T2D), reduces the autoregulation ability. In other words, in these patients the afferent arteriole is dilated for several reasons and/or cannot constrict properly to protect the glomerulus against the increased systemic BP load. Even minimal elevations in systemic BP are transformed into higher pulsatile energy transmitted to the kidney, with higher dissipation in the microcirculation. These hemodynamic alterations are considered as an important mediator of glomerular hyperfiltration, which in the long term would lead to elevated albuminuria and faster decline in kidney function, eventually resulting in glomerulosclerosis [21–23]. As such, arterial stiffness per se can start or accelerate kidney injury and this, in turn, can increase BP through established pathways. These data from mechanistic studies are in line with clinical studies showing that markers of arterial stiffness, such as PWV and augmentation index, are strong and independent determinants of the rate of eGFR decline in patients with or without established CKD, which are described below [1].

Studies Evaluating the Association Between Arterial Stiffness and Incident CKD/Albuminuria in Patients with Preserved Kidney Function

A number of observational studies aimed to investigate the longitudinal association of arterial stiffness with the initiation and progression of kidney injury in patients with preserved kidney function at study enrolment (Table 1). Bouchi et al. [13] evaluated prospectively 461 Japanese patients with type 2 diabetes (T2D) and eGFR 84.2 mL/min/1.73 m^2 over a median follow-up of 5.9 years. The analysis showed a significant association of aortic PWV with the annual rate of eGFR decline. Importantly, increased aortic PWV at the baseline was associated with 26% greater risk of progression from normo- to microalbuminuria [hazard ratio (HR): 1.26; 95% confidence interval (CI): 1.13–1.41] and with 25% greater risk of progression of micro- to macroalbuminuria (HR: 1.25; 95% CI: 1.11–1.40) [13]. A subsequent study evaluated the association of arterial stiffness with rapid kidney function decline (defined as eGFR loss >3 mL/min/1.73 m^2 per year) and with the risk of developing new-onset CKD (defined as an eGFR <60 mL/min/1.73 m^2) in 2129 older patients enrolled in the Health ABC study. The mean levels of eGFR at baseline were 79 mL/min/1.73 m^2 [16]. Over a median follow-up of 8.9 years, aortic PWV could not predict the outcome of rapid eGFR decline [odds ratio (OR): 1.16; 95 CI: 0.89–1.52], but was associated with 39% greater risk of incident CKD [incidence rate ratio (IRR): 1.39; 95% CI: 1.09–1.77]. In another study involving 2053 middle-aged Japanese people with preserved kidney function and normoalbuminuria at baseline, Tomiyama et al. [24] showed that brachial-ankle PWV (baPWV) was associated with a higher annual rate of eGFR decline. Furthermore, each 1 m/s increase in the levels of baPWV at baseline was shown to be associated with 36% greater risk of developing CKD over a follow-up period of 5.6 years (OR: 1.36; 95% CI: 1.09–1.70).

In contrast to the above, a prospective analysis incorporating data from 1675 third generation offspring participants in the Framingham Heart Study (mean age: 40 years) showed that the levels of aortic PWV at baseline had no clear association with the risk of developing CKD over a long-term follow-up period of 7–10 years (OR: 1.06; 95% CI: 0.89–1.26) [25]. Aortic PWV exhibited only a modest association with the risk of progression from normo- to microalbuminuria in the age- and gender-adjusted models (OR: 1.19; 95% CI: 1.01–1.40), an association that was not persistent after additional adjustment for multiple confounding factors (OR: 1.14; 95% CI: 0.94–1.42) [25]. The lack of significant associations in this study should be interpreted taking into consideration the limited statistical power of the analysis. The study included younger and low risk individuals and this resulted in a lower than expected incidence of adverse kidney outcomes during the observational period.

In a subsequent study, 577 patients with T2D and a mean eGFR of 91 mL/min/1.73 m^2 were prospectively followed over a period of 12 months. There was an inverse association of baPWV with the annual change in the levels of eGFR. baPWV was also an independent predictor of rapid kidney function decline (OR: 1.072; 95% CI: 1.011–1.136) [26]. In another study including 913 individuals with preserved kidney function (mean eGFR at baseline: 84 mL/min/1.73 m^2), neither aortic

Table 1 Studies evaluating the association between arterial stiffness and incident CKD/albuminuria in patients with preserved kidney function

Study ID	Population	Arterial stiffness assessment	Follow-up	Outcome
Upadhyay et al. [25] JASN 2009	1675 participants in the Framingham Offspring Cohort	Aortic PWV	7–10 years	Aortic PWV was associated with progression from normo- to micro-albuminuria (OR: 1.19; 95% CI: 1.01–1.40) but did not predict incident CKD (OR: 1.06; 95% CI: 0.89–1.26)
Tomiyama et al. [24] Atherosclerosis 2010	2053 middle-aged Japanese employees	baPWV	5.6 years	Each 1 m/s increase in baPWV was associated with 36% elevated risk for incident CKD (OR: 1.36; 95% CI: 1.09–1.70)
Bouchi et al. [13] Diabet Care 2011	461 type 2 diabetic patients	Aortic PWV	5.9 years	Aortic PWV was associated with annual change in eGFR (standardized estimate: −0.095, $P < 0.05$) and was predictor of albuminuria progression (HR: 1.23; 95% CI: 1.13–1.33)
Madero et al. [16] CJASN 2013	2129 older participants in the Health ABC study	Aortic PWV	8.9 years	Aortic PWV was associated with elevated risk of developing CKD (IRR: 1.39; 95% CI: 1.09–1.77)
Vasan et al. [28] Hypertension 2022	7283 participants in Framingham Offspring and Third Generation cohorts	Aortic PWV	15 years	Aortic PWV was associated with increased risk for incident CKD (HR: 1.19; 95% CI: 1.05–1.34)
Yao et al. [29] Am J Kidney Dis 2025	3161 participants in the community-based Atherosclerosis Risk in Communities study	Aortic PWV	6.6 years	Patients in the higher aortic PWV quartile had a faster eGFR annual decline than those in the lower quartile (eGFR slope, −0.44 mL/min/1.73 m^2/year [95% CI: −0.56 to −0.33] vs. −0.37 mL/min/1.73 m^2/year [95% CI: −0.48 to −0.26], respectively)

Abbreviations: *CKD* chronic kidney disease, *PWV* pulse wave velocity, *baPWV* brachial-ankle PWV, *eGFR* estimated glomerular filtration rate, *OR* odds ratio, *HR* hazard ratio, *IRR* incidence rate ratio, *CI* confidence interval

PWV nor baPWV were independently associated with a heightened risk of rapid eGFR decline over a median follow-up period of 3.2 years (OR: 1.39; 95% CI: 0.41–4.65 for aortic PWV and OR: 2.51; 95% CI: 0.66–9.46 for baPWV, respectively) [27]. However, each 10 mmHg increment in the levels of brachial PP was an independent prediction of a more rapid progression of kidney damage over the course of this study (OR: 1.22; 95% CI: 1.01–1.48) [27]. Notably, this study followed a retrospective design and therefore the possibility of recording bias cannot be excluded.

More clear evidence for the prognostic association of arterial stiffness with the risk for adverse health outcomes has been provided by a recent analysis from the Framingham Study [28]. The analysis included a total of 7283 participants, who had measurement of aortic PWV via applanation tonometry at one or more examinations. In multivariate-adjusted Cox-regression hazard models, over a long-term follow-up period of 15 years, each 1 standard deviation increment in the levels of aortic PWV was associated with significantly higher risk of developing hypertension (HR: 1.32; 95% CI: 1.21–1.44), diabetes (HR: 1.32; 95% CI: 1.11–1.58), CKD (HR: 1.19; 95% CI: 1.05–1.34), dementia (HR: 1.27; 95% CI: 1.06–1.53), cardiovascular disease (HR: 1.20; 95% CI: 1.06–1.36) and its components [28]. These prospective data from a large community-based observational study highlight that early vascular aging is an important predictor of the risk for multiple adverse health outcomes, inclusive of the risk of incident CKD.

Incorporating data from the Atherosclerosis Risk in Communities (ARIC) Study [29], a recent analysis included 3.161 patients without established CKD at visit 5. A secondary analysis included a larger sample of 4341 patients regardless of the levels of eGFR across visits 5–7. All patients had a priori assessment of stiffness in several arterial segments for their inclusion in the analysis. The primary outcome in the main analysis was incident CKD, defined as an eGFR <60 mL/min/1.73 m^2 accompanied by an at least 25 decrease in the levels eGFR or CKD-related hospitalization. In the secondary analysis, the outcome was the association of arterial stiffness with eGFR slope over time [29]. In the main analysis, over a median follow-up of 6.6 years, relative to the lowest tertile, patients stratified in the highest tertile of carotid-femoral PWV (HR: 1.53; 95% CI: 1.15–2.04), heart-femoral PWV (HR: 1.49; 95% CI: 1.12–1.99) and heart-ankle PWV (HR: 1.56; 95% CI: 1.16–2.08) had significantly higher risk of developing CKD [29]. Similarly, in the secondary analysis, patients with greater severity of arterial stiffness at baseline experienced a more rapid decline in eGFR over the follow-up period [29]. If these risk associations truly exist, then regression of arterial stiffness may be a measure for the prevention of CKD.

Studies Exploring the Association of Arterial Stiffness with Kidney Injury Progression in Patients with Preexisting CKD

Longitudinal studies have provided evidence that arterial stiffness is associated with faster progression of kidney injury decline and higher risk of initiating kidney replacement therapy in patients with preexisting CKD (Table 2). In an earlier small study, Ford et al. investigated the effect of aortic stiffness on the progression of kidney damage in 133 patients with stage 3–4 CKD (eGFR at baseline: 32 mL/min/1.73 m^2). Over a mean follow-up of 1.5 years, aortic PWV was associated with the gradient of reciprocal creatinine plot, a measure of the change in eGFR over time ($r = 0.46$, $P = 0.016$) and was an independent predictor of the

Table 2 Studies evaluating the association of arterial stiffness with the progression of kidney injury in patients with preexisting CKD

Study ID	Population	Arterial stiffness assessment	Follow-up	Outcome
Ford et al. [15] Hypertension 2010	133 patients with stage 3–4 CKD	Aortic PWV	1.5 years	Aortic PWV was independently associated with the combined renal outcome of >25% decline in eGFR or dialysis ($r = 0.48$, $P = 0.002$)
Weber et al. [30] Am J Hypertens 2011	111 patients with stage 3–4 CKD	AIx, AP	3.6 years	Each 10% increase in AIx and each 10 mm Hg elevation in AP were associated with 47% and 56% increased risks for the composite endpoint of doubling of serum creatinine, dialysis or transplantation (HR: 1.474; 95% CI: 1.020–2.030 and HR: 1.559; 95% CI: 1.015–2.394, respectively)
Chen et al. [31] CJASN 2011	145 patients with stage 3–4 CKD	baPWV	1.3 years	baPWV was independent predictor of the combined endpoint of >25% decline in eGFR or death (HR: 1.001; 95% CI: 1.000–1.001 for each 1 cm/s elevation in baPWV)
Chen et al. [29] Hypertens Res 2011	167 patients with stage 3 CKD	baPWV	2.6 years	baPWV was associated with increased risk of >25% decline in eGFR (HR: 1.001; 95% CI: 1.000–1.002 for each 1 cm/s increment in baPWV)
Su et al. [33] Am J Hypertens 2011	363 patients with stage 3–4 CKD	baPWV	3.1 years	Patients in the highest baPWV tertile had 5.93-fold elevated risk for the composite renal outcome of >25% decline in eGFR or dialysis than those in the lowest tertile (HR: 5.93; 95% CI: 2.94–11.99)
Lee et al. [34] Sci Rep 2018	1801 patients with stage 1–5 CKD	baPWV	2.2 years	Patients in the higher quintile of the baPWV had higher risk for a rapid decline in eGFR defined as a reduction >5 mL/min/1.73 m^2/year in comparison to the lower quintile (OR: 1.9; 95% CI: 1.141–3.129)
Townsend et al. [35] Hypertension 2018	2795 participants mainly with CKD 3–4 from the Chronic Renal Insufficiency Cohort study	Aortic PWV	4.1 years	Patients in the highest tertile of aortic PWV (>10.3 m/s) were at increased risk for ESRD in comparison to individuals in the lowest tertile (<7.7 m/s) (HR: 1.37; 95% CI: 1.05–1.80)

Abbreviations: *CKD* chronic kidney disease, *ESRD* end-stage renal disease, *PWV* pulse wave velocity, *baPWV* brachial-ankle PWV, *AIx* augmentation index, *AP* augmentation pressure, *eGFR* estimated glomerular filtration rate, *HR* hazard ratio, *CI* confidence interval

prespecified kidney outcome, defined as the composite of >25% decline in the levels of eGFR from baseline or initiation of dialysis ($r = 0.48$, $P = 0.002$) [15]. In a subsequent small study, Weber et al. showed that among 111 patients with stage 3 or 4 CKD, each 10% increment in the levels of augmentation index (AIx) and each 10 mmHg increment in the levels of augmentation pressure were associated with 47% and 56% greater risk for the combined kidney outcome of doubling of serum creatinine, initiation of kidney replacement therapy or transplantation over a median follow-up period of 3.6 years (HR: 1.474; 95% CI: 1.020–2.030 for AIx and HR: 1.559; 95% CI: 1.015–2.394 for augmentation pressure, respectively) [30]. Although AIx and augmentation pressure are indirect markers of arterial stiffness, these findings suggest that impaired cushioning of arterial function due to the premature arrival of the reflected waves back to the ascending aorta may be also mechanistically involved in the excessive delivery of pulsatile energy to the renal microcirculation.

In another study, Chen et al. [31] explored the association of baPWV with the rate of eGFR decline in 145 patients with stage 3–5 CKD (eGFR at baseline: 29.9 mL/min/1.73 m^2). Over a mean follow-up period of 1.2 years, baPWV was inversely associated with the eGFR slope and was an independent predictor of the composite outcome, defined as the progression of CKD to kidney failure or death from any cause (HR: 1.001; 95% CI: 1.000–1.001 for each 1 cm/s increment in baPWV) [31]. These findings were confirmed in a subsequent study, in which 167 patients with stage 3 CKD were prospectively followed for a mean period of 2.6 years. As compared to patients with a slower rate of kidney function decline, patients with faster progression of CKD tended to be older in age, had more commonly T2D, and had higher levels of baPWV and lower levels of left ventricular election fraction at baseline. In the prospective analysis, higher baPWV at baseline was independently associated with a higher risk for >25% decrease in eGFR during the follow-up (HR: 1.001; 95% CI: 1.000–1.002 per 1 cm/s increment in baPWV) [32]. Su at al [33]. explored the prognostic association of elevated arterial stiffness with the risk of kidney injury progression in 363 Taiwan patients with stage 3–4 CKD. Patients stratified in the highest tertile of baPWV at baseline had significantly higher annual rate of eGFR decline as compared with patients stratified in the lowest baPWV tertile (-2.68 ± 0.35 vs $+0.86 \pm 0.25$ mL/min/1.73 m^2/year, $P < 0.05$). Furthermore, increased baPWV was associated with a 5.93-fold higher risk of reaching the prespecified kidney outcome, defined as the composite of >25% decline in eGFR or initiation of dialysis over a follow-up period of 3.1 years (HR: 5.93; 95% CI: 2.94–11.99 for the comparison between the highest and the lowest baPWV tertile) [33].

A detailed examination of arterial remodeling in CKD was performed in the Nephrotest cohort study, in which aortic PWV and carotid stiffness parameters were assessed in 180 patients with stage 3–4 CKD [14]. Over a mean follow-up period of 3.1 years, stiffness of the carotid artery was progressively increased by 0.28 ± 0.05 m/s. In contrast, aortic stiffness was not substantially modified over time. Internal diameter of the carotid artery was increased, whereas intima-media thickness was significantly reduced over time. Absence of arterial wall thickening in response to the enlarged lumen diameter resulted in a significant elevation of 2.08 ± 0.43 kPa/year in the circumferential wall stress during the follow-up period. Most importantly, circumferential tensile stress was associated with 40% greater risk of progression of CKD to kidney failure (HR: 1.40; 95% CI: 1.08–1.83). In contrast, aortic PWV was not prognostically associated with the risk of progression of kidney damage [14]. Future studies including measurements of arterial stiffness in the aorta and in more peripheral segments of the arterial tree are needed to confirm or refute these observations.

Studies Showing Associations of Arterial Stiffness with Kidney Function Decline Independent from the Levels of Systemic BP

Evidence to support the notion that aortic stiffness influences the progression of CKD independently from BP has been provided by two larger longitudinal studies. In an analysis involving 1801 patients with predialysis CKD in Korea, the investigators explored the association of baPWV and heart-femoral PWV with the risk of rapid progression of kidney injury, defined as an annual rate eGFR change of at least −5 mL/min/1.73 m^2 [34]. Over a mean follow-up period of 2.2 years, the observed average change in eGFR was −3.6 mL/min/1.73 m^2, whereas 31.6 of participants met the prespecified criteria of rapid deterioration in kidney function. In the multivariate-adjusted analysis, the risk of rapid eGFR decline was 1.96-fold higher in the fifth quintile than in the first quintile of baPWV [34]. In a subgroup of 1182 patients who had concomitant measurement of heart-femoral PWV, high baPWV was associated with rapid eGFR decline only when accompanied by a simultaneously high heart-femoral PWV. Taken together, these data suggest that increased stiffness of central and peripheral (muscular-type arteries) possibly results in a substantially greater risk of progression of kidney damage in patients with CKD [34].

In the Chronic Renal Insufficiency Study (CRIC) [35], aortic PWV was measured in 2795 patients at baseline. The analysis explored the association of baseline aortic PWV with three prespecified outcomes: (i) incident end-stage kidney disease (ESKD); (ii) the composite of >50% decrease in the levels of eGFR from baseline or incident ESKD; (iii) death from any cause. Patients were stratified into tertiles, according to the levels of aortic PWV at baseline. During the follow-up period, as compared with the lowest tertile, patients in the highest tertile of aortic PWV had 37% greater risk of incident ESKD (HR: 1.37; 95% CI: 1.05–1.80), 25% greater risk of ESKD or halving of eGFR (HR: 1.25; 95% CI: 0.98–1.58) and 72% greater risk of all-cause mortality (HR: 1.72; 95% CI: 1.24–2.38) [35]. These risk associations were not modified in models adjusted for age, gender, BP levels and several additional confounding factors [35]. If these risk associations are causal, then the measurement of aortic stiffness may improve the stratification and reclassification of risk for adverse kidney outcomes in patients with CKD.

Conclusion

Mechanistically, arterial stiffness raises flow and pressure pulsatility and impairs cushioning function of the aorta and large central arteries, leading to elevation of systolic BP. Downstream transmission of enhanced pressure pulsatility to the level of microcirculation is long considered as an important contributor to the progression of end-organ damage in hypertension. In particular, increased arterial stiffness may be a major pathway, through which excessive pulsatile energy is transmitted to the low-impendence renal microvasculature, causing dynamic constriction of renal resistance vessels and promoting intra-glomerular hyper-perfusion. On this mechanistic basis, evidence from earlier and recent longitudinal studies suggests that increased arterial stiffness is possibly associated with the risk of incident CKD in patients with preserved kidney function and with faster progression of kidney damage in patients with preexisting CKD. If these risk associations are causal, then arterial stiffness is not simply a consequence of CKD, but a causal factor that increases the rate of progression of kidney impairment, and, thus, further worsens BP control. Future research, mainly randomized controlled trials, is now needed to investigate whether regression of arterial stiffness in response to treatment is translated into a long-term improvement in the risk of adverse cardiovascular and kidney outcomes.

Acknowledgements The authors report no specific funding in relation to this work.

Disclosure The authors have no conflicts of interest to disclose.

Conflicts of Interest None relevant to this work.

References

1. Georgianos PI, Sarafidis PA, Liakopoulos V. Arterial stiffness: a novel risk factor for kidney injury progression? Am J Hypertens. 2015;28:958–65.
2. Mancia G, Kreutz R, Brunstrom M, Burnier M, Grassi G, Januszewicz A, Muiesan ML, Tsioufis K, Agabiti-Rosei E, Algharably EAE, Azizi M, Benetos A, Borghi C, Hitij JB, Cifkova R, Coca A, Cornelissen V, Cruickshank JK, Cunha PG, Danser AHJ, Pinho RM, Delles C, Dominiczak AF, Dorobantu M, Doumas M, Fernandez-Alfonso MS, Halimi JM, Jarai Z, Jelakovic B, Jordan J, Kuznetsova T, Laurent S, Lovic D, Lurbe E, Mahfoud F, Manolis A, Miglinas M, Narkiewicz K, Niiranen T, Palatini P, Parati G, Pathak A, Persu A, Polonia J, Redon J, Sarafidis P, Schmieder R, Spronck B, Stabouli S, Stergiou G, Taddei S, Thomopoulos C, Tomaszewski M, Van de Borne P, Wanner C, Weber T, Williams B, Zhang ZY, Kjeldsen SE. 2023 ESH Guidelines for the management of arterial hypertension The Task Force for the management of arterial hypertension of the European Society of Hypertension: endorsed by the International Society of Hypertension (ISH) and the European Renal Association (ERA). J Hypertens. 2023;41:1874–2071.
3. Kidney Disease Outcomes Quality Initiative (K/DOQI). K/DOQI clinical practice guidelines on hypertension and antihypertensive agents in chronic kidney disease. Am J Kidney Dis. 2004;43:S1–290.
4. Briet M, Pierre B, Laurent S, London GM. Arterial stiffness and pulse pressure in CKD and ESRD. Kidney Int. 2012;82:388–400.

5. Laurent S, Cockcroft J, Van Bortel L, Boutouyrie P, Giannattasio C, Hayoz D, Pannier B, Vlachopoulos C, Wilkinson I, Struijker-Boudier H. Expert consensus document on arterial stiffness: methodological issues and clinical applications. Eur Heart J. 2006;27:2588–605.
6. Wallace SM, Yasmin, McEniery CM, Maki-Petaja KM, Booth AD, Cockcroft JR, Wilkinson IB. Isolated systolic hypertension is characterized by increased aortic stiffness and endothelial dysfunction. Hypertension. 2007;50:228–33.
7. Vlachopoulos C, Aznaouridis K, Stefanadis C. Prediction of cardiovascular events and all-cause mortality with arterial stiffness: a systematic review and meta-analysis. J Am Coll Cardiol. 2010;55:1318–27.
8. Georgianos PI, Sarafidis PA, Lasaridis AN. Arterial stiffness: a novel cardiovascular risk factor in kidney disease patients. Curr Vasc Pharmacol. 2015;13(2):229–38.
9. Safar ME, Nilsson PM, Blacher J, Mimran A. Pulse pressure, arterial stiffness, and end-organ damage. Curr Hypertens Rep. 2012;14:339–44.
10. O'Rourke MF, Safar ME. Relationship between aortic stiffening and microvascular disease in brain and kidney: cause and logic of therapy. Hypertension. 2005;46:200–4.
11. Mourad JJ, Pannier B, Blacher J, Rudnichi A, Benetos A, London GM, Safar ME. Creatinine clearance, pulse wave velocity, carotid compliance and essential hypertension. Kidney Int. 2001;59:1834–41.
12. Townsend RR, Wimmer NJ, Chirinos JA, Parsa A, Weir M, Perumal K, Lash JP, Chen J, Steigerwalt SP, Flack J, Go AS, Rafey M, Rahman M, Sheridan A, Gadegbeku CA, Robinson NA, Joffe M. Aortic PWV in chronic kidney disease: a CRIC ancillary study. Am J Hypertens. 2010;23:282–9.
13. Bouchi R, Babazono T, Mugishima M, Yoshida N, Nyumura I, Toya K, Hanai K, Tanaka N, Ishii A, Uchigata Y, Iwamoto Y. Arterial stiffness is associated with incident albuminuria and decreased glomerular filtration rate in type 2 diabetic patients. Diabetes Care. 2011;34:2570–5.
14. Briet M, Collin C, Karras A, Laurent S, Bozec E, Jacquot C, Stengel B, Houillier P, Froissart M, Boutouyrie P. Arterial remodeling associates with CKD progression. J Am Soc Nephrol. 2011;22:967–74.
15. Ford ML, Tomlinson LA, Chapman TP, Rajkumar C, Holt SG. Aortic stiffness is independently associated with rate of renal function decline in chronic kidney disease stages 3 and 4. Hypertension. 2010;55:1110–5.
16. Madero M, Peralta C, Katz R, Canada R, Fried L, Najjar S, Shlipak M, Simonsick E, Lakatta E, Patel K, Rifkin D, Hawkins M, Newman A, Sarnak M. Association of arterial rigidity with incident kidney disease and kidney function decline: the Health ABC study. Clin J Am Soc Nephrol. 2013;8(3):424–33.
17. Laurent S, Boutouyrie P. Arterial stiffness and hypertension in the elderly. Front Cardiovasc Med. 2020;7:544302.
18. Laurent S, Agabiti-Rosei C, Bruno RM, Rizzoni D. Microcirculation and macrocirculation in hypertension: a dangerous cross-link? Hypertension. 2022;79:479–90.
19. Carlstrom M, Wilcox CS, Arendshorst WJ. Renal autoregulation in health and disease. Physiol Rev. 2015;95:405–511.
20. Empana JP, Boutouyrie P, Lemogne C, Jouven X, van Sloten TT. Microvascular contribution to late-onset depression: mechanisms, current evidence, association with other brain diseases, and therapeutic perspectives. Biol Psychiatry. 2021;90:214–25.
21. Bidani AK, Griffin KA, Williamson G, Wang X, Loutzenhiser R. Protective importance of the myogenic response in the renal circulation. Hypertension. 2009;54:393–8.
22. Calabia J, Torguet P, Garcia I, Martin N, Mate G, Marin A, Molina C, Valles M. The relationship between renal resistive index, arterial stiffness, and atherosclerotic burden: the link between macrocirculation and microcirculation. J Clin Hypertens (Greenwich). 2014;16:186–91.
23. Fesler P, du Cailar G, Ribstein J, Mimran A. Glomerular hemodynamics and arterial function in normal individuals. J Hypertens. 2010;28:2462–7.

24. Tomiyama H, Tanaka H, Hashimoto H, Matsumoto C, Odaira M, Yamada J, Yoshida M, Shiina K, Nagata M, Yamashina A. Arterial stiffness and declines in individuals with normal renal function/early chronic kidney disease. Atherosclerosis. 2010;212:345–50.
25. Upadhyay A, Hwang SJ, Mitchell GF, Vasan RS, Vita JA, Stantchev PI, Meigs JB, Larson MG, Levy D, Benjamin EJ, Fox CS. Arterial stiffness in mild-to-moderate CKD. J Am Soc Nephrol. 2009;20:2044–53.
26. Sheen YJ, Lin JL, Li TC, Bau CT, Sheu WH. Peripheral arterial stiffness is independently associated with a rapid decline in estimated glomerular filtration rate in patients with type 2 diabetes. Biomed Res Int. 2013;2013:309294.
27. Kim CS, Kim HY, Kang YU, Choi JS, Bae EH, Ma SK, Kim SW. Association of pulse wave velocity and pulse pressure with decline in kidney function. J Clin Hypertens (Greenwich). 2014;16:372–7.
28. Vasan RS, Pan S, Xanthakis V, Beiser A, Larson MG, Seshadri S, Mitchell GF. Arterial stiffness and long-term risk of health outcomes: the Framingham Heart study. Hypertension. 2022;79:1045–56.
29. Yao Z, Ishigami J, Kim E, Ballew SH, Sang Y, Tanaka H, Meyer ML, Coresh J, Matsushita K. Arterial stiffness and subsequent incidence of CKD and kidney function decline in a large longitudinal community cohort: the Atherosclerosis in Communities (ARIC) study. Am J Kidney Dis. 2025;86:32–42.
30. Weber T, Ammer M, Gunduz D, Bruckenberger P, Eber B, Wallner M. Association of increased arterial wave reflections with decline in renal function in chronic kidney disease stages 3 and 4. Am J Hypertens. 2011;24:762–9.
31. Chen SC, Chang JM, Liu WC, Tsai YC, Tsai JC, Hsu PC, Lin TH, Lin MY, Su HM, Hwang SJ, Chen HC. Brachial-ankle pulse wave velocity and rate of renal function decline and mortality in chronic kidney disease. Clin J Am Soc Nephrol. 2011;6:724–32.
32. Chen SC, Lin TH, Hsu PC, Chang JM, Lee CS, Tsai WC, Su HM, Voon WC, Chen HC. Impaired left ventricular systolic function and increased brachial-ankle pulse-wave velocity are independently associated with rapid renal function progression. Hypertens Res. 2011;34:1052–8.
33. Su HM, Lin TH, Hsu PC, Chu CY, Lee WH, Tsai WC, Chen SC, Voon WC, Lai WT, Sheu SH. Brachial-ankle pulse wave velocity and systolic time intervals in risk stratification for progression of renal function decline. Am J Hypertens. 2012;25:1002–10.
34. Lee SW, Han SH, Yoo TH, Chung W, Park SK, Chae DW, Ahn C, Oh KH. Relationship between brachial-ankle and heart-femoral pulse wave velocities and the rapid decline of kidney function. Sci Rep. 2018;8:821.
35. Townsend RR, Anderson AH, Chirinos JA, Feldman HI, Grunwald JE, Nessel L, Roy J, Weir MR, Wright JT Jr, Bansal N, Hsu CY. Association of pulse wave velocity with chronic kidney disease progression and mortality: findings from the CRIC study (Chronic Renal Insufficiency Cohort). Hypertension. 2018;71:1101–7.

Serum Uric Acid and Hypertension in CKD

Elisa Russo, Giovanna Leoncini, Cecilia Barnini, Giovambattista Desideri, Claudio Borghi, Roberto Pontremoli, and Francesca Viazzi

Introduction

Hypertension and chronic kidney disease (CKD) are widespread in the general population, and hyperuricemia is a recognized risk factor for the development and progression of both conditions. Hyperuricemia is a metabolic disorder characterized by elevated serum uric acid (SUA) levels, which is biochemically defined as serum urate level ≥6.8 mg/dL based on the limit of urate solubility. It results from excessive urate production and/or absolute or relative impairment of renal uric acid (UA) excretion. Persistent hyperuricemia (usually defined as a male SUA greater than 7 mg/dL (420 μmol/L) and female SUA levels greater than 6 mg/dL (360 μmol/L)) promote the formation of monosodium urate crystals, which can deposit in joints and soft tissues, eventually leading to gout—a common form of inflammatory arthritis. Gout is thus the clinical manifestation of chronic hyperuricemia, but hyperuricemia itself is often asymptomatic and under-recognized.

E. Russo · G. Leoncini · R. Pontremoli · F. Viazzi (✉)
Department of Internal Medicine, University of Genoa and IRCCS Azienda Ospedaliera Metropolitana (IRCCS AOM) Plesso Ospedale San Martino, Genoa, Italy
e-mail: francesca.viazzi@unige.it

C. Barnini
Department of Internal Medicine IV, Nephrology and Hypertension, Medical University Innsbruck, Innsbruck, Tirol, Austria

G. Desideri
Department of Clinical, Internal Medicine, Anesthesiologic and Cardiovascular Sciences, Sapienza University of Rome, Rome, Italy

C. Borghi
Hypertension and Cardiovascular Disease Research Center, Medical and Surgical Sciences Department, Alma Mater Studiorum University of Bologna, Bologna, Italy

P. Sarafidis, R. Pontremoli (eds.), *Hypertension and Chronic Kidney Disease*, Updates in Hypertension and Cardiovascular Protection,
https://doi.org/10.1007/978-3-032-29564-4_6

Because the kidneys handle the majority of urate clearance (around two-thirds), while the gastrointestinal tract clears the rest, reduced kidney function significantly impairs urate excretion and contributes to the development of hyperuricemia. Moreover, hyperuricemia is common in type 2 diabetes and hypertension, which are conditions that cause CKD. CKD predisposes individuals to hyperuricemia, anemia, hypertension, and cardiovascular disease (CVD), which together greatly increase the risk of cardiovascular (CV) events.

Beyond being a marker of underlying metabolic and CV disorders, hyperuricemia may actively contribute to renal and CVD progression and has been linked to increased morbidity and mortality [1]. Notably, elevated SUA levels are associated not only with gout but also with a wide spectrum of cardiometabolic diseases, including hypertension, obesity, hypertriglyceridemia, atherosclerotic CVD, and metabolic syndrome. Recent epidemiological and experimental studies continue to support a potential causal role of hyperuricemia in the development and worsening of these conditions, particularly of CKD onset and progression. It is therefore important to understand how high UA levels modify kidney, CV, or metabolic outcomes.

Epidemiology: Asymptomatic Hyperuricemia and Gout in CKD

Despite the increasing prevalence of hyperuricemia and gout worldwide, their detailed epidemiology—particularly their relationship with comorbid conditions—remains incompletely characterized in many populations. The prevalence of hyperuricemia in patients with hypertension ranges from 20% to 40%, and a similar prevalence of hypertension has been reported in patients with gout (25%–50%) [2]. Data from the largest cohort studies clearly show an increasing prevalence of hyperuricemia and gout as the estimated glomerular filtration rate (eGFR) declines (Fig. 1).

Recent population-based cohorts, such as the NANHES [2], URRAH [1] and GCKD [3] studies, have reported varying prevalence figures, which also differ according to kidney function status. These discrepancies reflect the complex and multifactorial pathogenesis of hyperuricemia in individuals with impaired renal function—an aspect discussed in detail in subsequent chapters. Whether such differences in pathophysiology translate into distinct clinical outcomes or varied responses to therapy remains an active area of investigation.

GOUT

Study cohort	NHANHES Age standardized prevalence (%)	URRAH* unadjusted prevalence (%)
eGFR >90	13.5	20.1
CKD stage 2 eGFR 60-89	26.9	33.4
CKD stage 3 eGFR 30-59	60.1	50.1
		59.3
CKD stage 4 eGFR 15-29	57.4	53.9
CKD stage 5 eGFR <15		

ASYMPTOMATIC HYPERURICEMIA

Study cohort	NHANHES Age-standardized prevalence (%)	URRAH Unadjusted prevalence (%)	GCKD Prevalence (%)	CJASN 2017 3-yrs incidence (%)	
				F	M
eGFR >90	3.2	0.8	16.0	0.6	0.8
CKD stage 2 eGFR 60-89	4.8	1.7		0.7	1.2
CKD stage 3 eGFR 30-59	29.5	2.6	23.2	1.3	2.5
		3.3	27.6	2.2	3.7
CKD stage 4 eGFR 15-29	32.4	20.9	35.6	3.4	4.6
CKD stage 5 eGFR <15				2.0	2.9

Fig. 1 Unadjusted, age-adjusted prevalence and cumulative incidence of asymptomatic hyperuricemia (A) and gout (B) across CKD stages. CKD, chronic kidney disease, eGFR, estimated glomerular filtration rate (mL/min/1.73 m^2). Data from study cohorts: NHANHES, National Health and Nutrition Examination Surveys (cut off for defining hyperuricemia = 6 mg/dL for women and = 7 mg/dL for men) [2]. URRAH, URic acid Right for heArt Health (*cut off for defining hyperuricemia = 5.6 mg/dL) [1]. GCKD, German Chronic Kidney Disease (cut off for defining hyperuricemia = 6 mg/dL for women and = 7 mg/dL for men) [3]. The 3-year incidence of gout in elderly patients with CKD (CJASN 2017) (cut off for defining hyperuricemia = 6 mg/dL for women and = 7 mg/dL for men) [4]

Pathogenesis of Hyperuricemia and Kidney Role

Urate is the final metabolite produced from nucleic acid catabolism and also arises from the breakdown of high-energy nucleotides such as adenosine triphosphate (ATP). Its synthesis occurs intracellularly through the action of xanthine oxidoreductase (XOR) and it is subsequently transported into the circulation, where it predominantly exists as plasma sodium urate. Although intracellular urate levels are not precisely defined, they are believed to be significantly lower—potentially by several orders of magnitude—than serum concentrations. The primary drivers of renal urate reabsorption are the URAT1 (human urate transporter 1) and GLUT9 (glucose transporter member 9) transporters, while ABCG2 pumps UA into the urine.

Urate elimination occurs mainly via the kidneys (approximately two-thirds) and to a lesser extent through the gastrointestinal tract (approximately one-third). In addition, the molecular physiology of epithelial urate transport plays a key role in the genetic predisposition to hyperuricemia. The principal causes of hyperuricemia are summarized in Table 1.

Table 1 Causes of Hyperuricemia

	Purine overproduction	Decreased uric acid clearance
Genetic (Monogenic disorders)	Hypoxanthine-guanine phosphoribosyltransferase deficiency Phosphoribosylpyrophosphate synthetase overactivity Glucose-6-phosphatase deficiency (glycogen storage disease, type I)	Autosomal dominant tubulointerstitial kidney disease caused by UMOD pathogenic variants Glomerulocystic kidney disease Gene mutations of transporters that regulate renal or gut uric acid clearance: SLC2A9 (GLUT9), ABCG2, SLC22A11/A12 (URAT1/OAT4), SLC22A9 (OAT7), and SLC17A1-4 (NPT1-4)
Comorbid disease-related (Clinical disorders)	Myeloproliferative disorders Lymphoproliferative disorders Hemolytic disorders Psoriasis Tissue hypoxia Down syndrome Glycogen storage diseases (types III, V, VII)	Chronic kidney disease of any form Lead nephropathy (saturnine gout) Effective volume depletion (eg, fluid losses, heart failure) Diabetic or starvation ketoacidosis Lactic acidosis Preeclampsia Obesity and high circulating insulin
Environmental (Drug- or diet-induced)	Excessive ethanol ingestion Excessive dietary purine ingestion Excessive fructose ingestion Cytotoxic drugs	Diuretics (thiazides and loop diuretics) Cyclosporine and tacrolimus Low-dose salicylates Ethambutol Pyrazinamide Ethanol Levodopa Laxative abuse (alkalosis) Salt restriction

The most common causes are underlined

Hyperuricemia has been previously classified into the "UA overproduction type", "UA underexcretion type". and "combined type", and approximately 10%, 60%, and 30% of hyperuricemic patients have been classified into each type, respectively.

Regardless of the underlying cause of elevated plasma UA levels, UA has been shown to exert pathogenic effects both in vitro and in vivo. In cases where hyperuricemia results primarily from impaired renal excretion, its prognostic significance may be limited, as it does not reflect upstream activation of an inflammatory pathway such as xanthine oxidase (XO) overactivity. In contrast, in individuals without kidney dysfunction, hyperuricemia often indicates increased XO activity and thus serves as a marker of active oxidative stress and inflammation [5].

Increased XO activity not only produces more UA but also generates reactive oxygen species (ROS). Specifically, XO reduces oxygen to a superoxide anion, which is subsequently converted to hydrogen peroxide. Hydrogen peroxide is a ROS that, in excess, is toxic to cells and has been implicated in aging and several pathological conditions such as endothelial dysfunction, hypertension, kidney injury, and insulin resistance. These effects contribute to the development or worsening of CVD (Fig. 2).

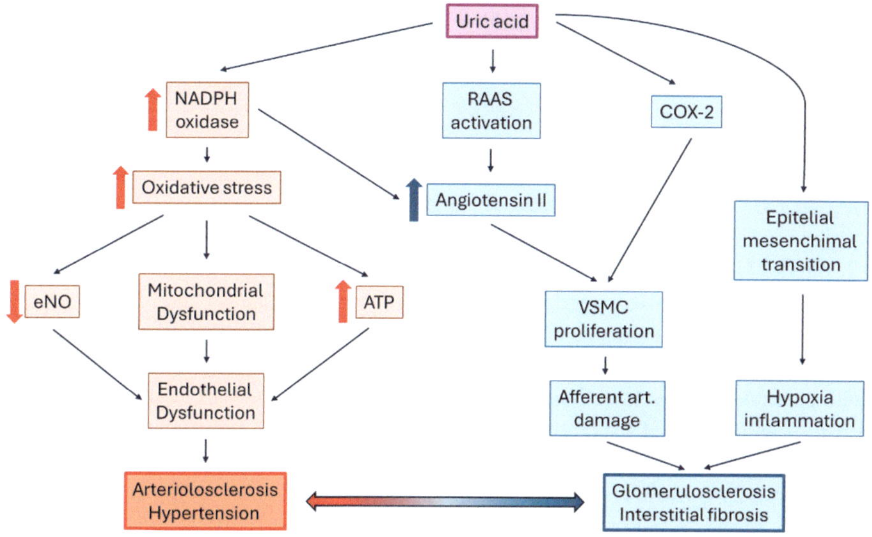

Fig. 2 Pathophysiological mechanisms of vascular and renal damage induced by hyperuricemia. NO, nitric oxide; COX-2, cyclooxygenase-2; RAAS, renin angiotensin aldosterone system; VSMC, vascular smooth muscle cells

UA is the final product of purine metabolism, produced by the XO-catalyzed oxidation of hypoxanthine to xanthine, and subsequently to UA. These substrates originate from the degradation of purine nucleotides, namely guanosine monophosphate (GMP) and adenosine monophosphate (AMP). XO thus plays a central role in purine catabolism, a continuous cellular process driven by both endogenous turnover and dietary intake.

XO is a key enzyme not only in UA production but also in the generation of ROS and promotion of inflammation [6]. Numerous experimental studies suggest that the pro-inflammatory and pathogenic effects of hyperuricemia are largely mediated by XO activity rather than by UA itself. This provides a strong rationale for the use of XO inhibitors not only to lower SUA levels but also as a strategy for CV and renal protection.

As with other enzymatic reactions, XO activity increases in the presence of higher substrate availability. A purine-rich diet or excessive fructose intake—by rapidly depleting ATP—can increase purine turnover and stimulate UA synthesis.

UA homeostasis is tightly regulated, with the kidney playing a central role. Several membrane transporters are involved in renal UA handling, both in tubular reabsorption and secretion. URAT1, located on the apical membrane of proximal tubular cells, is the main transporter responsible for urate reabsorption and a key therapeutic target in the management of hyperuricemia-related disorders [7]. SLC2A9, encoding the glucose transporter GLUT9, plays a crucial role in urate transport, mediating both reabsorption into the blood and excretion into the urine. Genetic variants of GLUT9 significantly affect SUA concentrations by altering this balance. Similarly, ABCG2, which encodes the ATP-binding cassette transporter

BCRP, contributes to UA elimination, particularly via the intestine and renal proximal tubules. Loss-of-function mutations in ABCG2 impair extra-renal UA clearance, leading to reduced intestinal and renal excretion and promoting hyperuricemia.

Impact of Serum Uric Acid on Hypertension

Elevated SUA levels have been consistently associated with an increased risk of developing hypertension, independent of traditional risk factors and renal function. Longitudinal studies and causal mediation analyses support a temporal relationship in which hyperuricemia precedes the onset of hypertension [8]. Notably, individuals with elevated UA levels exhibit a significantly higher relative risk of incident hypertension, as confirmed by large-scale epidemiological data and meta-analyses. For example, the PAMELA study found that each 1 mg/dL increase in UA was associated with a 29%–34% rise in the risk of new-onset hypertension [9]. In children at relatively high CV risk, UA shows a strong relationship with BP values and in children in the top UA quartile (ie, >5.0 mg/dL for boys and >4.7 mg/dL for girls) shows a twofold higher risk of being pre-hypertensive and hypertensive [10].

Animal models have been instrumental in elucidating pathophysiological mechanisms linking UA to elevated BP. Induction of moderate hyperuricemia in rats using oxonic acid results in a rapid increase in blood pressure within 4 weeks, independent of other risk factors. This hypertensive effect is directly proportional to SUA levels and is reversible with ULT such as xanthine oxidase (XO) inhibitors (e.g., allopurinol) or uricosurics (e.g., benzbromarone). Renal histology from these models reveals early signs of injury including interstitial fibrosis, macrophage infiltration, and tubular osteopontin expression, even in the absence of urate crystal deposition [11].

Mechanistically, UA contributes to hypertension through multiple pathways. It induces renal vasoconstriction and sodium retention via activation of the intrarenal renin–angiotensin system (RAS) and suppression of nitric oxide (NO) bioavailability, especially at the macula densa. Moreover, hyperuricemia is associated with increased vascular resistance at both afferent and efferent arterioles, suggesting a detrimental effect on glomerular perfusion and autoregulation. Intracellular UA can promote oxidative stress by stimulating NADPH oxidase, impairing NO signaling, and enhancing vascular smooth muscle cell proliferation, thereby contributing to arteriolosclerosis and glomerular hypertension [12].

In humans, hyperuricemia has been correlated with early renal microvascular damage in essential hypertension, as reflected by increased microalbuminuria, reduced kidney volume, and elevated intrarenal resistance indices [13]. UA further exacerbates renal and vascular injury by activating proinflammatory pathways, including Nuclear Factor kappa-light-chain-enhancer of activated B cells (NF-κB), and upregulating cytokines such as tumor necrosis factor alpha (TNF-α) and interleukin-1 (IL-1), as well as chemokines like monocyte chemoattractant protein 1 (MCP-1). Additionally, it may promote tubular epithelial-to-mesenchymal transition and subsequent fibrosis. Importantly, high dietary fructose intake accelerates intracellular ATP depletion, further amplifying UA synthesis and contributing to hypertension development.

Hyperuricemia is increasingly recognized as a key contributor to the development of hypertension, particularly within the framework of metabolic syndrome. UA enters renal tubular cells, vascular smooth muscle cells, and adipocytes via the URAT1 transporter, where it activates NADPH oxidase (NOX), promoting the generation of reactive oxygen species (ROS). This oxidative stress, coupled with decreased adiponectin levels and increased production of pro-inflammatory mediators such as MCP-1, induces a chronic low-grade inflammatory state. This response is mediated through Toll-like receptor 4 (TLR4) signaling and upregulation of NOX4, ultimately leading to endothelial dysfunction, sodium retention, vasoconstriction, and renal injury—all of which contribute to the onset and progression of hypertension [7].

Furthermore, as suggested by several epidemiological studies, hyperuricemia plays a significant role in the pathogenesis of metabolic disturbances, including visceral obesity, insulin resistance, type 2 diabetes, and non-alcoholic fatty liver disease (NAFLD) in turn, linked to the development of hypertension [14].

A large-scale study involving 96,863 Japanese adults demonstrated that the odds of hyperuricemia were significantly higher in obese individuals, as well as in those with central obesity despite normal weight. This underscores the need for targeted screening strategies using combined measures such as BMI and waist-to-height ratio, especially in middle-aged adults, to prevent hyperuricemia-related complications such as hypertension and CVD [15].

The interplay between UA, CKD, and CVD is intricate and continues to be a subject of ongoing research and debate. A meta-analysis of 44 prospective cohort studies confirmed a significant positive association between SUA levels and CV mortality, with a pooled hazard ratio (HR) of 1.45 (95% CI: 1.33–1.58; $I^2 = 79\%$). The association was non-linear, with risk increasing more sharply at higher UA concentrations ($r = 0.0709$, $p = 0.001$) [16]. Epidemiological studies have consistently observed an association between elevated SUA levels and increased CV risk, probably mediated by hypertension, metabolic syndrome, and organ damage. A mediation analysis on 322 children and adolescents suggest that SUA, through the effects of insulin resistance and BP may cause structural remodeling of the macrovascular wall, which may further trigger arteriolar narrowing and increased large artery stiffness [17]. Accordingly, a longitudinal association between SUA and PWV has been described in a community-dwelling population of elderly expanding the literature investigating a potential independent contribution of SUA to the progressive stiffening of the arterial tree [18]. However, whether UA is a true causal factor or merely a marker reflecting the underlying pathophysiology remains unclear.

One major challenge lies in the close relationship between UA levels and kidney function. The reduction in glomerular filtration rate (GFR) naturally lead to higher UA concentrations, introducing potential confounding in studies, as both elevated UA and reduced kidney function are independently associated with CV risk. In fact, adjusting for GFR in statistical models often attenuates the observed associations between UA and CV outcomes, raising the question of whether CKD mediates or confounds this relationship.

Prospective studies offer some support for a causal role of UA in both CKD and CVD. Higher baseline UA levels predicted a decline in GFR in healthy individuals, suggesting a possible role for UA in CKD progression. On the other hand, higher UA levels were associated with increased all-cause and CV mortality, in both high and low-risk individuals, even after adjustment for proteinuria and GFR. Adding further complexity, CKD itself is a well-established risk factor for CVD, and CVD can also accelerate the progression of kidney dysfunction, creating a bidirectional relationship. This makes it challenging to isolate the independent contribution of UA within this network of interrelated risk factors.

Despite the limitations of existing data—including reliance on single time-point UA measurements and imprecise estimates of GFR—the hypothesis that UA contributes directly to both CKD and CVD remains biologically plausible. Experimental studies have shown that UA can induce endothelial dysfunction, oxidative stress, and inflammation, mechanisms that are central to both kidney and vascular injury. Significant renal injury occurs only in the presence of UA crystalluria, which leads to tubular obstruction, inflammation, and interstitial fibrosis. This process is followed by the development of UA crystal granulomas, predominantly composed of proinflammatory M1-like macrophages, which actively contribute to disease progression. Notably, targeting these macrophages with adenosine attenuated granulomatous inflammation and GFR decline, whereas JAK/STAT pathway inhibition had no protective effect. These results suggest that crystal-induced macrophage-mediated inflammation, rather than hyperuricemia itself, is the primary driver of UA-associated kidney injury [19].

Importantly, hyperuricemia-induced hypertension in CKD may exacerbate renal function decline, establishing a vicious cycle where increased intraglomerular pressure accelerates nephron loss. This highlights the dual importance of addressing hyperuricemia in CKD: as a modifiable contributor to both hypertension and disease progression. While randomized data are mixed, observational and mechanistic evidence provide a compelling rationale for further studies targeting urate metabolism in this high-risk group.

Ultimately, while elevated UA is associated with increased CV and renal risk, causality has not been definitively established. Large, randomized controlled trials are needed to determine whether pharmacological reduction of UA can alter the course of CKD or reduce CV events. Until then, clinicians must interpret the role of UA within the broader context of an individual's risk profile, recognizing both its potential pathogenic role and its strong correlation with underlying renal function.

Uric Acid-Lowering Therapy (ULT) in CKD: Current Evidence and Clinical Considerations

Xanthine oxidase inhibitors (XOIs) represent the primary class of UA-lowering agents and constitute the cornerstone of pharmacological management in patients with CKD. The mechanism of action of XOIs is catalyzing the final steps in the degradation of purines to UA; thus, its inhibition effectively reduces UA production from both endogenous and dietary purine sources. This mechanism underlies the role of XOIs as first-line therapies for the management of hyperuricemia, even in the CKD context. These agents have demonstrated efficacy in reducing serum urate concentrations; however, their influence on BP regulation, metabolic homeostasis, and systemic inflammation remains an area of ongoing investigation. Current clinical practice guidelines recommend ULT predominantly in the context of gout [20], whereas the application of XOIs for reno-CV protection or anti-inflammatory effects remains a subject of debate.

Nevertheless, the rationale for targeting inflammation in CKD is robust, as the disease is characterized by a persistent low-grade inflammatory milieu. Within this framework, UA may act as a proinflammatory mediator and oxidative stress amplifier, potentially via enhanced xanthine oxidase activity. The pervasive use of diuretics in CKD further complicates the therapeutic landscape: although not directly proinflammatory, these agents frequently elevate serum urate levels, thereby influencing clinical decision-making regarding ULT.

Emerging evidence supports a broader role for urate-lowering strategies beyond gout, particularly in patients with diabetes mellitus, metabolic syndrome, elevated CV risk, other than CKD. Among these populations, CKD poses the greatest complexity, due to the multifactorial interplay of inflammation, metabolic dysregulation, and impaired renal urate excretion. This heterogeneity necessitates a personalized approach to ULT. A detailed overview of pharmacological agents and their use in the CKD setting is provided in Table 2.

In addition to XOIs, sodium–glucose cotransporter 2 (SGLT2) inhibitors have been shown to modestly lower SUA, potentially providing mechanistically complementary effects to conventional ULT. SGLT2i are now recognized as a cornerstone in CKD treatment due to their ability to reduce renal and CV events. Regarding UA, SGLT2 inhibitors decrease SUA by approximately 0.8–1.0 mg/dL ($p < 0.001$) through enhanced urinary uric acid excretion. This uricosuric effect is closely linked to glycosuria and differs mechanistically from XOIs that reduce UA production [21].

In the EMPA-KIDNEY trial [22], empagliflozin reduced mean serum UA by approximately 25 μmol/L (≈0.4 mg/dL; ≈6% relative reduction) over a median follow-up of 2 years in a heterogeneous CKD population, with the largest effect observed in patients with higher baseline eGFR (>45 mL/min/1.73 m^2) and without diabetes. The effect was attenuated in participants with poor glycemic control (mean HbA1c ≈ 8.3%), suggesting an interaction between insulin-mediated urate transporter regulation and SGLT2 inhibition. In posthoc subgroup analyses, the adjusted mean UA difference was −74 μmol/L in non-diabetic participants versus −59 μmol/L in those with diabetes ($p < 0.001$ for heterogeneity).

Table 2 Uric acid-lowering drugs and their use in CKD

	Dosing	Dose adjustment in kidney disease	Adverse effects	Contra-indications and warnings
Allopurinol	Initiation: 100 mg daily if eGFR >60 mL/min Titration: every 2–4 weeks to the minimum dose required to achieve and maintain the goal range Max: 800–900 mg/day	1.5 mg per mL/min of eGFR i.e. 50 mg daily for eGFR of 30 mL/min/1.73 m^2	Rash, hypersensitivity, and severe cutaneous reactions (Generalized rash, blistering skin patches, fever, flu-like symptoms, angioedema, photophobia, mucositis, peripheral eosinophilia), SCARs, DRESS syndrome.	Azathioprine and 6-MP (potentiate the immunosuppressive and cytolytic effects) Alkylating agents (bone marrow suppression) Ampicillin (rush)
Febuxostat	Initiation: 40 mg Titration: every 2 weeks to the minimum dose required to achieve and maintain the goal range Max: 80 mg (America) 120 mg (Europe)	No dose adjustment in kidney failure	Liver function test abnormalities, nausea, arthralgia, and rash	Azathioprine, mercaptopurine, and theophylline (decreased medication metabolism, bone marrow toxicity)
Uricosuric drugs				
Probenecid	Initiation: 250 mg twice daily Titration: maintenance dose of 500–1000 mg two or three times daily Not effective if GFR ≤30 mL/min Contraindicated in dialysis	Titration: 50 mg/day increments to achieve the desired level of serum urate Max: 200 mg/day	Precipitation of a gout flare, gastrointestinal intolerance, rash, uric acid urolithiasis and urinary calcium excretion in patients with gout, reinforcing the contraindication for its use in patients with prior nephrolithiasis.	Interference with the transport of other organic anions (prolongation of the half-lives of penicillin and ampicillin)
Benzbromarone	Initiation: 50 mg/day Titration: 50 mg/day increments to achieve the desired level of serum urate Max: 200 mg/day	Not effective if GFR ≤30 mL/min/1.73 m^2 Contraindicated in dialysis	Precipitation of a gout flare, gastrointestinal intolerance, uric acid urolithiasis and severe hepatotoxicity	Hepatotoxicity

Sulfinpyrazone	Initiation: 50 mg twice daily Titration: several weeks to 100–200 mg three or four times daily Max: 800 mg/day	Not effective if GFR ≤30 mL/min/1.73 m^2 Contraindicated in dialysis	Precipitation of a gout flare, gastrointestinal intolerance, uric acid urolithiasis	
Lesinurad	200 mg to be added to a XOi	Use with cautious in patients with eGFR between 30 and 45 mL/min. Contraindicated with eGFR <30 mL/min/1.73 m^2	Increased serum Creatinine, uric acid urolithiasis especially when used without XOI, precipitation of a gout flare	Not available in USA and Europe
Recombinant forms of uricase				
Pegloticase	Administration intravenously every 2 weeks as 8 mg of the agent diluted into 250 mL	No dose adjustment needed	Hypersensitivity (stridor, oral/lingual/pharyngeal edema, wheezing, or hemodynamic instability)	Contraindication in patients with glucose-6-phosphate dehydrogenase (G6PD) deficiency.
Rasburicase	Initiation: IV 3–6 mg as a single dose or 0.15–0.2 mg/kg (range: 1–7 days) for prevention/treatment of tumor lysis syndrome	No dosage adjustment necessary for any degree of kidney dysfunction	Cardiovascular (peripheral edema), skin rash, hypervolemia, hypophosphatemia, Gastrointestinal, Hyperbilirubinemia, Headache, fever	Contraindication in patients with glucose-6-phosphate dehydrogenase (G6PD) deficiency, or history of hemolytic reaction or methemoglobinemia associated with rasburicase

(continued)

Table 2 (continued)

	Dosing	Dose adjustment in kidney disease	Adverse effects	Contra-indications and warnings
Other drugs				
Losartan	Initiation: 50 mg, titration to desired effect on BP (max daily dose: 1.4 mg/kg/day or 100 mg/day)	No dose adjustment needed	Hypotension, rare cough, rare angioedema,	Avoid in pregnancy
Atorvastatin	10–80 mg/day	No dose adjustment needed	Muscle-related (e.g., myalgia, myopathy, myositis, rhabdomyolysis); headache; gastrointestinal (e.g., nausea, constipation, dyspepsia, diarrhea); sleep disturbance; elevations in hepatocellular enzymes and alkaline phosphatase.	Statins are dependent on CYP metabolism and/or transmembrane transporters (e,g.,OATP, BCRP) for clearance, subjecting them to a significant number of clinically relevant drug interactions.
Fenofibrate	35–105 mg once daily (tablets) or 67 mg, 134 mg, 200 mg once daily (capsules)	GFR >30–80 mL/min: Use lowest available tablet strength. Controindicated in GFR <30 mL/min/1.73 m^2 and dialysis	Hepatic (increased serum alanine aminotransferase and/or serum aspartate aminotransferase). Rabdomiolysis	Active liver disease, including unexplained, persistent liver function abnormality. Significant drug interactions exist, requiring dose/frequency adjustment or avoidance.
Gliflozins	Canagliflozin 100–300 mg/day Dapagliflozin 5–10 mg/day Empagliflozin 10–25 mg/day Ertugliflozin 5 mg/day Sotagliflozin 200–400 mg/day Bexagliflozin 20 mg/day	Initiation not recommended if GFR <20 mL/min/1.73 m^2	Genitourinary fungal infection, increased hematocrit, ketoacidosis (including diabetic ketoacidosis, euglycemia ketoacidosis)	Several case reports indicate increased risk of euglycemic diabetic ketoacidosis (DKA) with SGLT2 inhibitors after bariatric surgery. To consider temporary discontinuation at least 3 days prior to any surgery.

This magnitude of UA reduction is substantially lower than that achieved with XOIs such as allopurinol or febuxostat (≈30%–50%) or with potent URAT1 inhibitors such as verinurad (≈40%–60%) [23]. Moreover, mediation analyses demonstrated that the renoprotective effect of empagliflozin—slowing eGFR decline and reducing the risk of kidney disease progression—was not explained by on-treatment UA levels. Similarly, the modest UA reduction did not translate into a statistically significant decrease in clinical gout incidence, likely due to both the small effect size and the relatively low event rate [24].

The proposed mechanisms for UA lowering include increased urinary urate excretion via competitive inhibition of proximal tubular GLUT9b transport by glucosuria, direct modulation of urate transporters (GLUT9, ABCG2), and possibly reduced hepatic UA synthesis through downregulation of the pentose phosphate pathway [25, 26]. Interestingly, the uricosuric effect was observed even in participants already on ULT at baseline, implying an additive and non-saturable mechanism. Additionally, SGLT2 inhibitors may reduce the need for the loop or thiazide diuretics—agents that impair renal urate clearance and promote hyperuricemia—thus indirectly mitigating iatrogenic UA elevation in CKD patients.

Given their modest but consistent effect on UA, SGLT2 inhibitors should not be considered substitutes for dedicated ULT in hyperuricemic CKD patients. However, they may provide incremental benefit, particularly in individuals with concomitant diuretic therapy, metabolic syndrome, or preserved kidney function, where UA reduction is more pronounced. More broadly, this urate-lowering property appears to be a class effect of SGLT2 inhibitors, documented across all major cardiovascular and renal outcome trials, across substantial heterogeneity in study populations (e.g. diabetes prevalence), baseline GFR, and albuminuria levels, as summarized in Table 3.

Effects of ULT on Blood Pressure

There is a strong mechanistic rationale for the use of ULT as an adjunctive approach in managing hypertension, particularly in high-risk populations such as those with CKD or CV comorbidities. However, despite this theoretical foundation, the clinical efficacy of ULT in reducing BP remains uncertain due to limited and heterogeneous evidence.

Experimental and translational data support a pathogenic link between hyperuricemia and hypertension, encompassing epidemiological associations, in in vitro findings, animal models, and human studies.

- Animal models: in a widely cited rat model by Mazzali et al. [36], mild hyperuricemia induced by oxonic acid led to the development of hypertension and early renal interstitial fibrosis, with a direct correlation between UA levels and BP. This effect was prevented by either XOIs or uricosuric agents. Prolonged hyperuricemia in the same model resulted in irreversible arteriolosclerosis, further supporting the causal role of UA in vascular remodeling.

Table 3 Spectrum of uric acid and blood pressure lowering effects in SGLT2 inhibitor trials with cardiovascular and kidney end point

	N	Mean baseline eGFR	Inclusion criteria (eGFR/albuminuria)	% with DM (duration)	% with HT (mean baseline SBP)	Difference in UA[a]	Difference in SBP[b] (from baseline)	Effects on gout events alone (where reported)
Carviovascular primary end point								
EMPA-REG OUTCOME [27] (Empagliflozin)	7020	74 ± 21	eGFR >30	100%	SBP 135 ± 17	22.0	−7.8 (stage 2) −4.3 (stage 3) −11.2 (stage 4)	Time to first gout event: HR 0.81 (95% CI 0.56–1.16); 77 vs 47 events; 1.6% vs 2.0% (pooled empagliflozin vs placebo)
CANVAS [28] (Canagliflozin)	10,142	77 ± 20	eGFR >30 UACR >30	100% (>10 years)	90% SBP 137 ± 16	23.3	−3.9	Time to first gout event: HR 0.64 (95% CI 0.41–0.99); total 80 events; 2.0% vs 2.6% (canagliflozin vs placebo) Recurrent gout events: HR 0.54 (95% CI 0.38–0.76); total 125 events; 2.8% vs 4.3%
DAPA-HF [29] (Dapagliflozin)	4744	66 ± 20	eGFR >30	45%	122 ± 16	50.0	–	–
EMPEROR-reduced [30] (Empagliflozin)	3730	62 ± 22	eGFR >30	50%	72% SBP 123 ± 16	66.6	−1.8	Time to first gout event: HR 0.70 (95% CI 0.45–1.08); 36 vs 49 events; 1.9% vs 2.6% (empagliflozin vs placebo)
VERTIS-CV [31] (Ertugliflozin)	8246	76 ± 21	eGFR >30	100% (13 years)	100% SBP 133 ± 14	22.0	−2.1	–
EMPEROR-preserved [32] (Empagliflozin)	5988	61 ± 20	eGFR >20	49%	91% SBP 132 ± 16	59.5	−1.8	–

DELIVER [33]	6263	61 ± 19	eGFR >25	45%	88% SBP 128 ± 15	–	–	–
Kidney primary end point								
CREDENCE [34]	2131	56 ± 18	eGFR 30–90 UACR 300–5000	100% (15 years)	97% SBP 140 ± 16	13.1	−2.4	–
DAPA-CKD [35]	4304	43 ± 12	eGFR 25–75 UACR 200–5000	68%	– SBP 137 ± 17	–	−2.9	–
EMPA-KIDNEY [22]	6609	37 ± 14	eGFR 20–44 + any UACR or eGFR 45–90 + UACR >200	46%	– SBP 136 ± 18	25.6	−2.6	Time to first gout event: HR 0.87 (95% CI 0.74–1.02); total 869 events; 8.4% vs 9.6% (canagliflozin vs placebo) Recurrent gout events: HR 0.86 (95% CI 0.72–1.03); total 404 events; 12.2% vs 14.1%

Abbreviations: *eGFR* estimated glomerular filtration rate, expressed in mL/min/1.73 m^2, *SBP* systolic blood pressure (mmHg), *UACR* urine albumin/creatinine ratio (mg/g), *HR* hazard ratio, *CI* confidence interval

[a]Difference in serum uric acid levels between group (treatment versus placebo), expressed in umol/L. Where reported in mg/dL, approximately converted to μmol/L by multiplying by 59.48

[b]Difference in systolic blood pressure in the treated group (end of study—baseline, in mmHg)

- In vitro studies: it has revealed that UA can impair nitric oxide bioavailability and activate prohypertensive pathways such as the renin–angiotensin system, reactive oxygen species, thromboxane, and cyclooxygenase [37]. These mechanisms drive early, reversible vasoconstriction, which may evolve into persistent vascular remodeling marked by fibrosis, inflammatory signaling, and salt-sensitive hypertension.
- Human studies: although the exact mechanism remains unclear, UA has been associated with endothelial dysfunction, oxidative stress, and renal microvascular damage. Insulin resistance and reduced pressure natriuresis have also been observed in hyperuricemic individuals, often preceding the onset of hypertension.
- Genetic studies: while initial Mendelian randomization analyses were inconclusive, more recent genome-wide association studies have linked polymorphisms involved in UA metabolism—particularly those regulating xanthine oxidoreductase activity—with elevated BP and increased CV risk.

Clinically, several studies support a modest BP-lowering effect of ULT (Table 4). A large retrospective analysis from the UK showed significant reductions in systolic and diastolic BP with allopurinol in elderly hypertensive patients [38]. Febuxostat, another XOI, demonstrated systolic BP reduction in a subgroup of patients with preserved renal function [39]. Meta-analyses have confirmed these effects, especially with agents that achieve greater XO inhibition [40]. However, not all findings are consistent. The SURPHER trial, despite improving endothelial function, failed to show BP reductions, possibly due to the inclusion of normotensive individuals and suboptimal study design [41].

Overall, while ULT shows potential as an antihypertensive strategy, more rigorously designed trials with clearly defined high-risk populations are needed to validate its role in BP management.

Of note, SGLT2 inhibitors appear to exert CV and renal benefits at least in part through lowering both blood pressure and SUA—two key factors in the pathogenesis of renal and CV damage. Mechanistically, SGLT2 inhibitors block sodium–glucose cotransport in the renal proximal tubule, promoting glucosuria, natriuresis, and osmotic diuresis. Additional mechanisms proposed include inhibition of sympathetic nervous system overactivity via central autonomic regulation, reduction in arterial stiffness, and RAAS modulation. The BP reduces intravascular volume, arterial stiffness, and restores tubule-glomerular feedback, thereby lowering BP. Meta-analyses indicate that in patients with type 2 diabetes, SGLT2 inhibitors reduce systolic BP by an average of 2.46 mmHg (95% CI: −2.86 to −2.06) and diastolic BP by 1.46 mmHg (95% CI: −1.82 to −1.09), primarily via osmotic diuresis and natriuresis, which decrease plasma volume [45]. Importantly, these BP-lowering effects are independent of baseline glucose levels and have been observed in non-diabetic, prehypertensive, and normotensive populations as well. Consistent reductions in BP have been reported across major cardiovascular and renal outcome trials, as summarized in Table 3.

Table 4 Clinical evidence of blood pressure-lowering effects of urate-lowering therapy (ULT)

Study	Number of patients	Inclusion criteria	Effect on BP
Soletsky and Feig 2012 [42]	$N = 56$	Adolescents (11–17 years) with prehypertension (BP ≥90th percentile or odds ratio ≥120/80 mmHg) and obesity	SBP −10.2 mmHg DBP −9.0 mm Hg ($p < 0.01$ ULT compared to placebo)
Feig et al. 2008 [43]	$N = 30$	Adolescents (11–17 years) who had newly diagnosed, never-treated stage 1 hypertension and sUA ≥6 mg/dL	SBP −6.9 mmHg DBP −5.1 mmHg 24-h ambulatory SBP −6.3 mmHg ($p < 0.001$ Allopurinol compared to placebo)
Kanbay et al. 2011 [44]	$N = 67$	Adults: 37 with asymptomatic HU and no history of gout 30 normouricemic controls	SBP −10.7 mmHg DBP −0.2 mmHg ($p = 0.005$ Allopurinol compared to placebo for SBP; NS Allopurinol compared to placebo for DBP)
Beattie et al. 2014 [38]	$N = 626$	Patients with hypertension aged ≥65 years	SBP −2.2 mmHg DBP +0.2 mmHg (Allopurinol use was independently associated with a fall in both SBP and DBP on regression analysis; $p < 0.001$)
Gunawardhana et al. 2017 [39]	$N = 121$	Adults (≥18 years) with documented and stable hypertension	SBP −6.6 mmHg DBP −3.3 mmHg ($p = 0.05$ Febuxostat compared to placebo for SBP; NS Febuxostat compared to placebo for DBP)
Gaffo et al. 2021 [41]	$N = 82$	Adults (18–40 years) with baseline SBP ≥120 and <160 mm Hg or DBP ≥80 and <100 mmHg, and UA ≥5.0 mg/dL (M) or ≥4.0 mg/dL (F)	SBP −1.4 mmHg DBP −0.9 mmHg (NS Allopurinol compared to placebo)
Agarwal et al. 2013 [40] (metanalysis)	$N = 738$ (10 longitudinal studies)	Patients with 15 years to 72 years with HU (>6 to >7.6 mg/dL)	SBP −3.3 mmHg DBP −1.3 mmHg ($p < 0.05$ Allopurinol compared to placebo/no treatment)

Abbreviations: *DBP* diastolic blood pressure, *HU* hyperuricemia, *SBP* systolic blood pressure, *ULT* urate-lowering treatment

Effects of ULT on Kidney Outcomes

There is a strong pathophysiological rationale for the use of ULT to slow CKD progression. In humans, experimental evidence indicates that UA may induce kidney injury through mechanisms beyond crystal deposition. In vivo models have shown that XO inhibitors such as allopurinol and febuxostat can attenuate tubulointerstitial fibrosis, further supporting the nephrotoxic potential of hyperuricemia.

Despite this rationale, clinical evidence from RCTs remains inconclusive. The PERL [46] and CKD-FIX [47] trials, which investigated allopurinol in patients with diabetic and non-diabetic CKD respectively, achieved significant and sustained UA reductions but failed to demonstrate a difference in eGFR decline compared to placebo. These results align with the FEATHER trial [48], which also showed no benefit of febuxostat on kidney outcomes in stage 3 CKD. A meta-analysis of over 3900 participants, incorporating these RCTs, confirmed the lack of effect of XO inhibitors on major renal and CV outcomes. However, it suggested a modest potential to slow GFR decline, primarily in lower-quality or short-duration studies. Notably, these trials suffered from limitations including heterogeneous baseline renal function, varying UA levels, underpowered sample sizes, and high treatment discontinuation rates.

Some findings, however, leave room for further investigation. In the FREED trial, febuxostat appeared to delay progression of albuminuria and renal dysfunction over 36 months, particularly in patients with early-stage disease. Similarly, in the PERL study, a favorable trend for allopurinol was observed in patients with normal baseline albuminuria, but not in those with overt proteinuria. These results imply that ULT may exert renoprotective effects in earlier CKD stages or in specific subpopulations.

Interestingly, post hoc analyses from CV trials have also suggested associations between UA reduction and improved renal outcomes. In the RENAAL study [49], for instance, each 0.5 mg/dL decrease in UA with losartan—a drug with uricosuric properties—was linked to a 6% lower risk of doubling serum creatinine or progression to kidney failure, although causality could not be confirmed. Similarly, SGLT2 inhibitors and sacubitril–valsartan have shown beneficial renal effects partly attributed to their ability to reduce SUA levels [50, 51]. These observations, while indirectly, raise the possibility that UA lowering might be beneficial under certain pathophysiological contexts or in combination with other therapeutic agents.

One more possible explanation for the failure of recent RCTs to demonstrate renal benefit from ULT is the marked heterogeneity in enrolled populations. Variability in baseline SUA levels, CKD stage, presence of proteinuria, and background therapies such as RAAS inhibitors likely influenced outcomes. For example, in CKD-FIX, patients had advanced CKD (mean eGFR ~30 mL/min/1.73 m^2) and high baseline SUA (~8.2 mg/dL), a setting where the established structural damage may be less responsive to ULT. In contrast, trials like FREED and subgroup analyses from PERL and FEATHER suggest potential benefit in early-stage CKD, normoalbuminuric patients, or those with better preserved renal function (Fig. 3). This

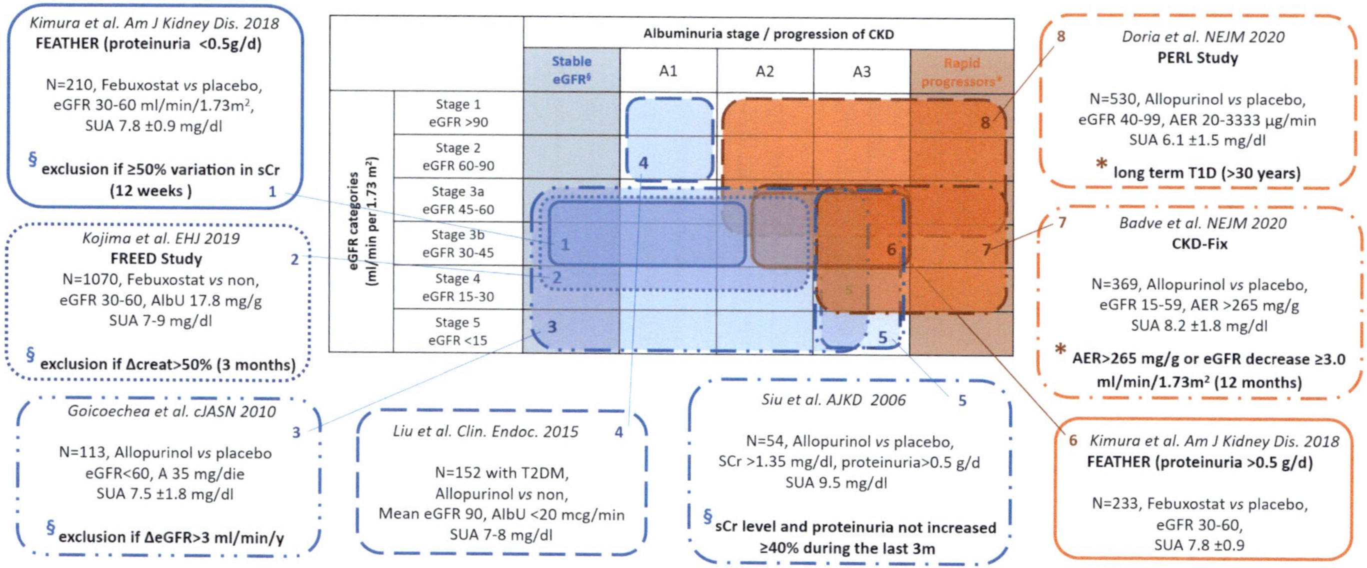

Fig. 3 Schematic presentation of clinical characteristics of randomized controlled trial (RCT) patients among chronic kidney disease (CKD) categories. Summary of all randomized controlled trials (≥12 months) evaluating urate-lowering therapy (ULT) versus placebo or no treatment, reporting renal outcomes such as GFR changes or kidney failure events. For each trial, baseline kidney function and albuminuria categories were classified according to NICE/KDIGO guidelines, along with the trajectory of kidney disease. Studies showing renal benefits from ULT are highlighted in blue, while those without a clear benefit are shown in maroon. (Adapted from Russo et al. [58])

highlights the importance of patient selection and timing, suggesting that ULT might be more effective before irreversible damage has occurred.

In summary, although various clinical guidelines support the assessment of serum urate levels for risk stratification [52], the extent to which UA contributes to organ damage may differ depending on both the severity and chronicity of the underlying condition. The role of UA in CKD progression seems to be more relevant in early disease stages, specific phenotypes, or as part of multifactorial intervention strategies.

Effects of ULT on CV Outcomes

There is a strong biological and epidemiological rationale supporting the use of ULT for CV risk reduction. SUA may exert CV effects through three interrelated but distinct mechanisms: (1) systemic inflammation from monosodium urate (MSU) crystal deposition, (2) soluble UA-mediated endothelial toxicity, and (3) XO-derived oxidative stress. Among these, XO activity may be the primary driver of CV risk, particularly in patients with high oxidative burden, making XO inhibitors a potentially useful tool in selected phenotypes. Mechanistic studies indicate that XO activity contributes to vascular oxidative stress, endothelial dysfunction, and myocardial ischemia, independent of urate levels. Small interventional trials have shown that high-dose allopurinol improves endothelial function, reduces BP, limits left ventricular hypertrophy, and enhances exercise tolerance in patients with ischemic heart disease. However, these findings have not been consistently reproduced, and several trials reported no benefit on CV parameters such as blood pressure, myocardial perfusion, or flow-mediated dilation.

The CARES trial, which compared febuxostat and allopurinol in >6000 patients with gout and established CV disease, showed no difference in composite CV outcomes. A post hoc analysis of CARES revealed that maintaining SUA <6 mg/dL was associated with improved kidney outcomes and potentially less CV deterioration, suggesting a benefit of tight urate control in high-risk subgroups [53].

The ALL-HEART trial [54], the largest prospective RCT of allopurinol in CV prevention, enrolled 5721 patients aged ≥60 with ischemic heart disease (but without gout). Over a mean follow-up of 4.8 years, allopurinol (up to 600 mg/day) failed to reduce the primary composite outcome of nonfatal MI, nonfatal stroke, or CV death compared to usual care (HR 1.04, 95% CI 0.89–1.21; $p = 0.65$), nor did it reduce all-cause mortality. These findings suggest that ULT may not confer CV protection in asymptomatic hyperuricemia or in patients without crystal deposition disease.

These findings contrast with the FAST trial [55], a European Medicines Agency-mandated non-inferiority study, which found febuxostat to be non-inferior to allopurinol for CV outcomes (adjusted HR 0.85; 95% CI 0.70–1.03) in over 6100 patients. Importantly, patients in FAST had less severe gout and fewer baseline CV comorbidities than in CARES, likely accounting for outcome discrepancies.

A recent meta-analysis of 28 RCTs involving 6458 patients reported no overall CV benefit from ULT on major adverse CV events (MACE; RR 0.93, 95% CI 0.74–1.18) or all-cause mortality (RR 1.04, 95% CI 0.78–1.39). However, ULT did significantly attenuate the decline in eGFR (+1.18 mL/min/1.73 m^2/year) and modestly reduced BP (systolic: −3.45 mmHg; diastolic: −2.02 mmHg). Similarly, a separate meta-analysis found that ULT significantly reduced MACE in patients with pre-existing CVD (OR 0.40, 95% CI 0.22–0.73), but not in unselected populations, emphasizing the importance of targeted therapy [56].

In conclusion, while each pathophysiological step is supported by strong scientific evidence and ULT—particularly XO inhibitors—shows promise in selected high-risk patients, the current evidence does not support widespread use for primary CV prevention. Similar SUA levels can reflect different phenotypes, distinguished by the predominant mechanisms linking UA metabolism to CVD. In particular, systemic inflammation related to UA deposits—whether clinically apparent or silent—likely accounts for only a small fraction of the CV burden associated with UA. The major underlying contributor appears to be CVD driven by both UA as a molecule and XO activity, which may represent the primary determinant of CV risk and the ideal target for preventive strategies using XO inhibitors. These pathophysiological mechanisms can overlap, but their relative importance varies among patient subgroups. While this phenotyping is less critical in patients with overt UA deposits and clear indications for ULT, assessing XO activity beforehand may help identify those at higher CV risk [57]. To advance CV prevention with XO inhibitors, precise patient characterization is essential. For this reason, future trials should adopt precision-medicine approaches, stratifying patients by SUA levels, XO activity, renal function, and inflammatory status to better define those most likely to benefit.

References

1. Virdis A, Masi S, Casiglia E, Tikhonoff V, Cicero AFG, Ungar A, et al. Identification of the uric acid thresholds predicting an increased total and cardiovascular mortality over 20 years. Hypertension. 2020;75(2):302–8. https://doi.org/10.1161/HYPERTENSIONAHA.
2. Zhu Y, Pandya BJ, Choi HK. Comorbidities of gout and hyperuricemia in the US general population: NHANES 2007–2008. Am J Med. 2012;125:679–687.e1. https://doi.org/10.1016/j.amjmed.2011.09.033.
3. Winitzki D, Zacharias HU, Nadal J, Baid-Agrawal S, Schaeffner E, Schmid M, et al. Educational attainment is associated with kidney and cardiovascular outcomes in the German CKD (GCKD) cohort. Kidney Int Rep. 2022;7(5):1004–15. https://doi.org/10.1016/j.ekir.2022.02.001.
4. Tan VS, Garg AX, McArthur E, Lam NN, Sood MM, Naylor KL. The 3-year incidence of gout in elderly patients with CKD. Clin J Am Soc Nephrol. 2017;12(4):577–84. https://doi.org/10.2215/CJN.06790616.
5. Sato Y, Feig DI, Stack AG, Kang DH, Johnson RJ, Khosla UM, et al. The case for uric acid-lowering treatment in patients with hyperuricaemia and CKD. Nat Rev Nephrol. 2019;15:767–75.
6. Nambu H, Takada S, Maekawa S, Matsumoto J, Kakutani N, Furihata T, et al. Inhibition of xanthine oxidase in the acute phase of myocardial infarction prevents skeletal muscle

abnormalities and exercise intolerance. Cardiovasc Res. 2021;117(3):805–19. https://doi.org/10.1093/cvr/cvaa127.
7. Verzola D, Ratto E, Villaggio B, Parodi EL, Pontremoli R, Garibotto G, et al. Uric acid promotes apoptosis in human proximal tubule cells by oxidative stress and the activation of NADPH oxidase NOX 4. PLoS One. 2014;9(12):e115210. https://doi.org/10.1371/journal.pone.0115210.
8. Perlstein TS, Gumieniak O, Williams GH, Sparrow D, Vokonas PS, Gaziano M, et al. Uric acid and the development of hypertension: the normative aging study. Hypertension. 2006;48:1031–6. https://doi.org/10.1161/01.HYP.0000248752.08807.4c.
9. Bombelli M, Ronchi I, Volpe M, Facchetti R, Carugo S, Dell'Oro R, et al. Prognostic value of serum uric acid: new-onset in and out-of-office hypertension and long-term mortality. J Hypertens. 2014;32(6):1237–44. https://doi.org/10.1097/HJH.0000000000000161.
10. Viazzi F, Antolini L, Giussani M, Brambilla P, Galbiati S, Mastriani S, et al. Serum uric acid and blood pressure in children at cardiovascular risk. Pediatrics. 2013;132(1):e93–9. https://doi.org/10.1542/peds.2013-0047.
11. Mazzali M, Hughes J, Kim YG, Jefferson JA, Kang DH, Gordon KL, et al. Elevated uric acid increases blood pressure in the rat by a novel crystal-independent mechanism. Hypertension. 2001;38(5):1101–6. https://doi.org/10.1161/hy1101.092839.
12. Perlstein TS, Gumieniak O, Hopkins PN, Murphey LJ, Brown NJ, Williams GH, et al. Uric acid and the state of the intrarenal renin-angiotensin system in humans. Kidney Int. 2004;66(4):1465–70. https://doi.org/10.1111/j.1523-1755.2004.00909.x.
13. Viazzi F, Leoncini G, Derchi LE, Pontremoli R. Ultrasound Doppler renal resistive index: a useful tool for the management of the hypertensive patient. J Hypertens. 2014;32(1):149–53. https://doi.org/10.1097/HJH.0b013e328365b29c.
14. Norvik JV, Storhaug HM, Ytrehus K, Jenssen TG, Zykova SN, Eriksen BO, et al. Overweight modifies the longitudinal association between uric acid and some components of the metabolic syndrome: the Tromsø Study. BMC Cardiovasc Disord. 2016;16:85. https://doi.org/10.1186/s12872-016-0265-8.
15. Shirasawa T, Ochiai H, Yoshimoto T, Nagahama S, Watanabe A, Yoshida A, et al. Cross-sectional study of associations between normal body weight with central obesity and hyperuricemia in Japan. BMC Endocr Disord. 2020;20(1):2. https://doi.org/10.1186/s12902-019-0481-1.
16. Rahimi-Sakak F, Maroofi M, Rahmani J, Kord-Varkaneh H, Alizadeh S, Clark CCT, et al. Serum uric acid and risk of cardiovascular mortality: a systematic review and dose-response meta-analysis of cohort studies of over a million participants. BMC Cardiovasc Disord. 2019;19(1):218. https://doi.org/10.1186/s12872-019-1215-z.
17. Genovesi S, Montelisciani L, Viazzi F, Giussani M, Lieti G, Patti I, et al. Uric acid and arterial stiffness in children and adolescents: role of insulin resistance and blood pressure. Front Cardiovasc Med. 2022;9:978366. https://doi.org/10.3389/fcvm.2022.978366.
18. Canepa M, Viazzi F, Strait JB, Ameri P, Pontremoli R, Brunelli C, et al. Longitudinal association between serum uric acid and arterial stiffness: results from the Baltimore Longitudinal Study of Aging. Hypertension. 2017;69(2):228–35. https://doi.org/10.1161/HYPERTENSIONAHA.116.08114.
19. Sellmayr M, Hernandez Petzsche MR, Ma Q, Krüger N, Liapis H, Brink A, et al. Only hyperuricemia with crystalluria, but not asymptomatic hyperuricemia, drives progression of chronic kidney disease. J Am Soc Nephrol. 2020;31(12):2773–92. https://doi.org/10.1681/ASN.2020040523.
20. Li Q, Li X, Wang J, Liu H, Kwong JS, Chen H, et al. Diagnosis and treatment for hyperuricemia and gout: a systematic review of clinical practice guidelines and consensus statements. BMJ Open. 2019;9:e026677. https://doi.org/10.1136/bmjopen-2018-026677.
21. Auberson M, Stadelmann S, Stoudmann C, Seuwen K, Koesters R, Thorens B, et al. SLC2A9 (GLUT9) mediates urate reabsorption in the mouse kidney. Pflugers Arch. 2018;470(12):1739–51. https://doi.org/10.1007/s00424-018-2190-4.

22. Herrington WG, Staplin N, Wanner C, Green JB, Hauske SJ, Emberson JR, EMPA-KIDNEY Collaborative Group, et al. Empagliflozin in patients with chronic kidney disease. N Engl J Med. 2023;388(2):117–27. https://doi.org/10.1056/NEJMoa2204233.
23. Heerspink HJL, Stack AG, Terkeltaub R, Stefánsson BV, Chertow GM, Correa-Rotter R, et al. Combination treatment with verinurad and allopurinol in CKD: a randomized placebo and active controlled trial. J Am Soc Nephrol. 2024;35:594–606. https://doi.org/10.1681/ASN.0000000000000326.
24. Mayne KJ, Sardell RJ, Staplin N, Judge PK, Zhu D, Sammons E, EMPA-KIDNEY Collaborative Group, et al. Empagliflozin lowers serum uric acid in chronic kidney disease: exploratory analyses from the EMPA-KIDNEY trial. Nephrol Dial Transplant. 2025;40(4):720–30. https://doi.org/10.1093/ndt/gfae203.
25. Lu YH, Chang YP, Li T, Wang Y, Zhao Z, Liu Y, et al. Empagliflozin attenuates hyperuricemia by upregulation of ABCG2 via AMPK/AKT/CREB signaling pathway in type 2 diabetic mice. Int J Biol Sci. 2020;16:529–42. https://doi.org/10.7150/ijbs.33007.
26. Toyoki D, Shibata S, Kuribayashi-Okuma E, Ishizawa K, Xu N, Ishizawa K, et al. Insulin stimulates uric acid reabsorption via regulating urate transporter 1 and ATP-binding cassette subfamily G member 2. Am J Physiol Renal Physiol. 2017;313:F826–34. https://doi.org/10.1152/ajprenal.00012.2017.
27. Zinman B, Wanner C, Lachin JM, Fitchett D, Bluhmki E, Hantel S, EMPA-REG OUTCOME Investigators, et al. Empagliflozin, cardiovascular outcomes, and mortality in type 2 diabetes. N Engl J Med. 2015;373(22):2117–28. https://doi.org/10.1056/NEJMoa1504720.
28. Neal B, Perkovic V, Mahaffey KW, de Zeeuw D, Fulcher G, Erondu N, CANVAS Program Collaborative Group, et al. Canagliflozin and cardiovascular and renal events in type 2 diabetes. N Engl J Med. 2017;377(7):644–57. https://doi.org/10.1056/NEJMoa1611925.
29. McMurray JJV, Solomon SD, Inzucchi SE, Køber L, Kosiborod MN, Martinez FA, DAPA-HF Trial Committees and Investigators, et al. Dapagliflozin in patients with heart failure and reduced ejection fraction. N Engl J Med. 2019;381(21):1995–2008. https://doi.org/10.1056/NEJMoa1911303.
30. Packer M, Anker SD, Butler J, Filippatos G, Pocock SJ, Carson P, EMPEROR-Reduced Trial Investigators, et al. Cardiovascular and renal outcomes with empagliflozin in heart failure. N Engl J Med. 2020;383(15):1413–24. https://doi.org/10.1056/NEJMoa2022190.
31. Cannon CP, Pratley R, Dagogo-Jack S, Mancuso J, Huyck S, Masiukiewicz U, VERTIS CV Investigators, et al. Cardiovascular outcomes with ertugliflozin in type 2 diabetes. N Engl J Med. 2020;383(15):1425–35. https://doi.org/10.1056/NEJMoa2004967.
32. Anker SD, Butler J, Filippatos G, Ferreira JP, Bocchi E, Böhm M, EMPEROR-Preserved Trial Investigators, et al. Empagliflozin in heart failure with a preserved ejection fraction. N Engl J Med. 2021;385(16):1451–61. https://doi.org/10.1056/NEJMoa2107038.
33. Solomon SD, McMurray JJV, Claggett B, de Boer RA, DeMets D, Hernandez AF, DELIVER Trial Committees and Investigators, et al. Dapagliflozin in heart failure with mildly reduced or preserved ejection fraction. N Engl J Med. 2022;387(12):1089–98. https://doi.org/10.1056/NEJMoa2206286.
34. Perkovic V, Jardine MJ, Neal B, Bompoint S, Heerspink HJL, Charytan DM, CREDENCE Trial Investigators, et al. Canagliflozin and renal outcomes in type 2 diabetes and nephropathy. N Engl J Med. 2019;380(24):2295–306. https://doi.org/10.1056/NEJMoa1811744.
35. Heerspink HJL, Stefánsson BV, Correa-Rotter R, Chertow GM, Greene T, Hou FF, DAPA-CKD Trial Committees and Investigators, et al. Dapagliflozin in patients with chronic kidney disease. N Engl J Med. 2020;383(15):1436–46. https://doi.org/10.1056/NEJMoa2024816.
36. Mazzali M, Kanellis J, Han L, Feng L, Xia YY, Chen Q, et al. Hyperuricemia induces a primary renal arteriolopathy in rats by a blood pressure-independent mechanism. Am J Physiol Renal Physiol. 2002;282:F991–7. https://doi.org/10.1152/ajprenal.00283.2001.
37. Joosten LAB, Crişan TO, Bjornstad P, Johnson RJ. Asymptomatic hyperuricaemia: a silent activator of the innate immune system. Nat Rev Rheumatol. 2020;16:75–86. https://doi.org/10.1038/s41584-019-0334-3.

38. Beattie CJ, Fulton RL, Higgins P, Padmanabhan S, McCallum L, Walters MR, et al. Allopurinol initiation and change in blood pressure in older adults with hypertension. Hypertension. 2014;64:1102–7. https://doi.org/10.1161/HYPERTENSIONAHA.114.03518.
39. Gunawardhana L, McLean L, Punzi HA, Hunt B, Palmer RN, Whelton A, et al. Effect of febuxostat on ambulatory blood pressure in subjects with hyperuricemia and hypertension: a phase 2 randomized placebo-controlled study. J Am Heart Assoc. 2017;6(11):e006683. https://doi.org/10.1161/JAHA.117.006683.
40. Agarwal V, Hans N, Messerli FH. Effect of allopurinol on blood pressure: a systematic review and meta-analysis. J Clin Hypertens (Greenwich). 2013;15(6):435–42. https://doi.org/10.1111/jch.12095.
41. Gaffo AL, Calhoun DA, Rahn EJ, Oparil S, Li P, Dudenbostel T, et al. Effect of serum urate lowering with allopurinol on blood pressure in young adults: a randomized, controlled, crossover trial. Arthritis Rheumatol. 2021;73(8):1514–22. https://doi.org/10.1002/art.41749.
42. Soletsky B, Feig DI. Uric acid reduction rectifies prehypertension in obese adolescents. Hypertension. 2012;60:1148–56.
43. Feig DI, Soletsky B, Johnson RJ. Effect of allopurinol on blood pressure of adolescents with newly diagnosed essential hypertension: a randomized trial. JAMA. 2008;300(8):924–32. https://doi.org/10.1001/jama.300.8.924.
44. Kanbay M, Huddam B, Azak A, Solak Y, Kadioglu GK, Kirbas I, Duranay M, Covic A, Johnson RJ. A randomized study of allopurinol on endothelial function and estimated glomular filtration rate in asymptomatic hyperuricemic subjects with normal renal function. Clin J Am Soc Nephrol. 2011;6(8):1887–94. https://doi.org/10.2215/CJN.11451210.
45. Mazidi M, Rezaie P, Gao HK, Kengne AP. Effect of sodium-glucose cotransport-2 inhibitors on blood pressure in people with type 2 diabetes mellitus: a systematic review and meta-analysis of 43 randomized control trials with 22 528 patients. J Am Heart Assoc. 2017;6(6):e004007. https://doi.org/10.1161/JAHA.116.004007.
46. Doria A, Galecki AT, Spino C, Pop-Busui R, Cherney DZ, Lingvay I, PERL Study Group, et al. Serum urate lowering with allopurinol and kidney function in type 1 diabetes. N Engl J Med. 2020;382(26):2493–503. https://doi.org/10.1056/NEJMoa1916624.
47. Badve SV, Pascoe EM, Tiku A, Boudville N, Brown FG, Cass A, CKD-FIX Study Investigators, et al. Effects of allopurinol on the progression of chronic kidney disease. N Engl J Med. 2020;382(26):2504–13. https://doi.org/10.1056/NEJMoa1915833.
48. Kimura K, Hosoya T, Uchida S, Inaba M, Makino H, Maruyama S, FEATHER Study Investigators, et al. Febuxostat therapy for patients with stage 3 CKD and asymptomatic hyperuricemia: a randomized trial. Am J Kidney Dis. 2018;72(6):798–810. https://doi.org/10.1053/j.ajkd.2018.06.028.
49. Brenner BM, Cooper ME, de Zeeuw D, Keane WF, Mitch WE, Parving HH, RENAAL Study Investigators, et al. Effects of losartan on renal and cardiovascular outcomes in patients with type 2 diabetes and nephropathy. N Engl J Med. 2001;345(12):861–9. https://doi.org/10.1056/NEJMoa011161.
50. Yang S, Hu Q, Liu K, Xiao B, Zhang B, Su N. Serum uric acid reduction through SGLT2 inhibitors: evidence from a systematic review and meta-analysis. Front Pharmacol. 2025;16:1551390. https://doi.org/10.3389/fphar.2025.1551390.
51. Kashiwagi Y, Nagoshi T, Kimura H, Tanaka Y, Oi Y, Inoue Y, et al. Effects of angiotensin receptor-neprilysin inhibitor on insulin resistance in patients with heart failure. ESC Heart Fail. 2023;10(3):1860–70. https://doi.org/10.1002/ehf2.14352.
52. Williams B, Mancia G, Spiering W, Rosei EA, Azizi M, Burnier M, et al. ESC/ESH guidelines for the management of arterial hypertension. Eur Heart J. 2018;39(33):3021–104. https://doi.org/10.1093/eurheartj/ehy339.
53. White WB, Saag KG, Becker MA, Borer JS, Gorelick PB, Whelton A, CARES Investigators, et al. Cardiovascular safety of febuxostat or allopurinol in patients with gout. N Engl J Med. 2018;378(13):1200–10. https://doi.org/10.1056/NEJMoa1710895.
54. Mackenzie IS, Hawkey CJ, Ford I, Greenlaw N, Pigazzani F, Rogers A, ALL-HEART Study Group, et al. Allopurinol versus usual care in UK patients with ischaemic heart disease

(ALL-HEART): a multicentre, prospective, randomised, open-label, blinded-endpoint trial. Lancet. 2022;400(10349):1195–205. https://doi.org/10.1016/S0140-6736(22)01503-0.
55. Mackenzie I, Ford I, Nuki G, Hallas J, Hawkey C, Walters M, et al. Long-term cardiovascular safety of febuxostat compared with allopurinol in patients with gout (FAST): a multicentre, prospective, randomised, open-label, non-inferiority trial. Lancet. 2020;396(10264):1745–57. https://doi.org/10.1016/S0140-6736(20)32234-0.
56. Chen Q, Wang Z, Zhou J, Chen Z, Li Y, Li S, et al. Effect of urate-lowering therapy on cardiovascular and kidney outcomes: a systematic review and meta-analysis. Clin J Am Soc Nephrol. 2020;15(11):1576–86. https://doi.org/10.2215/CJN.05190420.
57. Desideri G, Borghi C. Xanthine oxidase inhibition and cardiovascular protection: don't shoot in the dark. Eur J Intern Med. 2023;113:10–2. https://doi.org/10.1016/j.ejim.2023.04.006.
58. Russo E, Verzola D, Leoncini G, Cappadona F, Esposito P, Pontremoli R, Viazzi F. Treating Hyperuricemia: The Last Word Hasn't Been Said Yet. J Clin Med. 2021;10(4):819. https://doi.org/10.3390/jcm10040819.

The Heart in the Hypertensive Patient with Chronic Kidney Disease

Claudia Agabiti-Rosei, Carolina De Ciuceis, Giacomo Buso, Matteo Lemoli, and Maria Lorenza Muiesan

Abbreviations

ACEI	Angiotensin converting enzyme inhibitor
ARB	Angiotensin receptor blocker
ARNI	Angiotensin receptor neprilysin inhibitor
BP	Blood pressure
CAD	Coronary artery disease
CCB	Calcium channel blockers
CD	Cardiovascular disease
CKD	Chronic kidney disease
DM	Diabetes mellitus
eGFR	Estimated Glomerular filtration rate
HF	Heart failure
HFpEF	Heart failure with preserved ejection fraction
HFrEF	Heart failure with reduced ejection fraction
LVH	Left ventricular hypertrophy
MRA	Mineralcorticoid receptor antagonist
RAAS	Renin-angiotensin-aldosterone system
RCT	Randomized clinical trial
ROS	Reactive oxygen species
SGLT2	Sodium/glucose cotransporter 2
SNS	Sympathetic nervous system

C. Agabiti-Rosei · C. De Ciuceis · G. Buso · M. Lemoli · M. L. Muiesan (✉)
Department of Clinical and Experimental Sciences, University of Brescia, Brescia, Italy
e-mail: claudia.agabitirosei@unibs.it; carolina.deciuceis@unibs.it; giacomo.buso@unibs.it; m.lemoli@unibs.it; marialorenza.muiesan@unibs.it

P. Sarafidis, R. Pontremoli (eds.), *Hypertension and Chronic Kidney Disease*,
Updates in Hypertension and Cardiovascular Protection,
https://doi.org/10.1007/978-3-032-29564-4_7

Introduction

Chronic Kidney Disease (CKD) represents a growing global health burden, affecting approximately 10–20% of the adult population [1]. While its progressive impact on renal function is well recognized, an often underestimated consequence of CKD is its effect on cardiovascular health. Cardiovascular disease (CVD) and chronic heart failure (HF) remain the leading cause of morbidity and mortality in patients with CKD, across all stages of renal impairment [2].

The interplay between the heart and the kidneys is complex and bidirectional, giving rise to what is known as the cardiorenal syndrome. In CKD, a cascade of pathophysiological changes creates an environment that fosters structural and functional cardiac abnormalities.

Recently the relationship between heart health and CKD was addressed by Marx-Schütt K et al. [3] These authors highlight the elevated risk that CKD patients face in developing various forms of CVD, including coronary artery disease, HF, arrhythmias, sudden cardiac death, and stroke. Therefore, early detection and management of cardiovascular risk factors in CKD patients is mandatory to improve outcomes [3]. Finally, understanding the cardiovascular implications of CKD is essential to enhance management and treatment of these patients' categories.

The aim of this chapter is to describe the mechanisms by which CKD influences cardiac damage, to outline the major cardiovascular manifestations in this population of patients, and review current and emerging strategies for diagnosis and management.

Pathophysiology of the Heart–Kidney Interaction

The relationship between CKD and CVD is rooted in a shared and complex pathophysiological network. In patients with CKD, the deterioration of renal function triggers a cascade of systemic alterations that significantly compromise cardiac structure and performance. The progression of CVD in CKD is a complex and multifactorial process. It is driven not only by conventional risk factors such as hypertension, diabetes, and dyslipidemia, but also by CKD-specific contributors including persistent inflammation, oxidative stress, activation of the renin-angiotensin-aldosterone system (RAAS), fluid overload, hemodynamic disturbances, mineral and bone disorders, the buildup of uremic toxins, and CKD-related post-translational protein modifications [4].

Inflammation and oxidative stress are a key contributor to the progression CKD. As the kidney function deteriorates, levels of proinflammatory mediators rise, exerting direct effects on the vasculature by promoting endothelial dysfunction and attracting inflammatory cells to the vessel wall [5]. In patients with CKD, the progressive decline in renal function leads to elevated levels of proinflammatory cytokines and reactive oxygen species (ROS), contributing to endothelial dysfunction, myocardial remodeling, and vascular calcification [6]. These processes not only accelerate cardiovascular disease but also worsen renal injury through systemic effects. The pivotal role of inflammation is further highlighted by findings from the CANTOS trial, which showed that targeting interleukin-1β (IL-1β) with canakinumab significantly reduced cardiovascular risk, especially in patients with reduced estimated glomerular filtration rate (eGFR) [7]. Inflammation is increasingly acknowledged as a key mechanism contributing to the development of heart failure with preserved ejection fraction (HFpEF) [8].

Renin-Angiotensin-Aldosterone System (RAAS) and the Sympathetic Nervous System (SNS)

CKD significantly increases the risk of CVD through persistent activation of two key neurohormonal pathways: the renin-angiotensin-aldosterone system (RAAS) and the sympathetic nervous system (SNS). These neurohormonal pathways contribute significantly to disease progression in both organs.

In patients with CKD, impaired renal perfusion and sodium retention lead to persistent RAAS stimulation. This results in elevated levels of angiotensin II and aldosterone, promoting vasoconstriction, sodium and fluid retention, inflammation, and fibrosis, all of which contribute to hypertension, vascular remodeling, and adverse cardiac outcomes [9, 10]. Angiotensin II also promotes oxidative stress and endothelial dysfunction, enhancing cardiovascular risk and accelerating atherosclerosis and left ventricular hypertrophy (LVH) even in the early stages of CKD [11].

Independent of RAAS, CKD leads to sustained sympathetic overactivity, driven by increased afferent signaling from ischemic or damaged kidneys. This results in heightened norepinephrine release, which causes tachycardia, arterial vasoconstriction, and increased myocardial oxygen demand, all key contributors to CVD risk [12]. Chronic SNS activation is also implicated in arrhythmogenesis and worsened diastolic function contributing to the development of heart failure with preserved ejection fraction (HFpEF).

Moreover, RAAS and SNS systems are mutually reinforcing. Angiotensin II enhances sympathetic tone, while norepinephrine upregulates renin release. This synergy contributes to CKD's typical cardiac organ damage, including LVH and pathological fibrosis, arterial stiffness, with exacerbation of hypertension, volume overload, and structural cardiac injury, accelerating the progression of both CKD and CVD [9, 10, 13].

Anemia and Erythropoietin Deficiency in CKD-Related CVD

Anemia is a common and clinically significant complication of CKD and plays a key role in the development and progression of CVD. The primary cause of anemia in CKD is a deficiency of erythropoietin (EPO), caused by damaged peritubular fibroblasts in the kidney. This deficiency leads to reduced erythropoiesis and chronic hypoxia, which drive LVH, impaired myocardial contractility, HF, and heightened cardiovascular morbidity and mortality [14, 15]. Moreover, anemia exacerbates tissue ischemia and promotes oxidative stress and inflammation, which are central mechanisms in atherosclerosis and myocardial dysfunction [15]. The correction of anemia using erythropoiesis-stimulating agents (ESAs) has been shown to improve the quality of life and reduce transfusion requirements, although it has been observed that targeting higher hemoglobin levels may increase cardiovascular risk in some patients [16]. Emerging therapies such as hypoxia-inducible factor–prolyl hydroxylase inhibitors (HIF-PHIs) offer a promising alternative by enhancing endogenous EPO production and improving iron utilization, with potentially fewer adverse cardiovascular effects [17]. Beyond anemia, iron dysregulation and chronic inflammation, which are common in CKD, exacerbate these outcomes and contribute independently to atherosclerosis and HF.

Observational studies and clinical trials have demonstrated that transferrin saturation (TSAT) <20% is linked to increased cardiovascular mortality and hospitalization for HF, even in the absence of overt anemia [18]. Treatment with iron—especially via the intravenous (IV) route—has shown both hematologic and cardiovascular benefits. A recent meta-analysis analyzing data from 45 randomized controlled trials (RCTs) in adults with CKD to evaluate the effects of iron therapy (oral or intravenous) on cardiovascular, renal, and safety outcomes found that iron supplementation was associated with a 16% reduction in the composite risk of cardiovascular death or HF hospitalization in patients receiving iron therapy compared to placebo, particularly in non-dialysis CKD patients. Iron also reduced the need for erythropoiesis-stimulating agents (ESAs). No major safety concerns were identified [19].

According to the KDIGO guidelines, regular monitoring of ferritin and TSAT is recommended [20]. IV iron (e.g., ferric carboxymaltose, iron sucrose) is preferred in patients with poor oral absorption, those receiving erythropoiesis-stimulating agents (ESAs), or when rapid correction is needed. Moreover, restoring iron stores improves the erythropoietic response to ESAs, allowing for lower dosing and potentially reducing ESA-related cardiovascular risks [16].

Cardiovascular Manifestations in Chronic Kidney Disease

The onset of CVD in CKD involves a complex and multifactorial combination of traditional risk factors as well as CKD-related mechanisms described above, and CKD-related post-translational modifications. These processes collectively induce characteristic structural and functional alterations in both the vasculature and the myocardium (Fig. 1).

The most common and clinically relevant cardiovascular complications include LVH, HF (especially HFpEF), accelerated atherosclerosis, vascular calcification, arrhythmias, and sudden cardiac death.

LVH is present in roughly one-third of patients with CKD, its prevalence increasing to 70–80% in those with end-stage kidney disease [21]. In the LIFE study, hypertensive patients with higher degree of albuminuria, despite no difference in serum creatinine, had higher LV mass and concentric geometry, suggesting a higher risk of CV events [22]. LVH is usually recognized as an independent predictor of

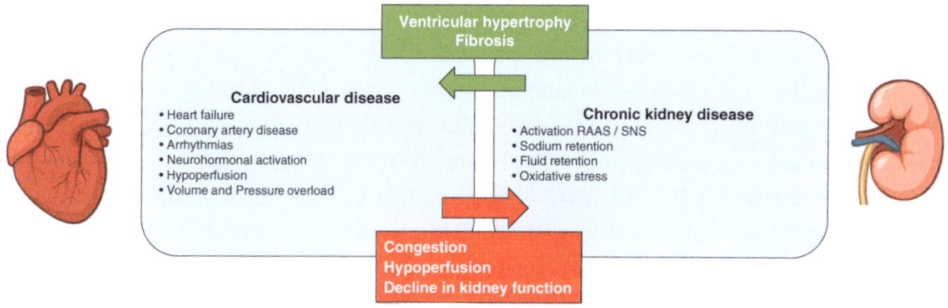

Fig. 1 Schematic interaction of cardiovascular disease and chronic kidney disease

mortality across all CKD stages. However, studies in the end-stage kidney disease population [23] and in patients with eGFR <45 mL/min/1.73 [24] have shown that left ventricular mass index (LVMI) conveys limited prognostic information.

Changes in LVH and in eGFR during treatment may imply a different prognostic influence in hypertensive patients; in a large group of hypertensive patients followed for more than 10 years a worse outcome was observed in those with persistence or development of LVH and CKD, as compared with those with absence or regression of both LVH and CKD and those with absence/regression of either LVH or CKD [25]. A CKD population of 3207 patients were followed for a median period of 9.9 years [26]. Renal replacement therapy (RRT) occurred in 883 patients and higher LVMI, left ventricular (LV) volume, left atrial (LA) area, peak tricuspid velocity, and lower EF were each statistically significantly associated with an increased risk of RRT and eGFR decrease [26]. The development and persistence of LVH is driven by afterload-related contributors, such as arterial stiffness and increased systemic vascular resistance, usually associated with the concentric LVH phenotype, while preload-related factors, particularly volume overload due to sodium and fluid retention and pressure overload (e.g., hypertension), promote eccentric ventricular remodeling [27].

Moody et al. [28] were able to demonstrate in living kidney donors, compared with healthy controls, that change in GFR after mono-lateral nephrectomy was independently associated with change in LV mass ($R^2 = 0.28$; $P = 0.01$), despite no changes in 24 h ambulatory blood pressure. The findings suggest that reduced GFR should be regarded as an independent causative cardiovascular risk factor; the role of other substances such as uric acid, parathyroid hormone, fibroblast growth factor-23, and hsC-reactive protein could have also contributed to changes in LV mass.

In a recent metanalysis [29], including 42 trials with duration ≥12 months (6 trials of erythropoietin stimulating agents, 10 trials with RAAS inhibitor vs. placebo or other BP lowering agents, 14 trials of modified hemodialysis regimens and 12 trials of other types of interventions) LV mass regression was associated with a statistically significant reduction of mortality risk (RR 0.71, 95% CI 0.57–0.92, $p = 0.005$) in patients with CKD; CV mortality reduction was similar to all-cause mortality, but did not reach statistical significance (RR 0.67, 95% CI 0.39–1.16).

Heart failure (HF) and CKD frequently coexist, amplifying morbidity and mortality. The presence of CKD in HF patients is associated with worse outcomes, including higher hospitalization and mortality rates [30]. Among CKD patients, both HFpEF and HFrEF are highly prevalent, but HFpEF appears to be more dominant, particularly in elderly individuals and those with diabetes or hypertension. Studies such as the CRIC and ASIAN-HF suggest that LVH, diastolic dysfunction, and increased ventricular stiffness, a common finding in patients with CKD, contribute to the reported higher incidence of HfpEF [31]. In contrast, HFrEF is more often associated with ischemic heart disease and overt volume overload. Recent therapeutic advances, particularly SGLT2 inhibitors (e.g., dapagliflozin, empagliflozin), have shown robust benefits in HFpEF and HFrEF populations, including those with moderate CKD (eGFR >20 mL/min/1.73 m^2) [32, 33]. Sacubitril/valsartan has shown a clear mortality benefit in HFrEF, but only modest symptomatic improvement in HFpEF [34]. Additionally, finerenone, a non-steroidal mineralocorticoid receptor antagonist, has shown promise in reducing cardiorenal events in patients with CKD and type 2 diabetes [35]. Despite these advancements, therapeutic inertia persists due to concerns over hyperkalemia and renal deterioration, especially in advanced CKD.

Cardiac valve calcification is significantly influenced by age, CRP, diabetes, coronary artery disease, and dialysis duration. In addition, the presence of cardiac valves (aortic and mitral) has been related to all cause and CV mortality, as shown by a recent metanalysis [36]. Calcific aortic stenosis is the most prevalent valvular alteration in patients with CKD and those on dialysis.

Vascular calcification is particularly prevalent and severe in CKD, due to disordered mineral metabolism (calcium-phosphate imbalance and elevated FGF23), and contributes to arterial stiffness, isolated systolic hypertension, and myocardial ischemia [4].

Atherosclerotic cardiovascular disease is often atypical in CKD patients. It occurs even in those without traditional risk factors, likely due to chronic inflammation and oxidative stress [37] and has an accelerated progression. In a large group of patients with moderate CKD. Huang et al. [38] demonstrated that CKD patients have more calcified plaques in the coronary arteries and further progression in calcified components of plaques over time, compared to individuals without CKD. In addition, in the same study, the decline in renal function was independently associated with plaque progression, with higher crude (54.1 ± 3.2 vs. 80.2 ± 9.0 mm^3/year, $P < 0.01$) or annualized (16.4 ± 0.9 vs. 23.9 ± 2.6 mm^3/year, $P < 0.01$) increase in total plaque volume.

Patients with CKD exhibit lower coronary flow reserve (CFR) than non-CKD patients, mainly because of increased resting coronary flow velocity [39] as observed in the Prognostic Impact of Cardiac Diastolic Function and Coronary Microvascular Function registry. Patients with CKD and those with reduced CFR, independently, showed higher prevalence of left ventricular wall thickness, left atrial volume index, increased E/e', and increased RV systolic pressure. The reduction of CFR in patients with CKD could result from diminished myocardial perfusion due to microvascular rarefaction distal to the level of smaller arterioles and endothelial dysfunction, but also to LV hypertrophy and LV diastolic dysfunction, known to induce compensatory vasodilation of arterioles, increased resting coronary flow, and depressed coronary circulatory reserve. Additionally, autonomic dysfunction and myocardial fibrosis increase the risk of atrial fibrillation and sudden cardiac death, which is a leading cause of mortality in advanced CKD and dialysis populations.

When the prognostic value of CKD or depressed CFR were assessed, each was independently associated with the increased risk of cardiac death or hospitalization for HF [39].

Diagnostic Tools for Cardiovascular Disease in CKD

Early and accurate identification of cardiovascular abnormalities in patients with CKD is crucial, given the high burden and often silent progression of the disease. Diagnosing CVD in patients with CKD is challenging due to overlapping symptoms, nontraditional risk factors, and the frequent presence of subclinical pathology. The main diagnostic tools for identifying cardiac organ damage in patients with CKD are summarized in Table 1.

In LVH, cardiac ischemia and HF, biomarkers are closely linked to neurohormonal activation, ventricular dysfunction, cardiac remodeling, and myocardial

Table 1 Diagnostic tools for identify cardiovascular damage in patients with CKD

Diagnostic Tool	Purpose	Key Findings
Electrocardiography (ECG)	LVH diagnosis	Low sensitivity in CKD
	Basic test for ischemia	LVH strain pattern confounding in acute ischemia, useful when compared to previous ECGs
	Diagnosis of arrhythmias	–
Troponins (T/I)	Biomarkers for myocardial injury	Troponin I-hs more reliable in CKD; serial measurements preferred, due to baseline elevation in CKD
NT-pro BNP	Diagnosis of HFpEF	Often elevated in CKD; if elevated worse prognostic value in CKD vs no CKD
Echocardiography (Echo)	Assessesment of LV mass index, LVH and LV geometry	Useful but limited prognostic value in more advanced CKD
	Assessment of systolic/diastolic function	Mandatory for HF subtypes speckle tracking for global longitudinal strain (GLS)
	Assessment of cardiac valves calcification	–
Cardiac MRI (CMR)	Precise assessment of LV mass index and LVH, function and fibrosis	High diagnostic accuracy; limited by cost; newer contrast-free methods under development

(continued)

Table 1 (continued)

Diagnostic Tool	Purpose	Key Findings
Stress Testing (ECG, Echo, SPECT, PET)	Detect myocardial ischemia	Variable sensitivity/specificity in CKD; Dobutamine echo preferred in transplant candidates
CT Angiography	Non-invasive coronary artery assessment	High sensitivity but low specificity; calcification may limit accuracy in CKD
Invasive Coronary Angiography	Gold standard for CAD	Most accurate; limited use due to contrast risk and cost
Ambulatory ECG (Holter, Loop recorders)	Detection of arrhythmias	High burden of arrhythmias in CKD; prolonged monitoring recommended
Blood Pressure Monitoring (Office, ABPM, Home)	Diagnose/manage hypertension	ABPM is gold standard; 44–48 h ABPM is recommended in dialysis; office BP prone to error

CKD chronic kidney disease, *LVH* left ventricular hypertrophy, *NT-proBNP* N-terminal pro-B-type natriuretic peptide, *HFpEF* heart failure with preserved ejection fraction, *LV* left ventricle, *MRI* magnetic resonance imaging, *SPECT* single photon emission computed tomography, *PET* positron emission tomography, *CT* computed tomography, *CAD* coronary artery disease, *ABPM* ambulatory blood pressure monitoring

injury. Their circulating levels often correlate with disease severity and prognosis. Furthermore, several biomarkers traditionally associated with the evaluation of CKD, have demonstrated diagnostic and prognostic relevance in HF, underscoring the interconnected nature of cardiorenal pathophysiology [40]. Troponins and natriuretic peptides may be chronically elevated in CKD due to reduced clearance, which may limit test specificity; however, trends and relative changes can still aid in diagnosing acute coronary syndromes or HF [37]. N-terminal pro-B-type natriuretic peptide (NT-proBNP) has emerged as a significant prognostic marker for kidney disease progression in nondiabetic patients with CKD. Additionally, other natriuretic and vasoactive peptides, including adrenomedullin (ADM) and A-type natriuretic peptide (ANP), have also demonstrated potential prognostic value in this patient population [41].

Electrocardiography may be used for the detection of LVH and cardiac ischemia and arrhythmias in patients with CKD. ECG sensitivity for LVH detection was lower as compared to echocardiography, despite high specificity, as shown in the AASK cohort and in a Swedish study [42, 43]. In dialysis patients ECG voltage may vary according to fluid removal and during the haemodialysis interval, demanding standardization of ECG timing in this group of patients.

In patients with CKD or kidney failure or on dialysis, ECG alterations such as the strain pattern may be frequently observed, making the diagnosis of cardiac ischaemia rather difficult. In addition, during ischemia about 30% of CKD patients do not present ST segment abnormalities.

Echocardiography remains the first-line imaging modality for assessing LVH, systolic and diastolic dysfunction parameters, and valvular disease in CKD patients, particularly given its non-invasive nature and accessibility [21]. Speckle tracking echocardiography can be used to measure left ventricular dysfunction and cardiac deformation. In addition to LVEF, LV global longitudinal strain may predict all-cause and cardiovascular mortality in patients with stage G3–4 CKD [44, 45].

Cardiac magnetic resonance imaging (CMRI) offers superior tissue characterization and is increasingly used to detect myocardial fibrosis, a common feature in advanced CKD that is associated with poor prognosis [4].

Coronary artery calcification (CAC) scoring using CT provides a sensitive marker of vascular calcification, which is highly prevalent in CKD and predictive of cardiovascular events, even in the absence of obstructive coronary artery disease [46]. Recent guidelines recommend multi-modality risk assessment, integrating imaging, biomarkers, and clinical scoring systems to better stratify cardiovascular risk in this high-risk population.

Management and Treatment Strategies

Lifestyle interventions—including smoking cessation, weight management, and regular physical activity—play a significant role in cardiovascular risk reduction and overall CKD management, in addition to pharmacologic therapy.

The coexistence of renal impairment may complicate pharmacologic therapy, limit clinical trial representation, and increase the risk of adverse effects. Recent advances in cardio-renal therapeutics and individualized care strategies have improved patient outcomes. A dual focus on cardiovascular risk reduction and renal protection is essential [47].

The cornerstone of therapy includes effective management of traditional cardiovascular risk factors, which is essential in patients with CKD to reduce both renal and cardiovascular morbidity. *Hypertension* control is fundamental, with a recommended target blood pressure of <130/80 mmHg, according to KDIGO 2024 [20] and ESH 2023 guidelines [48]. Angiotensin-converting enzyme inhibitors (ACEi) or angiotensin receptor blockers (ARBs) are preferred first-line agents, especially in patients with albuminuria, due to their demonstrated benefits in slowing CKD progression and reducing cardiovascular risk [49]. In advanced CKD (eGFR <30 mL/min/1.73 m^2), these agents require careful monitoring for hyperkalemia and increases in serum creatinine. However, the discontinuation of these classes of drugs in advanced CKD stages, does not seem to impact the long-term changes in eGFR or the incidence of renal replacement therapy [50].

Several studies have demonstrated that RAAS blockers reduce proteinuria, LVH, and cardiovascular mortality. The ARNI sacubitril/valsartan as compared with enalapril has demonstrated mortality and morbidity benefits in patients with HFrEF and CKD, but requires close monitoring of renal function and serum potassium [51]. Beta-blockers and loop diuretics remain essential in HF management; however, their use in CKD—especially in advanced stages—requires careful titration to avoid hypotension, bradycardia, or electrolyte imbalance [20, 52]. Among patients with advanced CKD and poorly controlled hypertension, treatment with chlorthalidone improved blood pressure control at 12 weeks as compared with placebo, although it induced hypokalemia, reversible increases in serum creatinine level, hyperglycemia, dizziness, and hyperuricemia more frequently as compared to placebo [53].

In *diabetes mellitus*, glycemic targets should be individualized, with a general goal of HbA1c around 7%, balancing the benefits of glycemic control against the risk of hypoglycemia, particularly in older adults and those with advanced CKD [54]. SGLT2 inhibitors have emerged as a transformative therapy in CKD patients, significantly lowering the risk of HF hospitalization and progression of kidney disease, independent of glycemic status [33]. SGLT2 inhibitors such as empagliflozin and dapagliflozin are now the standard of care in CKD patients, with or without diabetes, due to their robust cardiorenal protective effects demonstrated in landmark trials like DAPA-CKD and EMPA-KIDNEY [55, 56].

For *dyslipidemia*, statin therapy is recommended in all non-dialysis CKD patients aged ≥50 years, or in those with existing atherosclerotic cardiovascular disease (ASCVD), as per KDIGO lipid management guidelines [20]. In contrast, initiation of statins in patients already on dialysis has shown limited benefit and is not routinely recommended [57]. Lipid-lowering therapy with statins remains recommended for all non-dialysis CKD patients with atherosclerotic risk, while coronary revascularization decisions should be individualized based on symptoms burden and overall risk, as procedural risks are elevated in advanced CKD.

Emerging Therapies and Clinical Trials

Several recent and ongoing trials are expanding our understanding of how to manage cardiovascular risk in CKD.

The *non-steroidal mineralocorticoid* receptor antagonist finerenone has also shown cardiovascular and renal protective effects in diabetic CKD, as demonstrated in the FIDELIO-DKD and FIGARO-DKD trials [35, 58].

Glucagon-Like Peptide 1 (GLP-1) agonists originally developed for glycemic control in type 2 diabetes, are now being increasingly utilized for weight loss, cardiovascular protection, and potentially for CKD management. The FLOW trial assessed oral semaglutide in patients with type 2 diabetes and CKD. It was stopped early after 3.4 years due to positive results: semaglutide significantly reduced the risk of CKD progression and cardiovascular death [59]. The SOUL trial has demonstrated that oral semaglutide reduced the risk of major adverse cardiovascular events (MACE) in patients with diabetes mellitus type 2 and atherosclerotic CVD and/or CKD; in this trial no differences were observed in the occurrence of any major kidney disease between the oral semaglutide group, as compared with the placebo group [60].

In a recent metanalysis of 10 trials including 71,351 patients with type 2 diabetes, long-acting GLP-1RA reduced the incidence rate of MACE by 14%, HF hospitalization by 14%, the composite kidney outcome by 17%, and all-cause mortality by 12% [61].

Emerging therapies targeting inflammation, fibrosis, and vascular calcification are under investigation, aiming to further reduce the disproportionately high cardiovascular burden in this population.

Advances in genetic and proteomic profiling hold promise for the future of personalized therapy in patients with CKD who are at high cardiovascular risk. Ongoing research is exploring how specific genetic markers may predict susceptibility to complications such as LVH or vascular calcification, both of which significantly contribute to morbidity and mortality in this population [62]. In parallel, pharmacogenomic approaches aim to identify genetic variants that influence an individual's response to key therapeutic agents, including RAAS inhibitors and SGLT2 inhibitors, potentially optimizing efficacy while minimizing adverse effects [62].

Conclusions

Cardiovascular disease remains the leading cause of death and disability in patients with chronic kidney disease, underscoring the critical importance of understanding and managing the complex interplay between the heart and kidneys. CKD profoundly alters cardiovascular physiology through mechanisms such as neurohormonal activation, chronic inflammation, volume overload, and vascular calcification—leading to a unique and high-risk cardiac profile.

Prompt recognition of early cardiovascular complications, coupled with tailored diagnostics and evidence-based management strategies, is essential for improving patient outcomes. Recent advances—including the use of SGLT2 inhibitors, nonsteroidal mineralocorticoid receptor antagonists, and emerging biomarkers—have reshaped the therapeutic landscape, offering new hope for patients across the CKD spectrum.

Nonetheless, significant challenges remain, particularly in advanced CKD and dialysis populations, where data are limited and therapeutic options are constrained. Looking forward, a multidisciplinary, personalized approach—combining innovation, collaboration, and precision medicine—will be key to reducing the burden of cardiovascular disease in CKD and improving both quality and life expectancy.

References

1. Jha V, Garcia-Garcia G, Iseki K, et al. Chronic kidney disease: global dimension and perspectives. Lancet. 2013;382(9888):260–72.
2. Go AS, Chertow GM, Fan D, McCulloch CE, Hsu CY. Chronic kidney disease and the risks of death, cardiovascular events, and hospitalization. N Engl J Med. 2004;351(13):1296–305.
3. Marx-Schütt K, Cherney DZI, Jankowski J, Matsushita K, Nardone M, Marx N. Cardiovascular disease in chronic kidney disease. Eur Heart J. 2025;46(23):2148–60. https://doi.org/10.1093/eurheartj/ehaf167.
4. Jankowski J, Floege J, Fliser D, Böhm M, Marx N. Cardiovascular disease in chronic kidney disease: pathophysiological insights and therapeutic options. Circulation. 2021;143:1157–72.

5. Amdur RL, Feldman HI, Dominic EA, Anderson AH, Beddhu S, Rahman M, et al. Use of measures of inflammation and kidney function for prediction of atherosclerotic vascular disease events and death in patients with CKD: findings from the CRIC study. Am J Kidney Dis. 2019;73:344–53. https://doi.org/10.1053/j.ajkd.2018.09.012.
6. Stenvinkel P. Inflammation: A Key Driver in the Progression of CKD. Am J Kidney Dis. 2025;86(3):296–7. https://doi.org/10.1053/j.ajkd.2025.06.002. Epub 2025 Jul 18.
7. Ridker PM, Everett BM, Thuren T, MacFadyen JG, Chang WH, Ballantyne C, et al. Antiinflammatory therapy with Canakinumab for atherosclerotic disease. N Engl J Med. 2017;377:1119–31. https://doi.org/10.1056/NEJMoa1707914.
8. Borlaug BA, Sharma K, Shah SJ, Ho JE. Heart failure with preserved ejection fraction: JACC scientific statement. J Am Coll Cardiol. 2023;81:1810–34. https://doi.org/10.1016/j.jacc.2023.01.049.
9. Baaten C, Vondenhoff S, Noels H. The cardiorenal connection: molecular mechanisms linking kidney disease and cardiovascular risk. Circ Res. 2023;132(8):970–92. https://doi.org/10.1161/CIRCRESAHA.123.322467.
10. Cariddi A, et al. RAAS–SNS crosstalk in cardiorenal disease. Cardio Renal Metab Syndr. 2023. https://doi.org/10.1186/s44223-023-00025-1.
11. Schiffrin EL, Lipman ML, Mann JF. Chronic kidney disease: effects on the cardiovascular system. Circulation. 2007;116(1):85–97.
12. Schlaich MP, Socratous F, Hennebry S, et al. Sympathetic activation in chronic renal failure. J Am Soc Nephrol. 2009;20(5):933–9. https://doi.org/10.1681/ASN.2008060603.
13. Fisher JP, Fadel PJ. Therapeutic strategies to combat neurohumoral activation in chronic kidney disease. Clin Auton Res. 2010;20(4):229–38.
14. Babitt JL, Lin HY. Mechanisms of anemia in CKD. Nat Rev Nephrol. 2012;8(11):674–84.
15. Go AS, Chertow GM, et al. Chronic kidney disease and the risks of death, cardiovascular events, and hospitalization. N Engl J Med. 2004;351(13):1296–305.
16. Pfeffer MA, Burdmann EA, et al. A trial of darbepoetin alfa in type 2 diabetes and CKD. N Engl J Med. 2009;361(21):2019–32.
17. Ren S, Yao X, Li Y, Zhang Y, Tong C, Feng Y. Efficacy and safety of hypoxia-inducible factor-prolyl hydroxylase inhibitor treatment for anemia in chronic kidney disease: an umbrella review of meta-analyses. Front Pharmacol. 2023;14:1296702. https://doi.org/10.3389/fphar.2023.1296702.
18. Hasegawa T, Imaizumi T, Hamano T, Murotani K, Fujii N, Komaba H, Ando M, Maruyama S, Nangaku M, Nitta K, Hirakata H, Isaka Y, Wada T, Fukagawa M. Association between serum iron markers, iron supplementation and cardiovascular morbidity in pre-dialysis chronic kidney disease. Nephrol Dial Transplant. 2023;38(12):2713–22. https://doi.org/10.1093/ndt/gfad096.
19. Chan B, Varghese A, Badve SV, Pecoits-Filho R, Guedes M, Arnott C, Kozor R, O'Lone E, Jun M, Kotwal S, Block GA, Chertow GM, Solomon SD, Vaduganathan M, Perkovic V, Neuen BL. Systematic review of the effects of iron on cardiovascular, kidney, and safety outcomes in patients with CKD. Kidney Int Rep. 2025;10(4):1037–49. https://doi.org/10.1016/j.ekir.2025.01.029.
20. Kidney Disease: Improving Global Outcomes (KDIGO) CKD Work Group, Stevens PE, Ahmed SB, et al. KDIGO 2024 clinical practice guideline for the evaluation and management of chronic kidney disease. Kidney Int. 2024;105(4S):S117–314.
21. Graham-Brown MPM, et al. Cardiovascular disease in chronic kidney disease: pathophysiology and interventions. Nat Rev Cardiol. 2022;19(5):261–79. https://doi.org/10.1038/s41569-021-00611-1.
22. Wachtell K, Ibsen H, Olsen MH, Borch-Johnsen K, Lindholm LH, Mogensen CE, Dahlöf B, Devereux RB, Beevers G, de Faire U, Fyhrquist F, Julius S, Kjeldsen SE, Kristianson K, Lederballe-Pedersen O, Nieminen MS, Okin PM, Omvik P, Oparil S, Wedel H, Snapinn SM, Aurup P. Albuminuria and cardiovascular risk in hypertensive patients with left ventricular hypertrophy: the LIFE study. Ann Intern Med. 2003;139(11):901–6. https://doi.org/10.7326/0003-4819-139-11-200312020-00008.

23. Tripepi G, Pannier B, D'Arrigo G, Mallamaci F, Zoccali C, London G. Reappraisal in two European cohorts of the prognostic power of left ventricular mass index in chronic kidney failure. Kidney Int. 2017;91:704–10. https://doi.org/10.1016/j.kint.2016.10.012.
24. Tripepi G, D'Arrigo G, Mallamaci F, London G, Tangri N, Yenchih Hsu J, Feldman HI, Zoccali C. Prognostic values of left ventricular mass index in chronic kidney disease patients. Nephrol Dial Transplant. 2021;36(4):665–72. https://doi.org/10.1093/ndt/gfz254.
25. Salvetti M, Muiesan ML, Paini A, Monteduro C, Agabiti-Rosei C, Aggiusti C, Bertacchini F, Stassaldi D, Castellano M, Agabiti-Rosei E. Left ventricular hypertrophy and renal dysfunction during antihypertensive treatment adversely affect cardiovascular prognosis in hypertensive patients. J Hypertens. 2012;30(2):411–20. https://doi.org/10.1097/HJH.0b013e32834e90d8.
26. Ishigami J, Kansal M, Mehta R, Srivastava A, Rahman M, Dobre M, Al-Kindi SG, Go AS, Navaneethan SD, Chen J, He J, Bhat ZY, Jaar BG, Appel LJ, Matsushita K, CRIC Study Investigators. Cardiac structure and function and subsequent kidney disease progression in adults with CKD: the Chronic Renal Insufficiency Cohort (CRIC) study. Am J Kidney Dis. 2023;82(2):225–36. https://doi.org/10.1053/j.ajkd.2023.01.442.
27. Di Lullo L, Gorini A, Russo D, Santoboni A, Ronco C. Left ventricular hypertrophy in chronic kidney disease patients: from pathophysiology to treatment. Cardiorenal Med. 2015;5:254–66. https://doi.org/10.1159/000435838.
28. Moody WE, Ferro CJ, Edwards NC, Chue CD, Lin ELS, Taylor RJ, Cockwell P, Steeds RP, Townend JN, CRIB-Donor Study Investigators. Cardiovascular effects of unilateral nephrectomy in living kidney donors. Hypertension. 2016;67(2):368–77. https://doi.org/10.1161/HYPERTENSIONAHA.115.06608.
29. Maki KC, Wilcox ML, Dicklin MR, Kakkar R, Davidson MH. Left ventricular mass regression, all-cause and cardiovascular mortality in chronic kidney disease: a meta-analysis. BMC Nephrol. 2022;23(1):34. https://doi.org/10.1186/s12882-022-02666-1.
30. Damman K, Valente MA, Voors AA, et al. Renal impairment, worsening renal function, and outcome in patients with heart failure: an updated meta-analysis. Eur Heart J. 2014;35(7):455–69.
31. Bansal N, Zelnick LR, Bhat ZY, et al. Burden and outcomes of heart failure hospitalizations in CKD: findings from the CRIC study. J Am Coll Cardiol. 2019;73(21):2691–700.
32. McMurray JJV, Solomon SD, Inzucchi SE, et al. Dapagliflozin in patients with heart failure and reduced ejection fraction. N Engl J Med. 2019;381(21):1995–2008.
33. Anker SD, Butler J, Filippatos G, et al. Empagliflozin in heart failure with a preserved ejection fraction. N Engl J Med. 2021;385(16):1451–61.
34. Solomon SD, McMurray JJV, Anand IS, et al. PARAGON-HF trial: sacubitril/valsartan in HFpEF. N Engl J Med. 2019;381(17):1609–20.
35. Bakris GL, Agarwal R, Anker SD, et al. Effect of finerenone on chronic kidney disease outcomes in type 2 diabetes. N Engl J Med. 2020;383(23):2219–29.
36. Zhang J, Pang Q, Wang S, Leiyun W, Zhang A. Associated factors of cardiac valve calcification and its prognostic effects among patients with chronic kidney disease: a systematic review and meta-analysis. Front Cardiovasc Med. 2023;10:1120634. https://doi.org/10.3389/fcvm.2023.1120634.
37. Sarnak MJ, Levey AS, Schoolwerth AC, Coresh J, Culleton B, Hamm LL, McCullough PA, Kasiske BL, Kelepouris E, Klag MJ, Parfrey P, Pfeffer M, Raij L, Spinosa DJ, Wilson PW, American Heart Association Councils on Kidney in Cardiovascular Disease, High Blood Pressure Research, Clinical Cardiology, and Epidemiology and Prevention. Kidney disease as a risk factor for development of cardiovascular disease: a statement from the American Heart Association Councils on Kidney in Cardiovascular Disease, High Blood Pressure Research, Clinical Cardiology, and Epidemiology and Prevention. Circulation. 2003;108(17):2154–69. https://doi.org/10.1161/01.CIR.0000095676.90936.80.
38. Huang AL, Leipsic JA, Zekry SB, Sellers S, Ahmadi AA, Blanke P, Hadamitzky M, Kim Y-J, Conte E, Andreini D, et al. Effects of chronic kidney disease and declining renal function on coronary atherosclerotic plaque progression: a PARADIGM substudy. Eur Heart J Cardiovasc Imaging. 2021;22(9):1072–82. https://doi.org/10.1093/ehjci/jeab029.

39. Park S, Lee SH, Shin D, Hong D, Joh HS, Choi KH, Kim HK, Ha SJ, Park TK, Yang JH, et al. Prognostic impact of coronary flow reserve in patients with CKD. Kidney Int Rep. 2022;8(1):64–74. https://doi.org/10.1016/j.ekir.2022.10.003.
40. Sun RR, Lu L, Liu M, Cao Y, Li XC, Liu H, et al. Biomarkers and heart disease. Eur Rev Med Pharmacol Sci. 2014;18:2927–35.
41. Dieplinger B, Mueller T, Kollerits B, Struck J, Ritz E, von Eckardstein A, et al. Pro-A-type natriuretic peptide and pro-adrenomedullin predict progression of chronic kidney disease: the MMKD study. Kidney Int. 2009;75:408–14.
42. Esquitin R, Razzouk L, Peterson GE, Wright Jr JT, Phillips RA, De Backer TL, Baran DA, Kendrick C, Greene T, Reiffel J, Muntner P, Farkouh ME. Left ventricular hypertrophy by electrocardiography and echocardiography in the African American Study of Kidney Disease Cohort Study. J Am Soc Hypertens. 2012;6(3):193–200. https://doi.org/10.1016/j.jash.2012.01.004.
43. Cordeiro AC, Lindholm B, Sousa MG, Picotti JC, Nunes GJ, Santana MRO, Grimaldi Jr W, Amparo FC, Amodeo C, Carrero JJ. Reliability of electrocardiographic surrogates of left ventricular mass in patients with chronic kidney disease. J Hypertens. 2014;32(2):439–45. https://doi.org/10.1097/HJH.0000000000000026.
44. Kakiouzi V, Tsartsalis D, Aggeli C, Dimitroglou Y, Latsios G, Tsiamis E, Giannou P, Karampela M, Petras D, Vlachopoulos C, Tousoulis D, Tsioufis C. The prognostic value of speckle tracking echocardiography in patients with end stage renal disease on dialysis. Int J Cardiovasc Imaging. 2022;38(12):2605–14. https://doi.org/10.1007/s10554-022-02608-w.
45. Jahn L, Kramann R, Marx N, Floege J, Becker M, Schlieper G. Speckle tracking echocardiography and all-cause and cardiovascular mortality risk in chronic kidney disease patients. Kidney Blood Press Res. 2019;44(4):690–703. https://doi.org/10.1159/000501225.
46. Schlieper G, Schurgers L, Brandenburg V, Reutelingsperger C, Floege J. Vascular calcification in chronic kidney disease: an update. Nephrol Dial Transplant. 2016;31(1):31–9. https://doi.org/10.1093/ndt/gfv111.
47. Zoccali C, Mallamaci F, Adamczak M, de Oliveira RB, Massy ZA, Sarafidis P, Agarwal R, Mark PB, Kotanko P, Ferro CJ, Wanner C, Burnier M, Vanholder R, Wiecek A. Cardiovascular complications in chronic kidney disease: a review from the European Renal and Cardiovascular Medicine Working Group of the European Renal Association. Cardiovasc Res. 2023;119(11):2017–32. https://doi.org/10.1093/cvr/cvad083.
48. Mancia G, Kreutz R, Brunström M, Burnier M, Grassi G, Januszewicz A, Muiesan ML, Tsioufis K, Agabiti-Rosei E, Algharably EAE, et al. 2023 ESH Guidelines for the management of arterial hypertension The Task Force for the management of arterial hypertension of the European Society of Hypertension: endorsed by the International Society of Hypertension (ISH) and the European Renal Association (ERA). J Hypertens. 2023;41(12):1874–2071. https://doi.org/10.1097/HJH.0000000000003480.
49. Lewis EJ, Hunsicker LG, Bain RP, Rohde RD. The effect of angiotensin-converting-enzyme inhibition on diabetic nephropathy. The Collaborative Study Group. N Engl J Med. 1993;329(20):1456–62.
50. Bhandari S, Mehta S, Khwaja A, Cleland JGF, Ives N, Brettell E, Chadburn M, Cockwell P, STOP ACEi Trial Investigators. Renin-angiotensin system inhibition in advanced chronic kidney disease. N Engl J Med. 2022;387(22):2021–32.
51. McMurray JV, Packer M, Desai AS, Gong J, Lefkowitz MP, Rizkala AR, Rouleau JL, Shi VC, Solomon SD, Swedberg K, Zile MR, PARADIGM-HF Investigators and Committees. Angiotensin-neprilysin inhibition versus enalapril in heart failure. N Engl J Med. 2014;371(11):993–1004. https://doi.org/10.1056/NEJMoa1409077.
52. Heidenreich PA, Bozkurt B, Aguilar D, Allen LA, Byun JJ, Colvin MM, Deswal A, Drazner MH, Dunlay SM, Evers LR, Fang JC, Fedson SE, Fonarow GC, Hayek SS, Hernandez AF, Khazanie P, Kittleson MM, Lee CS, Link MS, Milano CA, Nnacheta LC, Sandhu AT, Stevenson LW, Vardeny O, Vest AR, Yancy CW, ACC/AHA Joint Committee Members. 2022 AHA/ACC/HFSA guideline for the management of heart failure: a report of the American College of

Cardiology/American Heart Association Joint Committee on Clinical Practice Guidelines. Circulation. 2022;145(18):e895–e1032. https://doi.org/10.1161/CIR.0000000000001063.
53. Agarwal R, Sinha AD, Cramer AE, Balmes-Fenwick M, Dickinson JH, Ouyang F, Tu W. Chlorthalidone for hypertension in advanced chronic kidney disease. N Engl J Med. 2021;385(27):2507–19. https://doi.org/10.1056/NEJMoa2110730.
54. American Diabetes Association. Standards of medical care in diabetes—2024. Diabetes Care. 2024;47(Supplement_1):S1–S291.
55. Heerspink HJL, Stefánsson BV, Correa-Rotter R, Chertow GM, Greene T, Hou FF, Mann JFE, McMurray JJV, Lindberg M, Rossing P, et al. Dapagliflozin in patients with chronic kidney disease. N Engl J Med. 2020;383(15):1436–46. https://doi.org/10.1056/NEJMoa2024816.
56. The EMPA-KIDNEY Collaborative Group, Herrington WG, Staplin N, Wanner C, Green JB, Hauske SJ, Emberson JR, Preiss D, Judge P, Mayne KJ, et al. Empagliflozin in nondiabetic kidney disease. N Engl J Med. 2023;388(2):117–27.
57. Fellström BC, Jardine AG, Schmieder RE, Holdaas H, Bannister K, Beutler J, Chae DW, Chevaile A, Cobbe SM, Grönhagen-Riska C, De Lima JJ, Lins R, Mayer G, AURORA Study Group, et al. Rosuvastatin and cardiovascular events in patients undergoing hemodialysis. N Engl J Med. 2009;360(14):1395–407. https://doi.org/10.1056/NEJMoa0810177.
58. Pitt B, Filippatos G, Agarwal R, Anker SD, Bakris GL, Rossing P, Joseph A, Kolkhof P, Nowack C, Schloemer P, Ruilope LM, FIGARO-DKD Investigators. Cardiovascular events with finerenone in kidney disease and type 2 diabetes. N Engl J Med. 2021;385(24):2252–63. https://doi.org/10.1056/NEJMoa2110956.
59. Rossing P, Baeres FMM, Bakris G, Bosch-Traberg H, Gislum M, Gough SCL, Idorn T, Lawson J, Mahaffey KW, Mann JFE, Mersebach H, Perkovic V, Tuttle K, Pratley R. The rationale, design and baseline data of FLOW, a kidney outcomes trial with once-weekly semaglutide in people with type 2 diabetes and chronic kidney disease. Nephrol Dial Transplant. 2023;38(9):2041–51. https://doi.org/10.1093/ndt/gfad009.
60. McGuire DK, Marx N, Mulvagh SL, Deanfield JE, Inzucchi SE, Pop-Busui R, Mann JFE, Emerson SS, Poulter NR, Engelmann MDM, Ripa MS, Hovingh GK, Brown-Frandsen K, Bain SC, Cavender MA, Gislum M, David JP, Buse JB, SOUL Study Group. Oral semaglutide and cardiovascular outcomes in high-risk type 2 diabetes. N Engl J Med. 2025;392(20):2001–12.
61. Lee MMY, Sattar N, Pop-Busui R, Deanfield J, Emerson SS, Inzucchi SE, Mann JFE, Marx N, Mulvagh SL, Poulter NR, Badve SV, Pratley RE, Perkovic V, Buse JB, McGuire DK, SOUL Trial Investigators. Cardiovascular and kidney outcomes and mortality with long-acting injectable and oral glucagon-like peptide 1 receptor agonists in individuals with type 2 diabetes: a systematic review and meta-analysis of randomized trials. Diabetes Care. 2025;48(5):846–59.
62. Ferro A, Segreti A, Crispino SP, Cricco R, Di Cristo A, Ciancio M, Gurrieri F, Ussia GP, Grigioni F. Exploring the role of genetic and genomic factors in therapeutic response to heart failure: a comprehensive analytical review. Genes. 2025;16:801. https://doi.org/10.3390/genes16070801.

Hypertension and Diabetic Kidney Disease

Giovanna Leoncini, Elisa Russo, Cecilia Barnini, Francesca Viazzi, and Roberto Pontremoli

Epidemiology and Natural History

The number of people with diabetes worldwide has recently surpassed 800 million, more than four times higher than in 1990 [1]. Diabetic kidney disease (DKD) is a major long-term complication of diabetes mellitus (DM) and implies an enormous burden in terms of financial costs and adverse health outcomes, such as decreased quality of life, frailty, end-stage kidney disease (ESKD), and premature mortality. DKD affects over one-third of patients with type 1 DM (T1DM) and approximately half of type 2 DM (T2DM) patients and represents the leading cause of end-stage kidney disease (ESKD) worldwide, accounting for 40% of new dialysis admissions [2]. Given the higher prevalence of T2DM, over 90% of diabetics on dialysis have this type of diabetes. Accordingly, in Europe, where people with diabetes are 2–5 times more likely to develop CKD than people without diabetes [3], using the criteria of eGFR <60 mL/min/1.73 m^2 or microalbuminuria or both, DKD was identified in 32% of people with type 1 diabetes and 46% of people with type 2 diabetes in the UK National Diabetes Audit [4].

Hypertension is a common feature in patients with chronic kidney disease (CKD) and diabetes mellitus and represents a risk factor for the development and progression of renal damage as well as for cardiovascular (CV) morbidity and mortality. Prevalence of hypertension is approximately twice in patients with diabetes

G. Leoncini (✉) · E. Russo · F. Viazzi · R. Pontremoli
Department of Internal Medicine, University of Genoa and IRCCS Azienda Ospedaliera Metropolitana, Genoa, Italy
e-mail: giovanna.leoncini@unige.it; elisa.russo@unige.it; francesca.viazzi@unige.it; roberto.pontremoli@unige.it

C. Barnini
Department of Internal Medicine IV, Nephrology and Hypertension, Medical University Innsbruck, Innsbruck, Tirol, Austria

P. Sarafidis, R. Pontremoli (eds.), *Hypertension and Chronic Kidney Disease*, Updates in Hypertension and Cardiovascular Protection,
https://doi.org/10.1007/978-3-032-29564-4_8

compared to the general population and increases significantly as kidney disease progresses and can reach nearly 90% in ESKD.

Many recent epidemiological studies have highlighted the great heterogeneity of the natural history of renal damage in the presence of diabetes both in T1DM and T2DM, suggesting the use of the term DKD to encompass the various forms. In fact, the traditional clinical presentation characterised by slowly worsening albuminuria that typically preceded a reduction in glomerular filtration rate (GFR), is often replaced by a different phenotype characterised by a progressive decline in renal function even in the absence of albuminuria. These findings suggest that the progression of DKD to ESKD may follow two distinct pathways, that of albuminuria and that of reduced GFR, which may appear and progress together or separately. In the classic albuminuric pathway, the loss of GFR is preceded and mainly caused by the onset and progression of albuminuria and, therefore, reducing albuminuria can significantly slow down GFR decline. In the emerging non-albuminuric pathway, the reduction in GFR is independent of the presence and progression of albuminuria and, therefore, may not benefit from its reduction. However, as CKD entails an increased incidence of cardiovascular events, albuminuria when present retains a powerful unfavourable predictive power, proportional to its magnitude and its reduction represents an independent goal of treatment.

Pathogenesis

DKD is one of the microvascular complications of diabetes and, in fact, the damage initially affects the small vessels. The pathophysiology is complex and is the result of a combination of hemodynamic and metabolic abnormalities with a central role of hyperglycaemia as the inducer. In addition to hyperglycaemia, arterial hypertension, dyslipidaemia, obesity and smoking are recognised as playing a key role in the pathogenesis of DKD. In particular, the relationship between DKD and hypertension is complex and bidirectional: high blood pressure can accelerate kidney damage, whereas impaired kidney function may worsen blood pressure regulation. The mechanisms of hypertension in diabetic nephropathy are complex and include excess sodium retention and volume expansion, sympathetic nervous system and renin-angiotensin-aldosterone system (RAAS) activation, endothelial dysfunction and increased oxidative stress.

Haemodynamic alterations are characterised by glomerular hypertension, as increased glomerular filtration of glucose leads to an increase of the expression of sodium-glucose cotransporters 2 (SGLT2) and, therefore, increased reabsorption of sodium and glucose. Concomitantly, passive reabsorption of chloride and water also increases, activating tubuloglomerular feedback from the macula densa which in turn leads to vasodilation of the afferent arteriole and, finally an increased intraglomerular pressure. Moreover, both metabolic and haemodynamic alterations, are associated with the generation of reactive oxygen species (ROS). Oxidative damage triggers inflammatory pathways, such as mitogen-activated protein kinases (MAPK), nuclear factor kappa-light chain-enhancer of activated B cells (NF-κB), and Janus kinase-signal transduction and transcription activation (JAK-STAT), as well as activating immune cells and promoting the release of pro-inflammatory cytokines, including transforming growth factor-beta (TGF-beta), platelet-derived growth factor (PDGF) and angiotensin II. Together, persistent inflammation and oxidative stress create a vicious cycle that promote kidney injury, leading to fibrosis and accelerating DKD progression [5].

In the diabetic kidney structural abnormalities can be observed at various levels [6]. Early glomerular changes include glomerular hypertrophy, podocyte injury with the effacement of foot processes, glomerular basement membrane (GBM) thickening and mesangial expansion. Tubular changes include renal tubular epithelial cells hypertrophy, tubular basement membrane thickening and tubular atrophy. Renal fibrosis is a severe consequence of a prolonged hyperglycaemic state and the consequent activation of a cascade of multiple pathogenic mechanisms, contributing towards the loss of renal function. The transition of renal tubular epithelial cells into mesenchymal cells, known as epithelial-mesenchymal transition has a key role in the progressive loss of functional renal parenchyma and the development of kidney fibrosis. One of the key elements of DKD is microangiopathy, characterised by aberrant angiogenesis in the early stages and glomerular capillary rarefaction in the advanced stages. This vascular dysfunction is closely linked to GBM thickening, glomerular hypertrophy, and mesangial expansion, which together exacerbate renal damage. The altered resistance of periglomerular arteries due to increased levels of vasoactive factors in DM further complicates glomerular hemodynamics.

As a matter of fact, the 'typical' diabetic nephropathy is predominantly a glomerular disease characterised, initially, by an increase in glomerular size, and over time by the nodular glomerular sclerosis (known as Kimmestiel-Wilson nodules) or diffuse sclerosis. There is also marked hyalinosis near the capillary loops or Bowman's capsule, as well as arteriosclerosis of the afferent and efferent arterioles, the latter being pathognomonic of diabetes. This is the histological picture that characterises kidney damage in most patients with T1DM, while in T2DM, which is much more prevalent, there is often an 'atypical' nephropathy with a clear predominance of tubulointerstitial and vascular lesions over glomerular lesions. It has been hypothesised that these lesions are actually the expression of repeated acute kidney injury (AKI), mostly subclinical and often not completely resolved (such as ischaemic, infectious, toxic or obstructive damage) [7] or of predominantly macrovascular damage, therefore more attributable to the concomitant presence of hypertension, dyslipidaemia and obesity rather than to the effects of hyperglycaemia. Furthermore, in some diabetic patients renal damage may be secondary to the concomitant presence of other well-known nephropathies (such as chronic glomerulonephritis etc), which should always be suspected and diagnosed by renal biopsy in the presence of atypical clinical features.

Clinical Presentation and Diagnosis

Clinically, diabetic nephropathy is characterised by the triad of proteinuria/albuminuria, reduced GFR and arterial hypertension.

Urine albumin excretion is usually assessed by 24 h urine collection or as the albuminuria/creatinine ratio (ACR) in spot urine. Based on the result of the test, albuminuria is classified as normoalbuminuria (albuminuria <30 mg/24 h or ACR <30 mg/g), moderate increase of albuminuria (albuminuria between 30 and 300 mg/24 h or RAC between 30 and 300 mg/g) or severe albuminuria (albuminuria >300 mg/24 h or RAC >300 mg/g). Albuminuria should be assessed on 3 samples over a period of 3–6 months to classify the patient based on the results of at least 2 out of 3 measurements, although a single measurement may be reliable.

As for GFR, which requires the determination of creatinine levels and the calculation of GFR using specific formulas, diabetic nephropathy often begins with a stage of glomerular hyperfiltration with an increase in GFR, which then returns to normal and subsequently decreases over time.

Arterial hypertension is usually secondary to kidney damage in T1DM, while it is usually primary and precedes the diagnosis of T2DM promoting the development of nephropathy.

The classic description of the natural history of diabetic nephropathy, described mainly, but not exclusively, in T1DM, involves five stages that occur in succession over time. It starts with a stage of hyperfiltration, characterised by an increase in GFR in the absence of urinary abnormalities, followed by a stage of silent nephropathy characterised by normoalbuminuria and normal GFR with episodes of moderate increase in albuminuria, followed by a stage of incipient nephropathy with persistent moderate increased albuminuria. The fourth stage, known as overt nephropathy, presents with severe albuminuria, reduced GFR and increased blood pressure. Increased urinary protein excretion is a signal of deteriorating kidney function and a prognostic factor of disease progression and a therapeutic target. The progressive reduction in GFR occurs at varying speeds until ESKD, the fifth and final stage of uraemia. However, various studies have shown that the natural history of DKD does not necessarily follow this pattern and is much more heterogeneous.

Firstly, microalbuminuria does not necessarily progress to macroalbuminuria but may remain stable in about one third of patients or even regress to normoalbuminuria in another third, in both T1DM and T2DM. In macroalbuminuric patients, regression to microalbuminuria or remission to normoalbuminuria is even possible and, at least in part, this phenomenon could be attributable to the increasing use of renin-angiotensin-aldosterone inhibitors (RAASi). Furthermore, the reduction and progression of GFR can occur independently of the presence and progression of albuminuria. In fact, in patients with T1DM and reduced GFR, about a quarter of them are normoalbuminuric, and even most patients with T2DM and GFR < 60 mL/min*1.73 m^2 have normal urinary albumin excretion. The non-albuminuric renal failure phenotype is more common in women and less correlated with retinopathy and with the duration and severity of hyperglycaemia. This increasingly common phenotype also seems to be influenced by the increasing use of RAASi inhibitors, which reduce albuminuria by altering renal haemodynamic. Furthermore, the few biopsy studies correlate this phenotype with a higher prevalence of atypical diabetic nephropathy with predominantly tubulointerstitial and vascular damage.

With regards to instrumental diagnostics, ultrasound can be useful to assess the presence, site and morphology of the kidneys by measuring their size and determining the cortico-medullary ratio. Combined with Doppler, it can also be a first-level test for the detection of nephrovascular diseases, which then require further investigation with CT angiography or MR angiography.

Although kidney biopsy is the gold standard to diagnose DKD, it is not routinely done in real-world clinical practice out of research setting, unless to rule out the presence of non-diabetic nephropathies in the presence of suspicious signs or symptoms, such as the presence of nephropathy within 5 years of the diagnosis of T1DM, rapid GFR worsening, the presence of active urinary sediment or the appearance of systemic manifestations suggestive of other nephropathy, and the absence of retinopathy in albuminuric forms [8].

Patients with T1DM, in the absence of a known kidney disease, should undergo initial screening for albuminuria 5 years after diagnosis and, subsequently, at least annually. Patients with type 2 diabetes should be screened at the time of diagnosis and every year thereafter.

Prevention and Treatment

Over a highly variable period of time, DKD tends in most cases to progress to ESKD requiring renal replacement treatment, a condition which has a profound adverse effect on the quality of life, morbidity as well as direct and indirect costs for health systems [9]. The rate of GFR decline appears to be greater in the presence of albuminuria, especially macroalbuminuria, but further studies are needed to confirm these observations on the long-term prognosis of different DKD phenotypes.

Treatment can slow progression, especially if started early. The use of nephrotoxic drugs or contrast media, urinary tract infections, obstructive urinary tract diseases or hypovolaemic states may accelerate the progression of nephropathy, causing overlapping episodes of AKI. Furthermore, it is not uncommon for patients to die from cardiovascular causes before reaching the ESKD stage, as CKD from any cause is associated with a marked increase in cardiovascular risk.

The treatment and prevention of DKD, its comorbidities and complications are challenging and require a multifactorial therapeutic strategy. Lifestyle changes, such as weight loss in cases of overweight/obesity, increased physical activity, smoking cessation, and a low-sodium diet, are the first step in managing DKD. In addition, an integrated pharmacological approach aimed at achieving careful glycaemic, blood pressure, and lipid control is necessary.

For approximately two decades the only drugs with evidence of nephroprotective effects in DKD were angiotensin-converting enzyme inhibitors (ACE-i) and angiotensin receptor blockers (ARBs), able to reduce or reverse albuminuria and slow the progression of nephropathy attenuating the RAAS activity and, therefore, reducing intraglomerular pressure [10–12]. Current guidelines recommend the use of ACE-i and ARBs for diabetic patients with albuminuria, while it is currently unclear whether these drugs also have a specific nephroprotective effect in non-albuminuric DKD, as there are no specific studies on patients with DKD with reduced GFR alone without albuminuria.

More recently, there has been a growing body of evidence on the efficacy of three other classes of drugs with nephroprotective effects in diabetic and non-diabetic patients: mineralocorticoid receptor antagonists (MRAs) and, among hypoglycaemic drugs, glucose-like peptide 1 receptor agonists (GLP1-RAs) and sodium/glucose co-transporter 2 inhibitors (SGLT2i). Hyperglycaemia stimulates the activation of mineralcorticoid receptors (MR) with a subsequent cascade of release of proinflammatory cytokines and pro-fibrotic mediators that lead to fibrosis at the cardiac, renal and vascular level. MRAs have been demonstrated to significantly reduce albuminuria when added to ACEIs or ARBs, but their use is limited by the risk of hyperkalaemia, especially in patients with renal failure. It has recently been shown that the anti-albuminuric effect in DKD achieved with finerenone, the first, non-steroidal, selective MRA, has less effect on potassium levels than other MRAs [13]. In the recently completed DKD outcome program comprising two randomized clinical trials, FIDELIO-DKD [14] and FIGARO-DKD [15], and in the FIDELITY [16] pooled analysis of both trials evaluating more than 13,000 patients, finerenone used on top of the maximally tolerated labelled dose of a RAS inhibitor demonstrated beneficial effects on the kidney and the heart across a broad spectrum of patients with CKD and T2D. In particular, the use of finerenone vs placebo conveyed a 14% lower risk of the composite CV outcome (time to CV death, nonfatal myocardial infarction, nonfatal stroke, or hospitalization for HF) and a 23% reduced risk of the composite kidney outcome (time to first onset of kidney failure, sustained decrease in eGFR of ≥57% from baseline over ≥4 weeks, or renal death) as well as a 20% reduced dialysis initiation Additionally, the discontinuation rate due to hyperkalaemia was higher with finerenone with respect to placebo (1.7% vs 0.6%) but lower than rates reported in previous trials using dual RAS blockade in patients with T2D and CKD [17, 18] and with steroid MRAs [19]. As a matter of fact, in patients with CKD it is imperative to assess serum potassium levels before starting finerenone therapy.

The choice of hypoglycaemic therapy in patients with T2DM is based on an overall assessment of the patient, the severity of hyperglycaemia and the available treatment options. Hypoglycaemic pharmacological interventions include both oral and injectable medications. Given the scientific evidence of recent years, glucagon-like peptide 1 receptor agonist (GLP1-RA) and sodium-glucose cotransporter 2 inhibitors (SGLT2i) should be considered the first choice in combination with metformin, when not contraindicated, in patients with T2DM and high cardiovascular risk and/or reduced renal function, preferring them to other classes such as dipeptidyl peptidase 4 (DPP4) inhibitors that degrade endogenous incretins or sulfonylureas [20]. As a matter of fact, there is such extensive data in the literature on the important nephroprotective effect exerted by SGLTIs in DKD in terms of reduction of albuminuria, as well as slowing the rate of GFR reduction and progression to

ESKD that SGLT2 inhibitors are now commonly recommended for the treatment of patients with DKD and an eGFR of ≥20 mL/min per 1.73 m^2, irrespective of the glycaemic control [21]. As a matter of fact, all SGLT2Is have demonstrated similar effects, and, therefore, it seems to be a class effect. The mechanisms of renal protection have not yet been fully clarified but are likely to be multiple (Table 1). They can exert indirect nephroprotective effects through improved glycaemic control, weight loss and improved insulin resistance. These effects are useful, but they are not sufficient to explain the nephroprotection also demonstrated in subjects without diabetes, and, therefore, non-glycaemic mechanisms are involved. In particular three large, randomised studies designed to investigate the nephroprotective effects of SGLT2i in diabetic and non-diabetic patients (CREDENCE with Canagliflozin, DAPA-CKD with Dapaglifozin and EMPA-KIDNEY with Empaglifozin) [22–24] have demonstrated the ability of SGLT2i to slow the progression of CKD regardless of the presence of diabetes and albuminuria. The non-glycaemic effects include stimulation of osmotic diuresis and natriuresis with reduction of blood pressure, reduction of intraglomerular pressure through action on local haemodynamic, reduction of pro-inflammatory and profibrotic factors, downregulation of the RAAS and increased oxygen bioavailability in the kidneys.

Similarly, the GLP1-RAs have been shown to reduce the incidence and progression of DKD [25–29]. Despite the overlapping benefit (Table 2), growing evidence indicates that SGLT2i and GLP-1 RA have distinct and separate roles in clinical practice and their combination therapy might be promising. More recently, the dual-action glucose-dependent insulinotropic polypeptide/glucagon-like peptide 1 (GIP/GLP-1) receptor agonist tirzepatide in the analysis of pooled SURPASS-1–5 trials

Table 1 SGLT2i: effects and potential mechanisms of nephroprotection

Metabolic Effects	Decreased plasma glucose levels
	Decreased body weight
	Decreased triglycerides and small-dense LDLc
	Increased HDLc
	Increased insulin sensitivity
	Decreased hepatic steatosis
	Decreased plasma uric acid levels
Hemodynamic Effects	Decreased blood pressure
	Modulation of tubuloglomerular feedback
	↓ Sympathetic nerve system activity
Direct Nephroprotective Effects	Inhibition of Na/H exchange
	Decreased endothelial dysfunction and oxidative stress
	Improvement of mitochondrial dysfuction
	Improvement of podocyte loss
	Decreased renal fibrosis
	Decreased inflammation
	Decreased albuminuria
	Decreased glomerular damage
	Increased erythropoiesis

Table 2 Nephroprotective effects of SGLT21 and GLP-1 RA in patients with CKD and diabetes

	CREDENCE [22]	DAPA-CKD [23]	EMPA-KIDNEY [24]	FLOW [29]
Intervention	Canaglifozin	Dapaglifozin	Empaglifozin	Semaglutide
Population	4401	4304	6609	3533
Inclusion criteria	T2DM; eGFR 30–<90 mL/min*1.73 m^2 and UACR >300 mg/g	eGFR 25–75 mL/min*1.73 m^2 and UACR >200 mg/g	eGFR 45–<90 mL/min*1.73 m^2 and UACR >200 mg/g or eGFR 20–<45 mL/min*1.73 m^2	T2DM; eGFR 50–75 mL/min*1.73 m^2 and UACR >300 mg/g or eGFR 25–<50 mL/min*1.73 m^2 and UACR >100 mg/g
Diabetes, %	100	67.5	46	100
RAASi use, %	99.9	98.1	85.2	95.1
Primary endpoint	Composite of ESKD, doubling of serum creatinine, or renal or CV death	Composite of ESKD, sustained eGFR decline ≥50%, or renal or CV death	Progression of kidney disease (ESKD, sustained eGFR decline <10 mL/min*1.73 m^2, sustained eGFR decline ≥40% or renal death) or CV death	Composite of kidney failure, sustained eGFR decline ≥50%, or kidney-related or CV death
HR (95% CI)	0.70 (0.59–0.82)	0.61 (0.51–0.72)	0.72 (0.64–0.82)	0.76 (0.66–0.88)
Between-group difference in UACR reduction, % (95% CI)[a]	31 (26–35)	29 (25–33)	19 (15–23)	32 (25–38)
Between-group difference in eGFR slope, mL/min*1.73 m^2/year (95% CI)[a]	1.52 (1.11–1.93)	0.93 (0.61–1.25)	0.75 (0.54–0.96)	1.16 (0.86–1.47)

[a]Favor active treatment over placebo

induced a clinically relevant decrease in albuminuria versus comparators, suggesting a potential renal benefit [30].

Moreover, the nephroprotective effect of targeting aldosterone overactivity with MRA provided the rationale to assess the effects of alternative pathways of aldosterone inhibition and, therefore, Aldosterone synthase inhibitors (ASi) have emerged as potential alternative to MRAs for aldosterone. Early phase II trials have demonstrated that ASIs decrease blood pressure in uncontrolled hypertension as well as urinary albumin excretion in proteinuric chronic kidney disease. Further long-term, double-blind placebo-controlled trial lo trials will evaluate their efficacy in cardiorenal protection when given alone or in combination with SGLT2 inhibitors in patients with and without diabetes [31, 32].

At present, it should be pointed out that no randomised clinical trial has specifically analysed the effect of these various classes of drugs on the various phenotypes of DKD, nor has it directly compared the renal and cardiovascular risk reduction effects of GLP1-RA and SGLT2i in diabetic patients based on the presence or absence of albuminuria as the primary outcome. For this reason, there are still no specific guidelines on the use of these drugs for different phenotypes, but they refer generically to diabetic patients with chronic kidney disease.

Future Directions

At present the main therapeutic milestones for DKD are RAS inhibitors, SGLT21, GLP-1 RAs and MRAs however, despite these therapeutic advances, a substantial residual risk of progression remain and DKD remains a leading cause of ESKD, underlining the need for research to identify new biomarkers and effective treatments. Future directions for preventing CKD and diabetes complication might involve targeting more specifically apoptosis, inflammation and fibrosis as well as regenerative medicine, specifically stem cell-based therapies and will also include combination therapies with complementary mechanism of action along with the identification of the phenotype most likely to benefit of specific interventions.

References

1. NCD Risk Factor Collaboration (NCD-RisC). Worldwide trends in diabetes prevalence and treatment from 1990 to 2022: a pooled analysis of 1108 population-representative studies with 141 million participants. Lancet. 2024;404(10467):2077–93. Erratum in: Lancet. 2025;405(10485):1146.
2. Ruiz-Ortega M, Rodrigues-Diez RR, Lavoz C, Rayego-Mateos S. Special Issue "Diabetic nephropathy: diagnosis, prevention and treatment". J Clin Med. 2020;9(3):813.
3. Brück K, Stel VS, Gambaro G, Hallan S, Völzke H, Ärnlöv J, Kastarinen M, Guessous I, Vinhas J, Stengel B, Brenner H, Chudek J, Romundstad S, Tomson C, Gonzalez AO, Bello AK, Ferrieres J, Palmieri L, Browne G, Capuano V, Van Biesen W, Zoccali C, Gansevoort R, Navis G, Rothenbacher D, Ferraro PM, Nitsch D, Wanner C, Jager KJ, European CKD Burden Consortium. CKD prevalence varies across the European general population. J Am Soc Nephrol. 2016;27(7):2135–47.
4. Hill CJ, Cardwell CR, Patterson CC, Maxwell AP, Magee GM, Young RJ, Matthews B, O'Donoghue DJ, Fogarty DG. Chronic kidney disease and diabetes in the national health service: a cross-sectional survey of the U.K. national diabetes audit. Diabet Med. 2014;31(4):448–54.
5. Tuttle KR, Agarwal R, Alpers CE, Bakris GL, Brosius FC, Kolkhof P, Uribarri J. Molecular mechanisms and therapeutic targets for diabetic kidney disease. Kidney Int. 2022;102(2):248–60.
6. Gupta S, Dominguez M, Golestaneh L. Diabetic kidney disease: an update. Med Clin North Am. 2023;107(4):689–705.
7. Lee K, He JC. AKI-to-CKD transition is a potential mechanism for non-albuminuric diabetic kidney disease. Fac Rev. 2022;11:21.

8. Yau A, Parikh SV, Almaani S. Diabetic kidney disease: the "silent" majority? Kidney Int Rep. 2021;6(12):2939–41.
9. Webster AC, Nagler EV, Morton RL, Masson P. Chronic kidney disease. Lancet. 2017;389(10075):1238–52.
10. Lewis EJ, Hunsicker LG, Bain RP, Rohde RD. The effect of angiotensin-converting-enzyme inhibition on diabetic nephropathy. The Collaborative Study Group. N Engl J Med. 1993;329(20):1456–62.
11. Lewis EJ, Hunsicker LG, Clarke WR, Berl T, Pohl MA, Lewis JB, Ritz E, Atkins RC, Rohde R, Raz I, Collaborative Study Group. Renoprotective effect of the angiotensin-receptor antagonist irbesartan in patients with nephropathy due to type 2 diabetes. N Engl J Med. 2001;345(12):851–60.
12. van Raalte DH, Bjornstad P, Cherney DZI, de Boer IH, Fioretto P, Gordin D, Persson F, Rosas SE, Rossing P, Schaub JA, Tuttle K, Waikar SS, Heerspink HJL. Combination therapy for kidney disease in people with diabetes mellitus. Nat Rev Nephrol. 2024;20(7):433–46.
13. Lv R, Xu L, Che L, Liu S, Wang Y, Dong B. Cardiovascular-renal protective effect and molecular mechanism of finerenone in type 2 diabetic mellitus. Front Endocrinol (Lausanne). 2023;14:1125693.
14. Bakris GL, Agarwal R, Anker SD, Pitt B, Ruilope LM, Rossing P, Kolkhof P, Nowack C, Schloemer P, Joseph A, Filippatos G, FIDELIO-DKD Investigators. Effect of finerenone on chronic kidney disease outcomes in type 2 diabetes. N Engl J Med. 2020;383(23):2219–29.
15. Pitt B, Filippatos G, Agarwal R, Anker SD, Bakris GL, Rossing P, Joseph A, Kolkhof P, Nowack C, Schloemer P, Ruilope LM, FIGARO-DKD Investigators. Cardiovascular events with finerenone in kidney disease and type 2 diabetes. N Engl J Med. 2021;385(24):2252–63.
16. Agarwal R, Filippatos G, Pitt B, Anker SD, Rossing P, Joseph A, Kolkhof P, Nowack C, Gebel M, Ruilope LM, Bakris GL, FIDELIO-DKD and FIGARO-DKD investigators. Cardiovascular and kidney outcomes with finerenone in patients with type 2 diabetes and chronic kidney disease: the FIDELITY pooled analysis. Eur Heart J. 2022;43(6):474–84. Erratum in: Eur Heart J. 2022;43(20):1989.
17. Fried LF, Emanuele N, Zhang JH, Brophy M, Conner TA, Duckworth W, Leehey DJ, McCullough PA, O'Connor T, Palevsky PM, Reilly RF, Seliger SL, Warren SR, Watnick S, Peduzzi P, Guarino P, VA NEPHRON-D Investigators. Combined angiotensin inhibition for the treatment of diabetic nephropathy. N Engl J Med. 2013;369(20):1892–903. Erratum in: N Engl J Med. 2014;158:A7255.
18. Parving HH, Brenner BM, McMurray JJ, de Zeeuw D, Haffner SM, Solomon SD, Chaturvedi N, Persson F, Desai AS, Nicolaides M, Richard A, Xiang Z, Brunel P, Pfeffer MA, ALTITUDE Investigators. Cardiorenal end points in a trial of aliskiren for type 2 diabetes. N Engl J Med. 2012;367(23):2204–13.
19. Zuo C, Xu G. Efficacy and safety of mineralocorticoid receptor antagonists with ACEI/ARB treatment for diabetic nephropathy: a meta-analysis. Int J Clin Pract. 2019;73:e13413.
20. Bae JH. SGLT2 inhibitors and GLP-1 receptor agonists in diabetic kidney disease: evolving evidence and clinical application. Diabetes Metab J. 2025;49(3):386–402.
21. American Diabetes Association Professional Practice Committee. 9. Pharmacologic approaches to glycemic treatment: standards of care in diabetes—2025. Diabetes Care. 2025;48(Supplement 1):S181–206.
22. Perkovic V, Jardine MJ, Neal B, Bompoint S, Heerspink HJL, Charytan DM, Edwards R, Agarwal R, Bakris G, Bull S, Cannon CP, Capuano G, Chu PL, de Zeeuw D, Greene T, Levin A, Pollock C, Wheeler DC, Yavin Y, Zhang H, Zinman B, Meininger G, Brenner BM, Mahaffey KW, CREDENCE Trial Investigators. Canagliflozin and renal outcomes in type 2 diabetes and nephropathy. N Engl J Med. 2019;380(24):2295–306.
23. Heerspink HJL, Stefánsson BV, Correa-Rotter R, Chertow GM, Greene T, Hou FF, Mann JFE, McMurray JJV, Lindberg M, Rossing P, Sjöström CD, Toto RD, Langkilde AM, Wheeler DC, DAPA-CKD Trial Committees and Investigators. Dapagliflozin in patients with chronic kidney disease. N Engl J Med. 2020;383(15):1436–46.

24. The EMPA-KIDNEY Collaborative Group, Herrington WG, Staplin N, Wanner C, Green JB, Hauske SJ, Emberson JR, Preiss D, Judge P, Mayne KJ, Ng SYA, Sammons E, Zhu D, Hill M, Stevens W, Wallendszus K, Brenner S, Cheung AK, Liu ZH, Li J, Hooi LS, Liu W, Kadowaki T, Nangaku M, Levin A, Cherney D, Maggioni AP, Pontremoli R, Deo R, Goto S, Rossello X, Tuttle KR, Steubl D, Petrini M, Massey D, Eilbracht J, Brueckmann M, Landray MJ, Baigent C, Haynes R. Empagliflozin in patients with chronic kidney disease. N Engl J Med. 2023;388(2):117–27.
25. Mann JFE, Ørsted DD, Brown-Frandsen K, Marso SP, Poulter NR, Rasmussen S, Tornøe K, Zinman B, Buse JB, LEADER Steering Committee and Investigators. Liraglutide and renal outcomes in type 2 diabetes. N Engl J Med. 2017;377(9):839–48.
26. Marso SP, Bain SC, Consoli A, Eliaschewitz FG, Jódar E, Leiter LA, Lingvay I, Rosenstock J, Seufert J, Warren ML, Woo V, Hansen O, Holst AG, Pettersson J, Vilsbøll T, SUSTAIN-6 Investigators. Semaglutide and cardiovascular outcomes in patients with type 2 diabetes. N Engl J Med. 2016;375(19):1834–44.
27. Gerstein HC, Colhoun HM, Dagenais GR, Diaz R, Lakshmanan M, Pais P, Probstfield J, Botros FT, Riddle MC, Rydén L, Xavier D, Atisso CM, Dyal L, Hall S, Rao-Melacini P, Wong G, Avezum A, Basile J, Chung N, Conget I, Cushman WC, Franek E, Hancu N, Hanefeld M, Holt S, Jansky P, Keltai M, Lanas F, Leiter LA, Lopez-Jaramillo P, Cardona Munoz EG, Pirags V, Pogosova N, Raubenheimer PJ, Shaw JE, Sheu WH, Temelkova-Kurktschiev T, REWIND Investigators. Dulaglutide and renal outcomes in type 2 diabetes: an exploratory analysis of the REWIND randomised, placebo-controlled trial. Lancet. 2019;394(10193):131–8.
28. Holman RR, Bethel MA, Mentz RJ, Thompson VP, Lokhnygina Y, Buse JB, Chan JC, Choi J, Gustavson SM, Iqbal N, Maggioni AP, Marso SP, Öhman P, Pagidipati NJ, Poulter N, Ramachandran A, Zinman B, Hernandez AF, EXSCEL Study Group. Effects of once-weekly exenatide on cardiovascular outcomes in type 2 diabetes. N Engl J Med. 2017;377(13):1228–39.
29. Perkovic V, Tuttle KR, Rossing P, Mahaffey KW, Mann JFE, Bakris G, Baeres FMM, Idorn T, Bosch-Traberg H, Lausvig NL, Pratley R, FLOW Trial Committees and Investigators. Effects of semaglutide on chronic kidney disease in patients with type 2 diabetes. N Engl J Med. 2024;391(2):109–21.
30. Apperloo EM, Tuttle KR, Pavo I, Haupt A, Taylor R, Wiese RJ, Hemmingway A, Cherney DZI, Sattar N, Heerspink HJL. Tirzepatide associated with reduced albuminuria in participants with type 2 diabetes: pooled post hoc analysis from the randomized active- and placebo-controlled SURPASS-1-5 clinical trials. Diabetes Care. 2025;48(3):430–6.
31. Tuttle KR, Hauske SJ, Canziani ME, Caramori ML, Cherney D, Cronin L, Heerspink HJL, Hugo C, Nangaku M, Rotter RC, Silva A, Shah SV, Sun Z, Urbach D, de Zeeuw D, Rossing P, ASi in CKD Group. Efficacy and safety of aldosterone synthase inhibition with and without empagliflozin for chronic kidney disease: a randomised, controlled, phase 2 trial. Lancet. 2024;403(10424):379–90.
32. Helmeczi W, Hundemer GL. Targeting aldosterone to improve cardiorenal outcomes: from nonsteroidal mineralocorticoid receptor antagonists to aldosterone synthase inhibitors. Curr Opin Nephrol Hypertens. 2025;34(3):241–6.

Preeclampsia and Hypertension in Pregnancy in Women Living with CKD

Massimo Torreggiani, Rosella Attini, Nora Schwotzer, Elisa Longhitano, and Giorgina Barbara Piccoli

Introduction

Chronic kidney disease (CKD) is an umbrella term encompassing all kidney diseases, with different etiologies and different levels of kidney function impairment. Hypertension is a frequent companion of CKD, especially in the presence of kidney function impairment or in glomerular diseases. During pregnancy, the presence of both CKD and hypertension can affect the developing fetus and the mother and has been associated with miscarriage, intrauterine death, fetal growth restriction, the full spectrum of hypertensive disorders of pregnancy (HDP), and prematurity. The risks increase as kidney function declines and are modulated by baseline hypertension and proteinuria [1]. The effects of pregnancy on maternal kidney function are variable, potentially leading to a progressive loss of kidney function, onset or worsening of hypertension with lifelong consequences. While evidence is scant, due also to the lack of studies with long-term maternal follow-up, it is conceivable that having developed an HDP is associated with faster CKD progression [2–4].

M. Torreggiani (✉) · G. B. Piccoli (✉)
Néphrologie et Dialyse, Centre Hospitalier Le Mans, Le Mans, France

R. Attini
Department of Obstetrics and Gynecology, Nuovo Ospedale degli Infermi, Ponderano, Biella, Italy

N. Schwotzer
Service de Néphrologie et d'Hypertension, Département de Médecine, Centre Hospitalier Universitaire Vaudois, and Université de Lausanne, Lausanne, Switzerland

E. Longhitano
Unit of Nephrology and Dialysis, Department of Clinical and Experimental Medicine, A.O.U. "G.Martino", University of Messina, Messina, Italy

P. Sarafidis, R. Pontremoli (eds.), *Hypertension and Chronic Kidney Disease*, Updates in Hypertension and Cardiovascular Protection,
https://doi.org/10.1007/978-3-032-29564-4_9

The exact prevalence of CKD in pregnancy is not known. In childbearing age, stage 1 and 2 CKD are estimated to affect around 3% of women and between 0.01% and 0.5% in later CKD stages [5–7]. However, since complex alterations of hormonal balance and fertility occur in the later CKD stages, the probability for a woman with advanced CKD to become pregnant may be lower, thus reducing the expected prevalence [8, 9].

In pregnancy, as also acknowledged by the recent KDIGO controversies conference, women with CKD should ideally be managed by maternal-fetal medicine specialists, and nephrologists trained in obstetric nephrology. Of note, a "sub-specialization" corresponding to what, in kidney medicine, is often referred to "obstetric nephrology" does not exist in obstetrics, perhaps due to the misconception that fertility is significantly reduced in women with CKD and that pregnancies in women with CKD are exceptional [8–10].

This chapter discusses the current evidence on hypertension in pregnancy in women with CKD, the recent advances in management, and the risks for the mother and the fetus.

Hypertensive Disorders of Pregnancy: A Mixed-Box of Diseases

Hypertension is a harbinger, a marker and a risk factor for adverse pregnancy outcomes (APOs).

The clinical course of CKD in pregnancy is strongly associated with its severity at presentation, including in this term the three main elements of kidney function impairment, proteinuria and hypertension. Developing hypertension, whether or not in the context of preeclampsia (PE), is associated with higher odds of persistent post-pregnancy hypertension and, at least in some diseases, like IgA nephropathy, to CKD progression [11, 12].

The definition of HDP is broad and includes pregestational chronic hypertension, gestational hypertension, preeclampsia (PE), superimposed PE and other categories, such as white coat hypertension or masked hypertension, with subtle differences among guidelines (Table 1) [13–19].

Of note, the term superimposed PE is often used in the nephrology setting to indicate PE occurring on the basis of CKD, but this relationship is not included in most international pregnancy guidelines, with the exception of the Japanese ones [19]. This is not just a semantic difference since superimposed PE seems to have different patterns, occurring later in pregnancy and being more compatible with an expectant management [20].

Interestingly, both masked and white coat hypertension, whose clinical relevance is not always clear, are associated with APOs, thus indirectly highlighting the importance of strict blood pressure control during pregnancy [21, 22].

The discussion whether HDP are separate diseases or belong to a continuum with different severity is still open. Figure 1 schematically reports the hypothesis of a continuum of disease, from pregnancy-induced hypertension to HELLP (hemolysis, elevated liver enzymes, low platelets) syndrome [23]. While the interpretation of a

Table 1 Definition of hypertensive disorders of pregnancy according to national and international guidelines

	SOCG, (2014) [14]	SOMANZ, (2014) [15]	ISSHP, (2018) [13]	RCOG, (2019) [16]	ACOG, (2020) [17]	JSSHP, (2021) [19]	FIGO, (2021) [18]
Chronic hypertension	HTN diagnosed before 20 GW Associated to comorbid conditions with superimposed PE	HTN diagnosed before 20 GW	Two measurement detection (hours apart during the same visit or in two consecutive visits) of HTN before 20 GW	HTN diagnosed before 20 GW or use of antihypertensive drugs when referred at first visit	Two measurement detection (at least 4 h apart) of HTN before 20 GW	HTN diagnosed before 20 GW, that persists beyond 12 weeks postpartum and no features of superimposed PE	Aligned with ISSHP criteria
Gestational hypertension	New-onset HTN diagnosed after 20 GW associated to comorbid conditions with evidence of PE	New-onset HTN diagnosed after 20 GW, followed by return of pregestational levels within 3 months postpartum	New-onset HTN diagnosed at or after 20 GW Absence of features of PE	New-onset HTN diagnosed after 20 GW and no proteinuria	Two measurement detection (at least 4 h apart) of new-onset HTN after 20 GW	De novo HTN that develops at or after 20 GW that normalizes by 12 weeks postpartum and no features of superimposed PE	Aligned with ISSHP criteria

(continued)

Table 1 (continued)

	SOCG, (2014) [14]	SOMANZ, (2014) [15]	ISSHP, (2018) [13]	RCOG, (2019) [16]	ACOG, (2020) [17]	JSSHP, (2021) [19]	FIGO, (2021) [18]
Preeclampsia (PE)	Gestational HTN with at least one of the following: New-onset proteinuria "Adverse conditions" (involvement of organ system)[a] "Severe adverse complications"[b]	New-onset HTN after 20 GW with at least one of the following: Proteinuria, AKI, thrombocytopenia, hemolysis, DIC, raised ALT and AST, epigastric or right upper quadrant pain, eclampsia, hyperreflexia with sustained clonus, persistent headache, visual disturbances, PRES, stroke, pulmonary edema, fetal growth restriction	Gestational hypertension with at least one of the following: Proteinuria Other maternal organ dysfunction[c] Uteroplacental dysfunction (such as fetal growth restriction, abnormal umbilical artery Doppler wave form analysis, or stillbirth)	Aligned with ISSHP criteria	New-onset HTN between 20 GW up to 2 weeks postpartum, with one or more of the following: Proteinuria ($\geq$0.3 g/24 h or PCR $\geq$ 0.3 g/g or dipstick 2+) AKI, AST or ALT doubling, pulmonary edema, thrombocytopenia, headache with visual symptoms or unresponsive to medications	Gestational HTN and one or more of the following new-onset conditions at or after 20 GW and normalize by 12 weeks postpartum: Proteinuria Other maternal organ dysfunction, including: Liver involvement without underlying diseases; progressive renal dysfunction; stroke, neurological complications; hematological complications Uteroplacental dysfunction (fetal growth restriction, abnormal umbilical artery doppler waveform analysis, or stillbirth)	Aligned with ISSHP criteria

Superimposed Preeclampsia	Chronic HTN with at least one of the following: Resistant HTN, new-onset or worsening of proteinuria, one or more "adverse conditions",[a] one or more "severe complications"[b]	Chronic HTN with, after 20 GW, at least one of the systemic signs of PE	PE developing on chronic hypertension or new-onset proteinuria in the setting of a rise in blood pressure	Aligned with ISSHP criteria	Chronic HTN and development of proteinuria	HTN diagnosed prior to pregnancy or before 20 GW followed after 20 GW by: Uteroplacental dysfunction developing after 20 GW; proteinuria; liver or renal involvement without any underlying diseases; stroke, neurological complications; hematological complications HTN and proteinuria diagnosed before pregnancy or before 20 GW, with one or both symptoms worsening after 20 GW Renal disease diagnosed prior to pregnancy or before 20 GW and HTN developing after 20 GW	Aligned with ISSHP criteria

(continued)

Table 1 (continued)

	SOCG, (2014) [14]	SOMANZ, (2014) [15]	ISSHP, (2018) [13]	RCOG, (2019) [16]	ACOG, (2020) [17]	JSSHP, (2021) [19]	FIGO, (2021) [18]
Other hypertensive categories	Aligned with ISSHP criteria		White coat HTN: Normal domiciliary pressure and detection at office/clinic of BP ≥140/90 mmHg Masked HTN: Normal at a clinic or office measurement, diagnosed by 24 h ABPM or HBPM.		White coat HTN: Normal domiciliary pressure and detection at office/clinic of BP ≥140/90 mmHg		

[a]CNS (headache, visual symptoms, seizure, etc.); –Cardiorespiratory (chest pain, hypoxia, poorly controlled HTN, etc.); –Hematologic (thrombocytopenia, elevated INR or PTT; –Renal (elevated uric acid, AKI); –Hepatic (elevated AST and/or ALT, right upper quadrant pain, hypoalbuminemia, etc.); –Feto-placental system (abnormal fetal heart rate, oligohydramnios, stillbirth, etc.)

[b]CNS (eclampsia, PRES, cortical blindness, Glasgow coma scale 13, stroke, TIA or RIND); –cardiorespiratory (uncontrolled severe HTN over 12 h, oxygen saturation < 90%, pulmonary edema, positive inotropic support, or myocardial ischemia or infarction); –hematologic (thrombocytopenia $<50 \times 10^9$/L or transfusion of any blood product); –renal (AKI or new indication for dialysis); –hepatic (INR.2 in the absence of DIC or warfarin); –Feto-placental system (abruption with evidence of maternal or fetal compromise, reverse ductus venosus A wave, or stillbirth)

[c]AKI; –liver involvement (ALT or AST > 40 IU/L) with or without right upper quadrant or epigastric abdominal pain; –neurological complications (eclampsia, altered mental status, blindness, stroke, clonus, severe headaches, persistent visual scotomata); –hematological complications (thrombocytopenia, DIC, hemolysis)

ACOG American College of Obstetricians and Gynecologists, *ACC/AHA* American College of Cardiology/American Heart Association, *DGGG* Deutsche Gesellschaft für Gynäkologie und Geburtshilfe, *ESC/ESH* European Society of Cardiology/European Society of Hypertension, *FIGO* The International Federation of Gynecology and Obstetrics, Hypertension Canada, *ISSHP* International Society for the Study of Hypertension in Pregnancy, *NICE* National Institute for Health and Care Excellence, Ireland, *SOMANZ* Society of Obstetric Medicine of Australia and New Zealand, *Queensland* Queensland Clinical Guideline, *JSSHP* Japan Society for the Study of Hypertension in Pregnancy, *AKI* acute kidney injury, *DIC* disseminated intravascular coagulation, *ALT* alanine aminotransferase, *AST* aspartate amino transferase, *GW* gestational week, *PE* preeclampsia, *BP* blood pressure, *HTN* hypertension, *ABPM* ambulatory blood pressure monitoring, *HBPM* home blood pressure monitoring

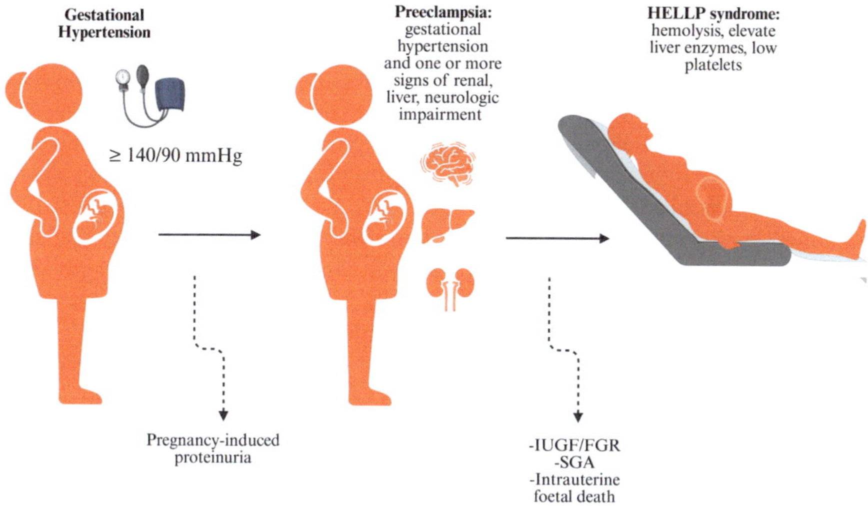

Fig. 1 Hypothesis of a continuum of severity of the hypertensive disorders of pregnancy. (Modified from Ref. 23). (Created in https://BioRender.com)

continuum with progressive endothelial damage is quite appealing, it should be noted that hypertension, albeit frequent, is not a constant finding in HELLP syndrome, nor is it implicit in its definition.

Preeclampsia and Its Relationship with CKD

Preeclampsia is the best known and studied among the HDP and it is estimated to affect between 2% and 5% of pregnancies, according to the clinical and demographic characteristics of the population. When assessed per woman, its prevalence increases to 5–7.5%. Indeed, its incidence may be as low as 1% in low-risk groups, such as kidney donors (pre-donation) and rise to over 20% after a previous HDP. The incidence of HDP in women living with CKD is less known, both on the account of their different definitions and of the heterogeneity of the available cohorts as for CKD cause, stage and prevalence of baseline hypertension [24–28].

Indeed, PE is a heterogeneous disorder whose definition changed over time. The classic definition of hypertension and proteinuria arising after 20 gestational weeks (GW) in a previously normotensive woman without proteinuria was expanded to hypertension, within the same time frame, associated to signs of end-organ damage, encompassing liver, kidneys, central nervous system and hematologic derangements, as well as fetal growth impairment (Table 1). Acknowledging its heterogeneity, there have been several attempts to classify PE, for instance according to its clinical presentation or time of onset: early versus late (before or after 34 GW); mild versus severe (according to blood pressure ≥ 160/110 mmHg and/or presence of organ damage). Moreover, a clinical syndrome mimicking PE can occur even within days or weeks after delivery, thus leading to the definition of postpartum PE (Table 2) [29]. No classification, however, fully corresponds to the clinical practice as, even if early PE is often more severe, late forms may still be life-threatening.

The placenta plays a central role in PE pathophysiology and impaired placentation is considered the key mechanism, which may be highlighted by an imbalance between angiogenic and anti-angiogenic factors, ultimately leading to endothelial dysfunction and impaired placental function. The two markers presently widely used in the clinical setting to monitor placental alterations are the anti-angiogenic soluble fsm-like tyrosine kinase-1 (sFLT-1), which is produced by the placenta and binds the angiogenic placenta growth factor (PlGF) and the vascular endothelial growth factor (VEGF). When sFLT1 binds to PlGF, this prevents the physiological binding to VEGF receptor 1 and 2, leading to endothelial dysfunction and altered

Table 2 Approaches to the classification of PE according to severity, time of onset, and pathogenesis

Classification based on severity	**Mild PE** 160/110 mmHg < BP ≤ 140/90 mmHg Proteinuria <5.0 g/24 h **Severe PE** Signs of impairment of CNS. Liver, Pulmonary edema, Kidney, with oliguria <500 ml/24 h, Uncontrolled hypertension, Biochemistry: Proteinuria > = 5 g/24 h, Thrombocytopenia <10⁹/L. IUGR
Classification based on the time of onset	**Early PE** Onset <34 gestation weeks, or < 32 weeks **Late PE** Onset ≥34 gestation weeks, or ≥ 32 weeks **Postpartum PE** Onset after delivery
Classification based on the proposed pathogenesis	**Placental PE** With signs of placental malperfusion **Maternal PE** With presence of maternal risk factors (obesity, diabetes, CKD, hypertension) **Angiogenic PE** With angiogenic factors imbalance (sFlt-1/PlGF, sEnd, etc) **Non-angiogenic PE** Without angiogenic imbalance (highly suggestive of CKD), or late angiogenic imbalance **Superimposed PE** PE onset in women affected by HTA or by CKD

Modified from Ref. (23)

placental function [30]. After the 20th week of gestation, the sFLT1-to-PlGF ratio has demonstrated a very high (about 95%) negative predictive value to rule out the development of PE within the next 4 weeks. The test is widely used in Europe, and has been recently granted approval of the Food and Drug Administration to assess the risk of PE in women hospitalized for HDP [31–33]. Nevertheless, as mentioned above, PE may present different clinical phenotypes, suggesting that other mechanisms, not necessarily of initial placental origin, can contribute to its development [34–38]. For example, animal studies have shown that an impaired regulation of L-kynurenine (a metabolite of L-tryptophan involved in maintaining immune tolerance and placental health during pregnancy) can mimic PE symptoms, especially in cases of reduced nephron mass [39, 40].

According to an interesting hypothesis, placental PE, primarily due to uteroplacental ischemia, differs from maternal PE, which is due to vascular dysfunction linked to maternal factors, including hypertension, diabetes or obesity [41]. Placental PE is characterized by the secretion of factors by the suffering placenta that, in turn, cause endothelial damage, leading to hypertension and multi-organ impairment. This presentation typically occurs early in pregnancy and is accompanied by fetal growth restriction and secretion of anti-angiogenic factors. Maternal PE, instead, is characterized by a normal initial placental anatomy and fetal growth, and late alteration of angiogenic-anti-angiogenic balance. Ultimately, the two forms converge to promote endothelial dysfunction. The final result can be either widespread (as in HELLP syndrome) or organ-specific damage such as acute kidney injury or eclampsia [23, 41].

Early-onset PE is overall characterized by a poor prognosis, high risk of fetal loss, early preterm delivery and severe maternal hypertension and proteinuria [41]. Maternal PE, instead, depends more on maternal comorbidities, such as CKD, and impacts on the last phase of fetal growth [42]. Noteworthy, even if it is usually thought that only severe forms of PE should be followed up after delivery to screen for kidney disease, women who experience late PE-HDP should benefit of a dedicated follow-up, in keeping with the association with maternal risk factors [43].

Alternative, and probably additive, pathogenetic mechanisms involve oxidative stress, inflammation, immune alterations and a pro-thrombotic state. All are common to PE and CKD and all potentially leading to endothelial activation and dysfunction (Fig. 2) [17, 44, 45].

At the kidney level, injured podocytes may detach from the glomerular basement membrane, leading to podocyturia and proteinuria. It has been reported that podocyturia anticipates the clinical onset of PE; however, beside the technical requirements for identifying podocytes in the urine, podocyturia is not a specific marker of PE as it has been described in women with chronic hypertension, diabetes, connective tissue disorders or CKD [46–48]. Lupus nephritis is an example of a situation in which the presence of podocyte in the urines is frequent, irrespective of pregnancy complications [49].

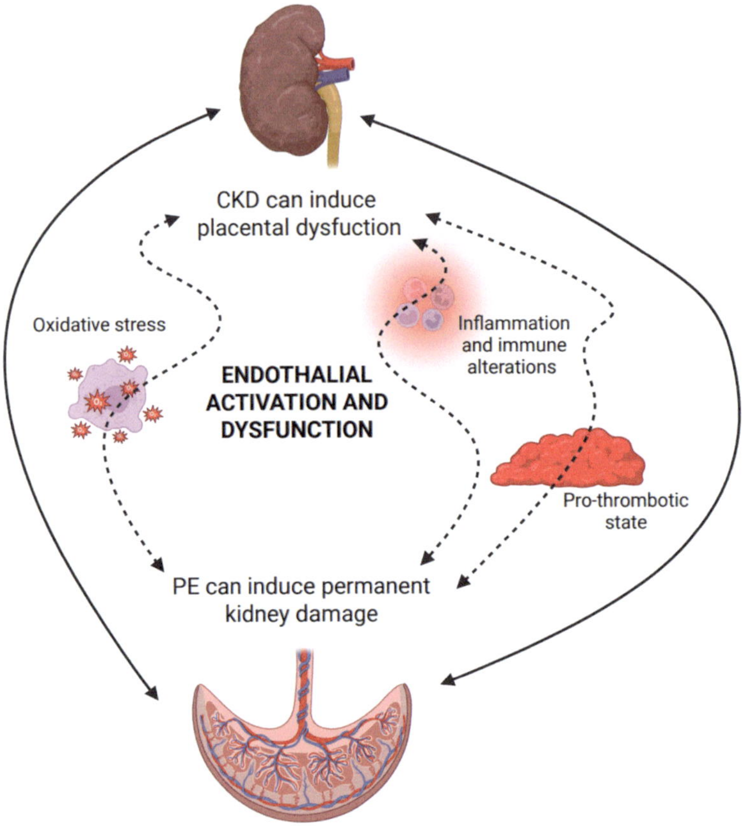

Fig. 2 From the placenta to the kidney and from the kidney to the placenta. (Modified from Ref. 45). (Created in https://BioRender.com)

Endotheliosis is considered the characteristic histopathological lesion associated with PE. However, in only 55% of women affected by PE endotheliosis is described at the kidney biopsy, while its presence has been reported also in a small series of kidney biopsies performed in normal pregnancies [50]. Podocyte swelling and intra-glomerular cell proliferation and activation of parietal epithelial cells in podocyte deprived areas may also be present [51]. Podocyte damage and defective podocyte turnover may explain why focal segmental glomerulosclerosis is the most prevalent lesion identified in kidney biopsies in women who had experienced PE [4, 52, 53]. Wider availability of data on podocyturia and placental angiogenic markers is needed to refine our understanding and classification of PE, in particular on the background of CKD [54].

Chronic Kidney Disease: Definitions and Diagnostic Indicators with Reference to Pregnancy

CKD is broadly defined as any disease affecting the kidneys, lasting for at least 3 months, characterized by one or more of the following: reduction in kidney function (assessed on the basis of an estimated glomerular filtration rate—eGFR) below 60 mL/min per 1.73 m^2 of body surface; anomalies in renal imaging (for example, single kidney or kidney scars); or persistent anomalies in the composition of blood and urine (proteinuria and hematuria). This wide definition also includes tubular disorders, such as renal tubular acidosis and hypercalciuria [44].

This definition of CKD, now employed for more than 20 years, highlights the importance of the initial phases of kidney disease, when kidney function is still normal [55]. Serum creatinine is the main marker of renal function. However, due to the large renal functional reserve, serum creatinine starts increasing only when more than 50% of the renal tissue has been damaged and, as a consequence, early CKD is not diagnosable if serum creatinine is the only parameter considered. Furthermore, while CKD with normal kidney function probably accounts for over 90% of kidney diseases in pregnancy, it is often asymptomatic in the absence of severe proteinuria, or of systemic involvement, as in lupus nephropathy. With respect to pregnancy, CKD is the most common cause of secondary hypertension in a young, non-obese woman, and its presence should always be excluded in the diagnostic work-up of juvenile hypertension, before or during pregnancy [56].

Pregnancy modifies blood pressure, kidney function, and renal imaging, and acknowledging these changes is important for early diagnosis and timely treatment.

Blood Pressure in Pregnancy

During pregnancy, following fine hormonal regulation, vasodilation occurs mainly due to elevated levels of progesterone, prostacyclin, nitric oxide (NO) and relaxin [8, 57, 58]. Consequently, increased activity of the renin-angiotensin-aldosterone system occurs [8, 59, 60]. Unexpectedly, a reduction in blood pressure and an increase in cardiac output occurs [58–60]. This probably occurs in a condition of reduced sensitivity to angiotensin II which allows the maintenance of low pressure levels despite volume expansion, the latter being necessary for placental perfusion [59–61]. As a result, since the early stages of pregnancy, blood pressure drops by 10–20 mmHg, as a normal physiological adaptation to support fetal growth and improve placental perfusion.

Interestingly, while the American Heart Association now lowered the threshold of hypertension to 130/80 mmHg, this new, albeit controversial, definition is not taken into account in pregnancy and the current guidelines still define new-onset hypertension as blood pressure (BP) $\geq$ 140/90 mmHg at or after 20 gestation weeks [10, 13, 15–17, 62–70]. According to these definitions, new-onset HDP are found in over 10% of pregnancies, and are experienced by at least 15% of women, but the prevalence would increase if the new definitions were applied. The prevalence of chronic hypertension is classically estimated as present in 1–2% of pregnancies, but once more according to the classic definitions [41]. Apart from the higher susceptibility of women of Afro-American ethnicity, the prevalence of chronic hypertension in pregnancy is rising, as shown by a population-based cross-sectional study of more than 150 million hospital deliveries in the United States, where its increase was strictly related to the higher maternal age and body mass index (BMI) [23].

Physiologically, blood pressure is expected to increase again to pre-pregnancy values after pregnancy, at difference with what is expected after pregnancy-induced hypertension or PE. This protective antihypertensive effect is present in isolated "essential" hypertension and in secondary forms, and its loss at delivery may at least partially explain the uncommon, but potentially severe event of "postpartum pre-eclampsia". Furthermore, anemia, that is frequent in the postpartum phase (up to 8 weeks postpartum), may mask hypertension, which may become evident only a few weeks later, once anemia is corrected [71].

Conversely, while hypertension normalizes shortly, usually within one month postpartum in most cases with HDP, normalization may be slower, in particular in the presence of comorbid factors, such as obesity or CKD, and up to 20% of previously normotensive (or considered as normotensive) women may remain hypertensive in the long term [72]. It is not known whether previously unrecognized HTA is the cause or the effect of this persistent hypertension, or the endothelial and renal damage induced by PE-HDP has reached a point of no return. In any case, the possibility of delayed resolution, or new-onset hypertension after delivery should be kept in mind, for timely identification and treatment of hypertensive women in childbearing age [72].

Kidney Function Assessment in Pregnancy

In women diagnosed with CKD, or at risk of CKD, kidney function should be assessed before the start of pregnancy, so that CKD stage can be determined. However, serum creatinine is not routinely performed at pregestational assessment and during pregnancy and, as far, only few nephrology societies advocated its inclusion amog other lab tests [73]. Since the start of pregnancy, renal plasma flow and glomerular filtration rate (GFR) increase, with a consequent reduction in serum creatinine that can mask mild renal insufficiency [5, 58]. There are currently no reference values for GFR in pregnancy and none of the formulas on which the estimation of GFR is currently based (Cockcroft and Gault, Modification of Diet in Renal Disease—MDRD—and Chronic Kidney Disease Epidemiology Collaboration—CKD-EPI) has been validated in pregnancy. While some authors still use a formula, generally CKD-EPI, others maintain that it is better to base evaluations on serum creatinine measurement [74]. Two recent systematic reviews indicates that the normal range of serum creatinine should decrease by about

20–30% starting in early pregnancy [57, 75]. Of note, the hyperfiltration response during pregnancy is usually preserved in CKD and a decrease in serum creatinine is a favorable prognostic marker even in advanced CKD stages and after kidney transplantation [76].

In women developing HDP or APOs, especially on a background of CKD, this physiological decrease is not always observed, and its abesence has a negative prognostic value. Even more, an increase in serum creatinine, up to the configuration of acute kidney injury (AKI) is now considered as a sign of PE, even in the absence of proteinuria. While AKI is usually reversible, its association with progressive kidney function impairment should be borne in mind [29].

Creatinine clearance, based on 24-h urine collection, is the gold standard for kidney function assessment in pregnancy [77]. While it is currently used in some countries (Italy, France), in others it is considered too demanding; the risk of pre-analytical errors needs to be considered, but the advantage of having a precise assessment of proteinuria and kidney function is valuable, especially in advanced CKD. Uric acid level decreases in physiological pregnancies, and the level is correlated with pregnancy outcomes, but this decrease is not always observed in CKD regardless of APOs, and the relationship is not strong enough to be considered a reliable biomarker of APOs.

On the account of the physiological glomerular hyperfiltration during pregnancy, the physiological upper limit of proteinuria is increased to 0.3 g per day; alternatives to 24-h urine collection include dipstick evaluation, the ratio between proteinuria and creatininuria (UPCR) or between albuminuria and creatininuria (UACR). The significance of proteinuria in the context of CKD is quite different from the setting of preeclampsia. In women with CKD proteinuria often increases in pregnancy, and may appear in the context of interstitial diseases, in which it is rare outside the context of pregnancy. Conversely, in immunological kidney diseases, an increase in proteinuria can be a sign of a disease flare [2]. In CKD, a significant relationship between baseline proteinuria and adverse pregnancy outcomes is well described [78]. However, an increase in proteinuria, even when associated with low albumin levels, should not be considered an indication for delivery per se, and should be discussed on a case-by-case basis, given the high heterogeneity of kidney diseases. Fetal growth and uteroplacental flows should prime the decision.

The issue of microhematuria is likewise complex. While pre-existing microhematuria defines the presence of CKD and is, as all CKDs, associated with an increased risk of APOs, microhematuria is found in up to 20% of low-risk pregnancies and is therefore of limited importance when first found in pregnancy [79].

The reversibility of both physiological and pathological functional changes is variable; in physiological pregnancies serum creatinine usually increases rapidly after delivery and decreases after AKI, while high-level proteinuria may take a few months to normalize, even if a drop in proteinuria is commonly observed shortly after delivery, especially in the absence of underlying CKD.

Renal Imaging in Pregnancy

Renal imaging is likewise modified by pregnancy. Kidney size increases on average by about 1 cm in longitudinal diameter [5]. Thus, small kidneys may appear normal in pregnancy. Even though the relationship between size and function varies, considering the normal non-pregnant range of kidney length of 9–13 cm, a measure below 10 cm in pregnancy should be regarded with concern. Similarly, the urinary tract increases in size and physiological pelvicalyceal dilatation is more pronounced (and often only evident) on the right side [80]. Conversely, bilateral or predominantly left dilatation are grounds for suspecting an obstruction, such as kidney stones, potentially predisposed by pregnancy-induced hypercalciuria, or malformations of the pyeloureteral junction exacerbated by pregnancy. In case of doubt, renal morphology should be re-assessed 4–6 months after delivery. Conversely, no difference in kidney Doppler flows has been reported in pregnancy and renal artery ultrasounds maintain their value in this context, potentially allowing for the diagnosis of renal artery stenosis, Finally, intrarenal resistance should drop in pregnancy and high levels maintain the role of marker of vascular kidney impairment in pregnancy [81, 82].

Obstetric-Nephrology Challenges in Women Living with CKD Who Have or Develop Hypertension in Pregnancy

Due to the specific sensitivity of the human brain in pregnancy, the risks of developing severe and possibly long-lasting complications of hypertension during pregnancy should be acknowledged.

Posterior reversible encephalopathy (PRES) syndrome is more common during pregnancy and may occur at lower blood pressure levels than usually observed outside of pregnancy. Cerebral vascular accidents are relatively rare in pregnancy, with an incidence rate that appears to increase during pregnancy, ranging from 4 to 34 cases per 100,000 pregnancies. The highest peak occurs in the first 3 days of postpartum. Mortality is high, accounting for more than 12% of maternal deaths. Among the risk factors we find hypertensive disorders of pregnancy [83].

Acknowledging this increased susceptibility, non-controlled hypertension is one of the reasons why delivery should be promoted to preserve maternal health. Table 3 summarizes the recommendations for delivery of major obstetric guidelines (ACOG, NICE, International Society for the Study of Hypertension in Pregnancy) in the course of HDP [84–87].

While severe hypertension is expected to be more frequent in women living with CKD, none of the current guidelines and recommendations take the presence of CKD into consideration in this regard.

Table 3 Recommendations for the timing of delivery in HDP

	ACOG [84]		International society for the study of hypertension in pregnancy [87]	NICE [85, 86]
Chronic hypertension	*Isolated, uncomplicated, controlled, not requiting medications*	Delivery can be offered at 38^0 to 39^7 GW	Initiation of delivery can be offered at 38^0 to 39^6 GW, but should be advised from 40^0 GW (conditional, low)	Do not offer planned early birth before 37 GW to women with chronic hypertension whose blood pressure is lower than 160/110 mmHg, with or without antihypertensive treatment, unless there are other medical indications After 37 weeks timing of birth should be agreed between the woman and the senior obstetrician
	Isolated, uncomplicated, controlled on medications	Delivery can be offered at 37^0 to 39^7 GW		
	Difficult to control	Delivery can be offered at 36^0 to 37^7 GW		
Gestational hypertension	*Without severe-range blood pressure*	Delivery can be offered at 37^0 GW or at diagnosis if diagnosed later	Initiation of delivery can be offered at 38^0 to 39^6 GW, but should be advised from 40^0 GW (conditional, low) For women who are already at 37^0 GW or later and present with gestational hypertension, initiation of delivery should be discussed (strong, moderate)	Do not offer planned early birth before 37 GW to women with chronic hypertension whose blood pressure is lower than 160/110 mmHg, with or without antihypertensive treatment, unless there are other medical indications After 37 GW timing of birth should be agreed between the woman and the senior obstetrician
	With severe-range blood pressures	Delivery can be offered at 34^0 GW or at diagnosis if diagnosed later		

(continued)

Table 3 (continued)

	ACOG [84]		International society for the study of hypertension in pregnancy [87]	NICE [85, 86]
Preeclampsia	*Without severe features*	Delivery can be offered at 37^0 GW or at diagnosis if diagnosed later	At 34^0–35^6 GW gestation, initiation of delivery should be discussed At 36^0–36^6 GW, initiation of delivery should be considered (strong, moderate) At 37^0 GW or later, initiation of delivery is recommended (strong, high)	Thresholds for considering scheduled preterm birth (before 37 GW) could include (but are not limited to) any of the following known features of severe PE: inability to control maternal blood pressure despite the use of 3 or more classes of antihypertensives in appropriate doses maternal pulsoximetry less than 90% progressive deterioration of liver function, kidney function, hemolysis, or platelet count persistent neurological features, such as severe intractable headache, repeated visual scotomas, or eclampsia placenta detachment inverted end-diastolic flow in umbilical artery Doppler velocimetry, a non-reassuring cardiotocograph, or fetal death.
	With severe features, stable maternal and fetal conditions after fetal viability (includes superimposed)	Delivery can be offered at 34^0 GW or at diagnosis if diagnosed later		
	With severe features, unstable or complicated, after fetal viability (includes superimposed and HELLP)	Soon after maternal stabilization		
	With severe features, before viability	Soon after maternal stabilization		

ACOG American College of Obstetricians and Gynecologists, *NICE* National Institute for Health and Care Excellence, *GW* gestational week, *PE* preeclampsia, *HELLP* hemolysis, elevated liver enzymes, low platelet count syndrome

Effect of Pregnancy and Hypertensive Disorders on CKD

In the early CKD stages, progression of CKD during and after an uncomplicated pregnancy is exceptional, and although immunologic nephropathies may flare in pregnancy, due to the overall better treatment of these conditions, flares are increasingly rare [88]. Conversely, underlining the entangled relationship between APOs and CKD, a faster progression of CKD was reported in the case of IgA nephropathy in women who have experienced PE-HDP, but has not been observed after kidney transplantation, possibly for the overlap between graft dysfunction and PE, both potentially characterized by appearance or increase in proteinuria and appearance of hypertension or worsening in its control [11, 89–91].

Differential Diagnosis Between PE and CKD

Hypertension, proteinuria and impaired kidney function are markers of both PE and CKD, making a differential diagnosis difficult, and sometimes impossible on clinical grounds only. The lack of a clear definition of superimposed PE should also be kept in mind (Table 1) [23].

If PE is clinically diagnosed because of onset or worsening of hypertension and proteinuria, the overlap between PE and CKD is very high. However, if the definition of PE is based on placental health, including fetal growth, Doppler flows and angiogenic-anti-angiogenic patterns (soluble Fms-like tyrosine kinase-1 [sFlt-1] and placental growth factor [PIGF]) the overlap with CKD is considerably reduced (Fig. 3). Of note, a biochemical signature of PE superimposed on CKD has been described, with late and milder alterations in angiogenic marker balance [2, 44, 51, 92, 93]. Although further studies are needed to establish a role for the sFlt-1/PIGF ratio in the differential diagnosis between PE and CKD, their role in ruling out PE in the presence of a normal ratio has been acknowledged by European guidelines and best practices. The differences have a deep clinical importance for allowing

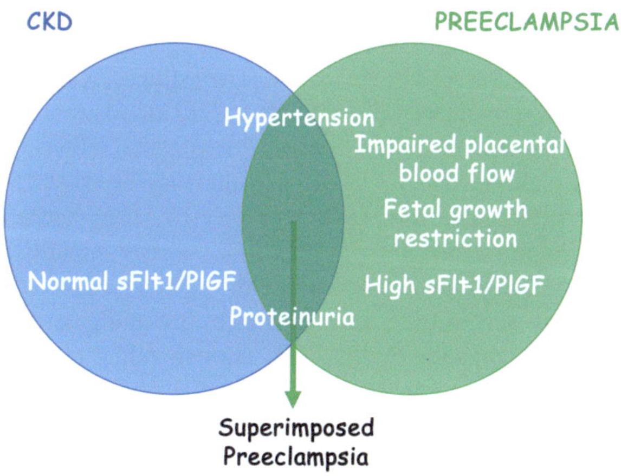

Fig. 3 Overlapping CKD-PE

pregnancy to continue in the absence of, or in case of minimal placental dysfunction [31, 94–96]. Indeed, hypertension and proteinuria due to recurrence of the original disease, chronic allograft nephropathy or reduced nephron mass usually have a better materno-fetal prognosis than PE, at least under careful nephrologic surveillance [10].

In keeping with the association between CKD and late-maternal PE, according to most of the large series, fetal growth restriction is not a predominant feature of early-stage CKD, but is associated with the presence of baseline hypertension and increases in advanced CKD and women undergoing dialysis.

Antihypertensive Treatments in Pregnancy in Women with CKD, HPD and During Breastfeeding

As previously mentioned, blood pressure targets and when to start treatment in the case of hypertension in pregnancy are still a matter of controversy (Table 4).

Indeed the main concern in pregnancy is related to hypercorrection, since hypotension may cause placental hypoperfusion with detrimental effects on the fetus. The issue is similar to diabetes control, as also in these cases hypercorrection and frequent hypoglycaemic episodes may exert negative effects on pregnancy outcomes [97–99].

Of note, no randomized controlled trial was targeted to blood pressure control in pregnant women living with CKD. As recently discussed in the KDIGO controversies conference on women and kidney health, Nephrology societies adopt since at least 20 years lower BP targets, basically the same one adopted in young women out of pregnancy, but none, as far, considers the physiological decrease of blood pressure in pregnancy in setting even lower targets, as acknowledged in the general non-pregnat population [10, 58–60]. Indeed, out of the pregnancy context, the recent results of the ACCORD-BP trial in the CKD subgroup demonstrated, along with the benefits on reduction of cardiovascular events and mortality, a higher risk of AKI [100]. No such data are available in CKD pregnancy.

Once hypertension is diagnosed, the focus is shifted to treatment and monitoring. The Control of Hypertension In Pregnancy Study (CHIPS) and the Chronic Hypertension And Pregnancy (CHAP) studies, respectively in 2015 and 2022, modified the previous nihilist attitude toward blood pressure control, with firstly (CHIPS trial) the demonstration of lack of detrimental effects of optimal BP control in pregnancy, and secondly (CHAP trial) showing the association between strict BP control and better materno-fetal outcomes [101, 102]. Once more these studied are not related to women living with CKD, but their conclusions were widely and rapidly transferred in the nephrology field.

However, to mitigate enthusiasms, no antihypertensive drug is labeled as fully safe in pregnancy by the FDA, corresponding to the old label "C", i.e., drugs in which animal studies showed a potentially harmful effect on the fetus, but for which there were not enough well-controlled studies in humans and the potential benefits in pregnant women may justify their use despite the potential associated risks, and their use or combination is not devoid of side effecst.

Table 4 Classic indications for antihypertensive medication initiation in pregnancy and blood pressure goals in hypertensive disorder of pregnancy according to national and international guidelines

Guideline	Recommended Medication Initiation (mmHg)	Target BP (mmHg)
KDIGO Controversies Conference, 2025 [10]	SBP ≥ 140 DBP ≥ 90	<130 <80
The Netherlands, 2022 [62]	SBP > 140 DBP > 90	130–140 80–90
DGGG, OEGGG, DGfN, 2022 [63]	SBP > 135 DBP > 85	110–135 70–85
Best practice, Italy 2015–2022 [64, 65]	SBP > 140 DBP > 90	130 80
ACOG, 2020 [17]	SBP ≥ 160 DBP ≥ 110	<160 <110
NICE, 2020 [85, 86]	SBP ≥ 140 DBP ≥ 90	135 85
Royal College of Physicians of Ireland, 2019 [66]	SBP ≥ 150 DBP ≥ 100	<150 80–100
ISSHP, 2018 [13]	SBP ≥ 140 DBP ≥ 90	110–140 85
Hypertension Canada, 2018 [67]	SBP ≥ 140 DBP ≥ 90	DBP < 85
ESC/ESH, 2018 [68]	SBP ≥ 150 DBP ≥ 95	<140 <90
Brazilian Guideline of Arterial Hypertension, 2016 [69]	SBP > 150 DBP > 100	130–150 80–100
Queensland, 2016 [70]	SBP ≥ 140 DBP ≥ 90	<140 <90
SOMANZ, 2014 [15]	SBP ≥ 160 DBP ≥ 110	<160 <110

ACOG American College of Obstetricians and Gynecologists, *ACC/AHA* American College of Cardiology/American Heart Association, *DGGG* Deutsche Gesellschaft für Gynäkologie und Geburtshilfe, *ESC/ESH* European Society of Cardiology/European Society of Hypertension, *FIGO* The International Federation of Gynecology and Obstetrics, Hypertension Canada, *ISSHP* International Society for the Study of Hypertension in Pregnancy, *NICE* National Institute for Health and Care Excellence, Ireland, *SOMANZ* Society of Obstetric Medicine of Australia and New Zealand, *Queensland* Queensland Clinical Guideline, *SBP* systolic blood pressure, *DBP* diastolic blood pressure

Three main issues have to be discussed with regard to pharmacological treatment: in patients with pre-existing hypertension, when to discontinue antihypertensive drugs that are at risk of teratogenicity, which drugs choosing as first option in pregnancy and how to combine optimal blood pressure control, nephroprotection and breastfeeding (Table 5).

The teratogenicity of angiotensin-converting enzyme inhibitors (ACEi) and angiotensin II receptor blockers (ARBs) is still a matter of debate, and while some recent reports have even challenged the risk, caution is mandatory. The timing of discontinuation is however still debated: while some groups support pre-emptive discontinuation of ACEi and ARBs, others prefer early discontinuation at the first

Table 5 Antihypertensive drugs in pregnancy: benefit, risk and safety according to FDA

Drugs	Benefit	Risk	Safety according to FDA
Allowed—First choice			
Alpha-methyl dopa	Safety and efficacy	Neuro-depressant side effects. Not be able to correct severe hepertension	B (*no evidence of risk in humans)*
Long acting Niphedipine	No effect in umbelical artery flow	Increase in peripheral edema may be a relevant side effect in CKD patients	C (*risk cannot be ruled out)*
Labetalole	Safety and efficacy (should be avoided in subjects with asthma). May be use for hypertensive urgency	Fetal bradicardia, neonatal hypoglycemia, decresed uteroplacental flow	C (*risk cannot be ruled out)*
Allowed—Second choice			
Pindolole	More effective than alpha-methyldopa in severe hypertension	Hypoglycaemia, hypotension and bradycardia (usually mild and transient)	B (*no evidence of risk in humans)*
Metoprolol	More effective than alpha-methyldopa in severe hypertension	Hypoglycaemia, hypotension and bradycardia (usually mild and transient)	C (*risk cannot be ruled out)*
Clonidine	Efficacy	Unproven safety. Side effects and rebounds at discontinuation are common. Fetal growth impairment also reported	C (*risk cannot be ruled out)*
Alpha blockers	Efficacy	Controlled studies are missing.	C (*risk cannot be ruled out)*
To be avoided			
Atenolole	NA	Intrauterine growth restriction. May induce hypoglycaemia, hypotension and bradycardia at delivery	D (*positive evidence of risk)*
Short acting niphedipine	NA	Sudden hypotension with detrimental effects on placental flow	D (*positive evidence of risk)*
ACE-I and ARB	NA	Increment risk for congenital malformation	C (*risk cannot be ruled out) first trimester* D (*positive evidence of risk) second third trimester*

Note: Diuretics should be used with care due to the risk of hypovolemia and placental hypoperfusion. Anti-aldosteronics can be used in case of documented hyperaldosteronism but should be avoided in the first 20 GW due the risk of feminization of male genitalia

positive pregnancy test (4th–6th gestational week) in particular in patients with relevant proteinuria, or needing nephroprotection [10, 103]. In our practice, prefer discontinuation at a positive pregnancy test, at least in women with good understanding and adherence to the indication of performing timely pregnancy tests in case of doubt [10, 64, 65].

Data about breastfeeding in women CKD are scant and scattered, however, a large body of evidence indirectly supports breastfeeding advantages in particular in fragile babies and in preterm infants. These advantages should induce a broader adoption of breastfeeding practices also in patients with advanced CKD or after a severe HDP, provided that they are not being treated with potentially toxic drugs [104].

Antihypertensives are the most commonly involved drugs in this context. As for nephroprotection, the ACEi of old generation (enalapril, captopril or quinalapril) can be resumed after delivery, as they are compatible with breastfeeding; limited data are however available with other ACEi and until more data are published, known and safer alternatives may be preferable [105–107]. Conversely ARBs, except for candesartan, for which preliminary evidence suggests it passes poorly into milk and is barely detectable in the plasma of breastfed infants, little information is available on the use of sartans during lactation, so that an alternative drug may be preferable, especially during the lactation of a newborn or premature infant [105–108].

In the absence of data, other increasingly used nephroprotective agents, such as sodium/glucose cotransporter 2 inhibitors (SGLT2i) are not advised during breastfeeding.

There is no advantage of a high protein diet in breastfeeding and even women with high urea levels or on dialysis have been reported to successfully breastfeed. A balanced, eventually moderately protein-restricted diet, with avoidance of ultra-processed food is an important add-on strategy to contribute to the preservation of the kidney function. Furthermore, since ultra-processed food is usually rich in salt, such a diet is expected to exert a negative effect on blood pressure control, as widely reported outside of the context of pregnancy and breastfeeding [109, 110].

Some data on the most commonly used antihypertensive drugs and breastfeeding are reported in Table 6. Due to the rapid development of drugs aimed at treating CKD and its complications, and to the increasing experience with older drugs in breastfeeding, no list can be considered exhaustive and regularly updated databanks should be used in case of doubt (such as www.ncbi.nlm.nih.gov/books/NBK501922 o www.lecrat.fr).

Table 6 Comparison of recent international guidelines (UK 2019, DGGG 2022, Netherlands 2022, KDIGO 2025) on breastfeeding and medication compatibility in women with CKD

Guideline	Recommendation	Medication compatibility	Other drugs
UK 2019 [74]	Women with CKD should be supported in their wish to breastfeed. Prescribe only medications safe in lactation.	Contraindicated: Mycophenolate mofetil Compatible: Prednisolone, azathioprine, ciclosporin, tacrolimus, avoid NSAIDs	Enalapril, captopril, amlodipine, nifedipine, labetalol, atenolol, LMWH
DGGG 2022 [63]	Encourage breastfeeding for at least 4 months. Provide support to ensure continuation. All postpartum medications must be safe for the infant.	Contraindicated: Mycophenolate mofetil	NSAIDs not recommended (use paracetamol) Compatible: Captopril, enalapril, quinapril, dihydralazine Not recommended: Ramipril, losartan Adjust all treatments with nephrologist
Netherlands 2022 [62]	Prescribe only medications considered safe during breastfeeding		Antihypertensives in lactation: Preferred → enalapril (esp. with proteinuria/diabetes) Safe β-blockers: Labetalol, metoprolol, pindolol, propranolol (favorable PK) Avoid α-blockers (safety unknown)
KDIGO controversies 2025 [10]	Lactation should be supported if desired		Some ACE inhibitors compatible with breastfeeding, preferred to ARBs (lack data) Safety of newer drugs (SGLT2i, GLP-1 receptor agonists) unknown → refer to updated sources

DGGG Deutsche Gesellschaft für Gynäkologie und Geburtshilfe, *NSAIDs* non-steroidal anti-inflammatory drugs, *LMWH* low molecular weight heparin, *PK* pharmacokinetics, *ACE* angiotensin-converting enzyme, *SGLT2i* sodium/glucose cotransporter 2 inhibitors, *GLP-1* glucagon-like peptide 1

Long-Term Follow-Up After Hypertensive Disorders of Pregnancy (With or Without Residual Hypertension)

The old tenet that PE and other HDP were transitory events healed by delivery, with the obvious exception of pre-existing chronic hypertension, has been completely dispelled in the last decades, and HDP are presently considered as a window on future maternal cardiovascular and kidney health [111–114].

Over 20% of women who experience new-onset HDP remain hypertensive after delivery, and the prevalence may be higher in some high-risk cohorts, or applying the lower blood pressure cut-offs supported by the American Heart Association. Even when normotensive, these women frequently remain at upper normal blood pressure levels and have a high risk of recurrence of HDP (up to 50% of the cases of PE, or even more according to the series, and the case-mix) [115]. As expected, repeated exposure to HDP increases the long-term risk of CKD, cardiovascular diseases and hypertension. Hence, the most important cardiology societies are presently supporting universal referral after HDP to correct risk factors, identify secondary causes of hypertension, establish a long-term follow-up and if needed treatment plan. While the position of many nephrology societies is still rather nihilist, the importance of diagnosis and follow-up after PE has been clearly highlighted by the recent WHO document supporting kidney care as a health priority ("Reducing the burden of noncommunicable diseases through promotion of kidney health and strengthening prevention and control of kidney disease") [116].

Children exposed in utero to PE and HDP have a higher risk of cardiometabolic and kidney diseases and, while these risks are higher in the case of preterm birth or low birth-weight, being exposed even to "term" PE is associated with increased susceptibility in early adulthood. For females, being born small or small for gestational age is likewise associated with a 4–6 higher risk of developing PE or other HDP once pregnant [117]. Due to the recent advances in neonatal care, an increasing number of "small babies" are presently reaching adulthood. Future studies will highlight their contribution to the global burden of hypertension, HDP and CKD.

Conclusions

Hypertension is a relatively frequent finding in pregnancy; chronic hypertension is found in 2–3% of pregnant women and incidence of HDP is estimated at over 10% if calculated per pregnancy and over 15–20% if calculated per woman.

Hypertension is both a risk factor for APOs, if pre-existing, and an APO in itself if developed in pregnancy. The relationship with CKD is strict: CKD is the most frequent cause of secondary hypertension in a young woman, hypertension is a cause of CKD, and the risk of developing HDP is higher in pregnancies occurring on a CKD background. While having developed HDP is a risk factor for postpartum and long-term hypertension, whether or not linked to CKD, the risk is transgenerational and children exposed to HDP have a higher lifetime risk of developing hypertension and CKD, often at relatively early ages. These risks have been acknowledged in the recent WHO declaration acknowledging the need for prioritizing CKD care.

Blood pressure control is fundamental since the preconception phase, as normalization of blood pressure is associated with better pregnancy outcomes; during pregnancies the current targets are lower than in the past, and basically reproduce those agreed in young women with CKD. The limited number of drugs available is a potential problem, but wise combinations are usually sufficient to reach the targets. After delivery, careful drug review is needed for promoting breastfeeding while ensuring nephroprotection.

Further studies, targeted to women living with CKD, are needed to better tune general policies in these specific cases.

Disclosure Statement All authors report no conflict of interest for the present contribution.

References

1. Piccoli GB, Cabiddu G, Attini R, Vigotti FN, Maxia S, Lepori N, et al. Risk of adverse pregnancy outcomes in women with CKD. J Am Soc Nephrol. 2015;26(8):2011–22.
2. Fakhouri F, Schwotzer N, Cabiddu G, Barratt J, Legardeur H, Garovic V, et al. Glomerular diseases in pregnancy: pragmatic recommendations for clinical management. Kidney Int. 2023;103(2):264–81.
3. Vikse BE, Irgens LM, Leivestad T, Skjaerven R, Iversen BM. Preeclampsia and the risk of end-stage renal disease. N Engl J Med. 2008;359(8):800–9.
4. Cabiddu G, Longhitano E, Cataldo E, Lepori N, Chatrenet A, Torreggiani M, et al. History of preeclampsia in patients undergoing a kidney biopsy: a biphasic, multiple-hit pathogenic hypothesis. Kidney Int Rep. 2022;7(3):547–57.
5. Williams D, Davison J. Chronic kidney disease in pregnancy. BMJ. 2008;336(7637):211–5.
6. Vrijlandt WAL, de Jong MFC, Prins JR, Bramham K, Vrijlandt P, Janse RJ, et al. Prevalence of chronic kidney disease in women of reproductive age and observed birth rates. J Nephrol. 2023;36(5):1341–7.
7. Al Khalaf SY, O'Reilly EJ, McCarthy FP, Kublickas M, Kublickiene K, Khashan AS. Pregnancy outcomes in women with chronic kidney disease and chronic hypertension: a National cohort study. Am J Obstet Gynecol. 2021;225(3):298 e1–20.
8. Wiles KS, Nelson-Piercy C, Bramham K. Reproductive health and pregnancy in women with chronic kidney disease. Nat Rev Nephrol. 2018;14(3):165–84.
9. Burgner A, Hladunewich MA. Women's reproductive health for the nephrologist. Am J Kidney Dis. 2019;74(5):675–81.
10. Piccoli GB, Ahmed SB, Fakhouri F, Garovic VD, Hladunewich MA, Jesudason S, et al. Women and kidney health: conclusions from a Kidney Disease: Improving Global Outcomes (KDIGO) controversies conference. Kidney Int. 2025;108(3):355–79.
11. Wang F, Lu JD, Zhu Y, Wang TT, Xue J. Renal outcomes of pregnant patients with immunoglobulin a nephropathy: a systematic review and meta-analysis. Am J Nephrol. 2019;49(3):214–24.
12. Cheung CK, Barratt J. Pregnancy in IgA nephropathy: an effect on renal outcome? Am J Nephrol. 2019;49(3):212–3.
13. Brown MA, Magee LA, Kenny LC, Karumanchi SA, McCarthy FP, Saito S, et al. The hypertensive disorders of pregnancy: ISSHP classification, diagnosis & management recommendations for international practice. Pregnancy Hypertens. 2018;13:291–310.

14. Magee LA, Pels A, Helewa M, Rey E, von Dadelszen P, Canadian Hypertensive Disorders of Pregnancy Working G. Diagnosis, evaluation, and management of the hypertensive disorders of pregnancy. Pregnancy Hypertens. 2014;4(2):105–45.
15. Lowe SA, Bowyer L, Lust K, McMahon LP, Morton MR, North RA, et al. The SOMANZ guidelines for the Management of Hypertensive Disorders of Pregnancy 2014. Aust N Z J Obstet Gynaecol. 2015;55(1):11–6.
16. National Institute for Health and Care Excellence Hypertension in Pregnancy: Diagnosis and Management. NICE Guideline
17. Gestational Hypertension and Preeclampsia. ACOG Practice Bulletin, Number 222. Obstet Gynecol. 2020;135(6):e237–e60.
18. Poon LC, Magee LA, Verlohren S, Shennan A, von Dadelszen P, Sheiner E, et al. A literature review and best practice advice for second and third trimester risk stratification, monitoring, and management of pre-eclampsia: compiled by the Pregnancy and Non-Communicable Diseases Committee of FIGO (the International Federation of Gynecology and Obstetrics). Int J Gynaecol Obstet. 2021;154(Suppl 1):3–31.
19. Takagi K. A review of the best practice guide 2021 for the diagnosis and Management of Hypertensive Disorders of Pregnancy (HDP). Hypertension Research In Pregnancy; 2022.
20. Cabiddu G, Mannucci C, Fois A, Maxia S, Chatrenet A, Osadolor S, et al. Pre-eclampsia is a valuable opportunity to diagnose chronic kidney disease: a multicentre study. Nephrol Dial Transplant. 2022;37(8):1488–98.
21. Mussarat N, Biggio J Jr, Martin J, Morgan J, Tivis R, Elmayan A, et al. Masked pregnancy-associated hypertension as a predictor of adverse outcomes. Am J Obstet Gynecol MFM. 2023;5(7):100976.
22. Fang Y, Zuo L, Li J, Shi H, Zhang R, Han C, et al. Optimization of ambulatory blood pressure monitoring during pregnancy: a path toward risk stratification improvement and management of hypertensive disorders. Rev Cardiovasc Med. 2025;26(5):27235.
23. Longhitano E, Siligato R, Torreggiani M, Attini R, Masturzo B, Casula V, et al. The hypertensive disorders of pregnancy: a focus on definitions for clinical nephrologists. J Clin Med. 2022;11(12)
24. Webster P, Lightstone L, McKay DB, Josephson MA. Pregnancy in chronic kidney disease and kidney transplantation. Kidney Int. 2017;91(5):1047–56.
25. Pippias M, Skinner L, Noordzij M, Reisaeter AV, Abramowicz D, Stel VS, et al. Pregnancy after living kidney donation, a systematic review of the available evidence, and a review of the current guidance. Am J Transplant. 2022;22(10):2360–80.
26. Barton JR, Sibai BM. Prediction and prevention of recurrent preeclampsia. Obstet Gynecol. 2008;112(2 Pt 1):359–72.
27. Hernandez-Diaz S, Toh S, Cnattingius S. Risk of pre-eclampsia in first and subsequent pregnancies: prospective cohort study. BMJ. 2009;338:b2255.
28. Ukah UV, Platt RW, Auger N, Lisonkova S, Ray JG, Malhame I, et al. Risk of recurrent severe maternal morbidity: a population-based study. Am J Obstet Gynecol. 2023;229(5):545 e1–11.
29. Piccoli GB, Zakharova E, Attini R, Ibarra Hernandez M, Covella B, Alrukhaimi M, et al. Acute kidney injury in pregnancy: the need for higher awareness. A pragmatic review focused on what could be improved in the prevention and care of pregnancy-related AKI, in the year dedicated to women and kidney diseases. J Clin Med. 2018;7(10)
30. Levine RJ, Maynard SE, Qian C, Lim KH, England LJ, Yu KF, et al. Circulating angiogenic factors and the risk of preeclampsia. N Engl J Med. 2004;350(7):672–83.
31. Verlohren S, Brennecke SP, Galindo A, Karumanchi SA, Mirkovic LB, Schlembach D, et al. Clinical interpretation and implementation of the sFlt-1/PlGF ratio in the prediction, diagnosis and management of preeclampsia. Pregnancy Hypertens. 2022;27:42–50.
32. Thadhani R, Lemoine E, Rana S, Costantine MM, Calsavara VF, Boggess K, et al. Circulating angiogenic factor levels in hypertensive disorders of pregnancy. NEJM Evid. 2022;1(12):EVIDoa2200161.
33. Food and Drug Administration. FDA Roundup; 2023.

34. Chappell LC, Cluver CA, Kingdom J, Tong S. Pre-eclampsia. Lancet. 2021;398(10297):341–54.
35. Magee LA, Nicolaides KH, von Dadelszen P. Preeclampsia. N Engl J Med. 2022;386(19):1817–32.
36. Garovic VD, White WM, Vaughan L, Saiki M, Parashuram S, Garcia-Valencia O, et al. Incidence and long-term outcomes of hypertensive disorders of pregnancy. J Am Coll Cardiol. 2020;75(18):2323–34.
37. Garovic VD, Dechend R, Easterling T, Karumanchi SA, McMurtry Baird S, Magee LA, et al. Hypertension in pregnancy: diagnosis, blood pressure goals, and pharmacotherapy: a scientific statement from the American Heart Association. Hypertension. 2022;79(2):e21–41.
38. Santos JSM, Garovic VD. Early identification of individuals at risk for hypertensive disorders of pregnancy. JAMA Netw Open 2023. 2023.
39. Dupont V, Berg AH, Yamashita M, Huang C, Covarrubias AE, Ali S, et al. Impaired renal reserve contributes to preeclampsia via the kynurenine and soluble fms-like tyrosine kinase 1 pathway. J Clin Invest. 2022;132(20)
40. Broekhuizen M, Danser AHJ, Reiss IKM, Merkus D. The function of the kynurenine pathway in the placenta: a novel pharmacotherapeutic target? Int J Environ Res Public Health. 2021;18(21)
41. Yagel S, Cohen SM, Admati I, Skarbianskis N, Solt I, Zeisel A, et al. Expert review: preeclampsia type I and type II. Am J Obstet Gynecol MFM. 2023;5(12):101203.
42. Kariori M, Katsi V, Tsioufis C. Late vs. early preeclampsia. Int J Mol Sci. 2025;26(22)
43. Lewey J, Levine LD, Yang L, Triebwasser JE, Groeneveld PW. Patterns of postpartum ambulatory care follow-up care among women with hypertensive disorders of pregnancy. J Am Heart Assoc. 2020;9(17):e016357.
44. Kidney Disease: Improving Global Outcomes CKDWG. KDIGO 2024 clinical practice guideline for the evaluation and Management of Chronic Kidney Disease. Kidney Int. 2024;105(4S):S117–314.
45. Piccoli GB, Attini R, Torreggiani M, Cabiddu G. Pregnancy and kidney diseases: multidisciplinary follow-up and the vicious circles involving pregnancy and CKD, preeclampsia, preterm delivery and the kidneys. J Clin Med. 2022;11(9)
46. Garovic VD, Wagner SJ, Turner ST, Rosenthal DW, Watson WJ, Brost BC, et al. Urinary podocyte excretion as a marker for preeclampsia. Am J Obstet Gynecol. 2007;196(4):320 e1–7.
47. Jim B, Jean-Louis P, Qipo A, Garry D, Mian S, Matos T, et al. Podocyturia as a diagnostic marker for preeclampsia amongst high-risk pregnant patients. J Pregnancy. 2012;2012:984630.
48. Jim B, Mehta S, Qipo A, Kim K, Cohen HW, Moore RM, et al. A comparison of podocyturia, albuminuria and nephrinuria in predicting the development of preeclampsia: a prospective study. PLoS One. 2014;9(7):e101445.
49. Nakamura T, Ushiyama C, Suzuki S, Hara M, Shimada N, Sekizuka K, et al. Urinary podocytes for the assessment of disease activity in lupus nephritis. Am J Med Sci. 2000;320(2):112–6.
50. Fisher KA, Luger A, Spargo BH, Lindheimer MD. Hypertension in pregnancy: clinical-pathological correlations and remote prognosis. Medicine (Baltimore). 1981;60(4):267–76.
51. Weissgerber TL, Milic NM, Milin-Lazovic JS, Garovic VD. Impaired flow-mediated dilation before, during, and after preeclampsia: a systematic review and meta-analysis. Hypertension. 2016;67(2):415–23.
52. Vikse BE, Hallan S, Bostad L, Leivestad T, Iversen BM. Previous preeclampsia and risk for progression of biopsy-verified kidney disease to end-stage renal disease. Nephrol Dial Transplant. 2010;25(10):3289–96.
53. Oliverio AL, Zee J, Mariani LH, Reynolds ML, O'Shaughnessy M, Hendren EM, et al. Renal complications in pregnancy preceding glomerulonephropathy diagnosis. Kidney Int Rep. 2019;4(1):159–62.

54. Gilani SI, Anderson UD, Jayachandran M, Weissgerber TL, Zand L, White WM, et al. Urinary extracellular vesicles of podocyte origin and renal injury in preeclampsia. J Am Soc Nephrol. 2017;28(11):3363–72.
55. National Kidney F. K/DOQI clinical practice guidelines for chronic kidney disease: evaluation, classification, and stratification. Am J Kidney Dis. 2002;39(2 Suppl 1):S1–266.
56. Charles L, Triscott J, Dobbs B. Secondary hypertension: discovering the underlying cause. Am Fam Physician. 2017;96(7):453–61.
57. Lopes van Balen VA, van Gansewinkel TAG, de Haas S, Spaan JJ, Ghossein-Doha C, van Kuijk SMJ, et al. Maternal kidney function during pregnancy: systematic review and meta-analysis. Ultrasound Obstet Gynecol. 2019;54(3):297–307.
58. Cheung KL, Lafayette RA. Renal physiology of pregnancy. Adv Chronic Kidney Dis. 2013;20(3):209–14.
59. Irani RA, Xia Y. Renin angiotensin signaling in normal pregnancy and preeclampsia. Semin Nephrol. 2011;31(1):47–58.
60. Ouzounian JG, Elkayam U. Physiologic changes during normal pregnancy and delivery. Cardiol Clin. 2012;30(3):317–29.
61. Gant NF, Worley RJ, Everett RB, MacDonald PC. Control of vascular responsiveness during human pregnancy. Kidney Int. 1980;18(2):253–8.
62. de Jong MFC, van Hamersvelt HW, van Empel IWH, Nijkamp EJW, Lely AT, Dutch Guideline Working Group on Pregnancy in CKD. Summary of the Dutch practice guideline on pregnancy wish and pregnancy in CKD. Kidney Int Rep. 2022;7(12):2575–88.
63. Schmidt M, Stracke S, Schneider U, Kuschel B, Feldkamp T, Habbig S, et al. Chronic kidney disease and pregnancy. Guideline of the DGGG, OEGGG, DGfN (S2k Level, AWMF Registry No. 015–090). Geburtshilfe Frauenheilkd. 2022;82(8):795–830.
64. Cabiddu G, Castellino S, Gernone G, Santoro D, Moroni G, Giannattasio M, et al. A best practice position statement on pregnancy in chronic kidney disease: the Italian Study Group on Kidney and Pregnancy. J Nephrol. 2016;29(3):277–303.
65. Piccoli GB, Cabiddu G, Castellino S, Gernone G, Santoro D, Moroni G, et al. A best practice position statement on the role of the nephrologist in the prevention and follow-up of preeclampsia: the Italian study group on kidney and pregnancy. J Nephrol. 2017;30(3):307–17.
66. Guideline. IoOaGRCoPoIatCSaPDHSECP. The Management of Hypertension in Pregnancy.
67. Butalia S, Audibert F, Cote AM, Firoz T, Logan AG, Magee LA, et al. Hypertension Canada's 2018 guidelines for the Management of Hypertension in Pregnancy. Can J Cardiol. 2018;34(5):526–31.
68. Williams B, Mancia G, Spiering W, Agabiti Rosei E, Azizi M, Burnier M, et al. 2018 ESC/ESH guidelines for the management of arterial hypertension. Eur Heart J. 2018;39(33):3021–104.
69. Malachias MV. 7th Brazilian guideline of arterial hypertension: presentation. Arq Bras Cardiol. 2016;107(3 Suppl 3):0.
70. Queensland Health Maternity and Neonatal Clinical Guidelines.
71. Milman N. Postpartum anemia I: definition, prevalence, causes, and consequences. Ann Hematol. 2011;90(11):1247–53.
72. Xu J, Li T, Wang Y, Xue L, Miao Z, Long W, et al. The association between hypertensive disorders in pregnancy and the risk of developing chronic hypertension. Front Cardiovasc Med. 2022;9:897771.
73. Piccoli GB, Chatrenet A, Cataldo M, Torreggiani M, Attini R, Masturzo B, et al. Adding creatinine to routine pregnancy tests: a decision tree for calculating the cost of identifying patients with CKD in pregnancy. Nephrol Dial Transplant. 2023;38(1):148–57.
74. Wiles K, Chappell L, Clark K, Elman L, Hall M, Lightstone L, et al. Clinical practice guideline on pregnancy and renal disease. BMC Nephrol. 2019;20(1):401.
75. Wiles K, Bramham K, Seed PT, Nelson-Piercy C, Lightstone L, Chappell LC. Serum creatinine in pregnancy: a systematic review. Kidney Int Rep. 2019;4(3):408–19.

76. Park S, Lee SM, Park JS, Hong JS, Chin HJ, Na KY, et al. Midterm eGFR and adverse pregnancy outcomes: the clinical significance of gestational hyperfiltration. Clin J Am Soc Nephrol. 2017;12(7):1048–56.
77. Gao M, Vilayur E, Ferreira D, Nanra R, Hawkins J. Estimating the glomerular filtration rate in pregnancy: the evaluation of the Nanra and CKD-EPI serum creatinine-based equations. Obstet Med. 2021;14(1):31–4.
78. Kervella D, Torreggiani M. Baseline proteinuria level and adverse outcomes in pregnant women with chronic kidney disease: new evidence and a note of caution. Clin Kidney J. 2023;16(10):1550–2.
79. Brown MA, Holt JL, Mangos GJ, Murray N, Curtis J, Homer C. Microscopic hematuria in pregnancy: relevance to pregnancy outcome. Am J Kidney Dis. 2005;45(4):667–73.
80. Ciciu E, Pasatu-Cornea AM, Petcu LC, Tuta LA. Early diagnosis and management of maternal ureterohydronephrosis during pregnancy. Exp Ther Med. 2022;23(1):27.
81. Bahser N, Godehardt E, Hess AP, Blume C. Examination of intrarenal resistance indices indicate the involvement of renal pathology as a significant diagnostic classifier of preeclampsia. Am J Hypertens. 2014;27(5):742–9.
82. Zimmermann P, Ranta T. Doppler assessment of the maternal interlobar renal and uterine arteries in mid-pregnancy in women at low and high risk for pregnancy-induced hypertension. J Clin Ultrasound. 1998;26(5):239–45.
83. Shainker SA, Edlow JA, O'Brien K. Cerebrovascular emergencies in pregnancy. Best Pract Res Clin Obstet Gynaecol. 2015;29(5):721–31.
84. The American College of Obstetricians and Gyncecologists. Medically indicated late-preterm and early-term deliveries; 2021.
85. National Institute for Health and Care Excellence. Caesarean birth. NICE guideline [NG192].
86. National Institute for Health and Care Excellence. Inducing labour. NICE guideline [NG207].
87. Magee LA, Smith GN, Bloch C, Cote AM, Jain V, Nerenberg K, et al. Guideline No. 426: hypertensive disorders of pregnancy: diagnosis, prediction, prevention, and management. J Obstet Gynaecol Can. 2022;44(5):547–71 e1.
88. Moroni G, Ponticelli C. Pregnancy in women with systemic lupus erythematosus (SLE). Eur J Intern Med. 2016;32:7–12.
89. Piccoli GB, Kooij IA, Attini R, Montersino B, Fassio F, Gerbino M, et al. A systematic review on Materno-Foetal outcomes in pregnant women with IgA nephropathy: a case of "Late-maternal" preeclampsia? J Clin Med. 2018;7(8)
90. Park S, Yoo KD, Park JS, Hong JS, Baek S, Park SK, et al. Pregnancy in women with immunoglobulin A nephropathy: are obstetrical complications associated with renal prognosis? Nephrol Dial Transplant. 2018;33(3):459–65.
91. Spotti D. Pregnancy in women with diabetic nephropathy. J Nephrol. 2019;32(3):379–88.
92. Beers K, Patel N. Kidney physiology in pregnancy. Adv Chronic Kidney Dis. 2020;27(6):449–54.
93. Purswani JM, Gala P, Dwarkanath P, Larkin HM, Kurpad A, Mehta S. The role of vitamin D in pre-eclampsia: a systematic review. BMC Pregnancy Childbirth. 2017;17(1):231.
94. Suresh S, Mueller A, Salahuddin S, Naseem H, Dhir R, Rana S. Evaluation of angiogenic factors in the decision to admit women with suspected preeclampsia. Pregnancy Hypertens. 2020;21:124–31.
95. Peguero A, Herraiz I, Perales A, Melchor JC, Melchor I, Marcos B, et al. Placental growth factor testing in the management of late preterm preeclampsia without severe features: a multicenter, randomized, controlled trial. Am J Obstet Gynecol. 2021;225(3):308 e1–14.
96. Duhig KE, Myers JE, Gale C, Girling JC, Harding K, Sharp A, et al. Placental growth factor measurements in the assessment of women with suspected preeclampsia: a stratified analysis of the PARROT trial. Pregnancy Hypertens. 2021;23:41–7.
97. Long PA, Abell DA, Beischer NA. Importance of abnormal glucose tolerance (hypoglycaemia and hyperglycaemia) in the aetiology of pre-eclampsia. Lancet. 1977;1(8018):923–5.

98. Nayak AU, Vijay AMA, Indusekhar R, Kalidindi S, Katreddy VM, Varadhan L. Association of hypoglycaemia in screening oral glucose tolerance test in pregnancy with low birth weight fetus. World J Diabetes. 2019;10(5):304–10.
99. Langer O, Damus K, Maiman M, Divon M, Levy J, Bauman W. A link between relative hypoglycemia-hypoinsulinemia during oral glucose tolerance tests and intrauterine growth retardation. Am J Obstet Gynecol. 1986;155(4):711–6.
100. Margolis KL, O'Connor PJ, Morgan TM, Buse JB, Cohen RM, Cushman WC, et al. Outcomes of combined cardiovascular risk factor management strategies in type 2 diabetes: the ACCORD randomized trial. Diabetes Care. 2014;37(6):1721–8.
101. Sanusi AA, Sinkey RG, Tita ATN. Clinical trials that have changed obstetric practice: the chronic hypertension and pregnancy (CHAP) trial. Clin Obstet Gynecol. 2024;67(2):411–7.
102. Magee LA, Singer J, von Dadelszen P, Group CS. Less-tight versus tight control of hypertension in pregnancy. N Engl J Med. 2015;372(24):2367–8.
103. Cooper WO, Hernandez-Diaz S, Arbogast PG, Dudley JA, Dyer S, Gideon PS, et al. Major congenital malformations after first-trimester exposure to ACE inhibitors. N Engl J Med. 2006;354(23):2443–51.
104. Parnizari P, Hladunewich MA, Zipursky J. Safety of drugs in breastfeeding women with CKD. Kidney Int Rep. 2025;10(7):2189–201.
105. Anderson PO. Drugs in lactation. Pharm Res. 2018;35(3):45.
106. Drugs and Lactation Database (LactMed®).
107. Rowe H, Baker T, Hale TW. Maternal medication, drug use, and breastfeeding. Child Adolesc Psychiatr Clin N Am. 2015;24(1):1–20.
108. Coberger ED, Jensen BP, Dalrymple JM. Transfer of candesartan into human breast milk. Obstet Gynecol. 2019;134(3):481–4.
109. Barbosa SS, Sousa LCM, de Oliveira Silva DF, Pimentel JB, Evangelista K, Lyra CO, et al. A systematic review on processed/ultra-processed foods and arterial hypertension in adults and older people. Nutrients. 2022;14(6)
110. Juul F, Vaidean G, Parekh N. Ultra-processed foods and cardiovascular diseases: potential mechanisms of action. Adv Nutr. 2021;12(5):1673–80.
111. Ying W, Catov JM, Ouyang P. Hypertensive disorders of pregnancy and future maternal cardiovascular risk. J Am Heart Assoc. 2018;7(17):e009382.
112. Poon LC, Nguyen-Hoang L, Smith GN, Bergman L, O'Brien P, Hod M, et al. Hypertensive disorders of pregnancy and long-term cardiovascular health: FIGO best practice advice. Int J Gynaecol Obstet. 2023;160(Suppl 1):22–34.
113. Malek AM, Hunt KJ, Turan TN, Mateus J, Lackland DT, Lucas A, et al. Hypertensive disorders of pregnancy with and without prepregnancy hypertension are associated with incident maternal kidney disease subsequent to delivery. Hypertension. 2022;79(4):844–54.
114. Piccoli GB, Orozco A, Shemies R, Attini R, Cabiddu G, Toreggiani M, et al. Postpartum counseling and interventions to reduce the risk of chronic kidney disease: back to the future. Kidney Int. 2025;108(2):160–6.
115. De Marco O, Ruotolo C, Njanjo L, Mariani C, Maze B, Santagati G, et al. Recurrence of preeclampsia is common, even during rigorously controlled multidisciplinary follow-up: a pilot experience. Clin Kidney J. 2025;18(4):sfaf070.
116. World Health Organization. Reducing the burden of noncommunicable diseases through promotion of kidney health and strengthening prevention and control of kidney disease. Available at https://apps.who.int/gb/ebwha/pdf_files/EB156/B156_CONF6-en.pdf. Last accessed on 2 Aug 2025.
117. Piccoli GB, Torreggiani M, Crochette R, Cabiddu G, Masturzo B, Attini R, et al. What a paediatric nephrologist should know about preeclampsia and why it matters. Pediatr Nephrol. 2022;37(8):1733–45.

Prevention and Treatment of Hyperkalemia in CKD: The Role of New Potassium Binders

Francesca Rivela, Clorinda Rossi, Sara Elsaman, and Mario Cozzolino

Introduction

Potassium (K^+) is an essential mineral, fundamental for maintaining the cell membrane potential, the regulation of cell volume and the ion and solute transportation.

Hyperkalemia is an elevation of the blood potassium level, usually defined as a concentration $[K^+] > 5/5, 5$ mmol/L. Hyperkalemia is a relatively common metabolic complication which leads to a partial depolarization of the cell membrane which can result in muscle weakness, paralysis, and life-threatening arrhythmias such as ventricular fibrillation causing sudden cardiac arrest.

The human body has a variety of homeostatic mechanisms to avoid hyperkalemia, but it is well known that in patients with chronic kidney disease (CKD) the compensation mechanisms do not work the same compared to people with a normal renal function [1].

Pathophysiology of Hyperkalemia

Potassium is the most abundant intracellular cation; roughly 98% of the total body potassium is stored within the cells, the majority of which is stocked in the skeletal muscle cells. The intracellular potassium concentration is approximately 140 mmol/L, compared with 4–5 mmol/L in the extracellular space. The difference in intra and extracellular potassium concentration creates a transmembrane potential that is responsible for neuromuscular activities [2].

F. Rivela · C. Rossi · S. Elsaman · M. Cozzolino (✉)
Renal Division, ASST Santi Paolo e Carlo, Department of Helath Sciences, University of Milan, Milan, Italy
e-mail: mario.cozzolino@unimi.it

P. Sarafidis, R. Pontremoli (eds.), *Hypertension and Chronic Kidney Disease*, Updates in Hypertension and Cardiovascular Protection,
https://doi.org/10.1007/978-3-032-29564-4_10

Serum potassium concentration is maintained at a relatively constant concentration by a variety of homeostatic mechanisms: Potassium enters the cells due to the action of the Na^+/K^+/ATPase pump which moves the potassium in the cell and the sodium out in a ratio of 2:3. These movements generate an electric gradient which leads to an action potential that is vital for cell function, nerve conduction, and muscular contraction.

Potassium enters the body via oral intake (120 mmol/day), and it is then absorbed in the gastrointestinal system (80% by the small intestine) and excreted via the urinary tract (90%) and the colon (10%) [3].

Physiologically, potassium is freely filtered in the glomerulus; here, the concentration of potassium in the filtrate is nearly the same as that in the blood plasma. Most of the filtered potassium (about 80%) is then passively reabsorbed in the proximal convoluted tubule through paracellular transport driven by osmotic gradients. In the Loop of Henle, the remaining 20% of the filtered potassium is reabsorbed via a $Na^+/K^+/2Cl$ – symporter. This transporter actively transports sodium, potassium, and chloride from the lumen of the tubule into the cell's lining, contributing to the renal concentration gradient that is essential for urine concentration. In the collecting duct, the remaining potassium is reabsorbed via the luminal H^+/K^+/ATPase and other paracellular pathways.

The primary site of potassium secretion is the distal convoluted tubule and the collecting duct. Here, potassium is actively secreted from the blood into the tubular lumen via specialized potassium channels (ROMK—Renal Outer Medullary Potassium channel). This last secretion mechanism is mediated by aldosterone, which increases the expression of the luminal epithelial sodium channel and the Na^+/K^+/ATPase leasing to an increase of Na^+ reabsorption and consequently to K^+ secretion [4–7].

Potassium concentration may increase due to a combination of factors such as increased oral intake, reduced urinary excretion, and redistribution from cell damage (e.g., tumor lysis syndrome, rhabdomyolysis and crush syndrome). In people with normal renal function, the excretion rate can increase to avoid hyperkalemia. In addition, the extracellular K^+ are buffered by K^+ moving into the cells: the most important factors regulating this movements in normal conditions are insulin and catecholamines [8].

In CKD, these mechanisms do not work the same, leading to a much greater chance of symptomatic hyperkalemia. It has been established that the most common factors associated with hyperkalemia were chronic kidney disease, type 2 diabetes, hypertension, heart failure, and use of angiotensin-converting enzyme inhibitors (ACEi), mineralocorticoid receptor antagonists (MRA), and angiotensin receptor blockers (ARB) [7].

Hyperkalemia is one of the most common complications of chronic kidney disease. More than 50% of people with CKD have hyperkalemia, and moreover a decline in renal function corresponds to a significant increase in prevalence [9]; hyperkalemia is observed in about 26% of patients with stage V, 22% in stage IV, and 5% in stage III [10]. Hyperkalemia in CKD is associated with an increased risk of cardiovascular events and mortality also caused by the limited use of kidney and cardioprotective therapies that are known to increase the serum concentration of potassium.

In CKD, several factors are known to have a crucial role in the pathophysiology of hyperkalemia: Lifestyle habits and pharmacological treatments are known to increase potassium concentration, but the main mechanism is related to an increase of extracellular extrusion associated with a decreased renal function. This is mainly caused by four pathological conditions:

1. Reduced urine output which compromises K^+ secretion.
   The ability to excrete potassium is usually maintained until advanced renal failure (GFR < 15–20 mL/min) due to the ability of the remaining nephrons to enhance their ability to secrete K^+ through the upregulation of the entire machinery mediating its secretion along the distal nephron, including the Na^+/K^+ ATPase, the ENaC, and ROMK channels [11].
2. Metabolic acidosis that favors the release of K^+ in the extracellular space.
   The potassium release in the extracellular space depends on the type of acid present: An excess of mineral acid (NH_4Cl or HCl) rather than organic acidosis such as ketoacidosis or lactic acidosis causes a decrease of extracellular pH and limits the activity of the Na^+/K^+ exchange. This leads to a decrease of the activity of the Na^+/K^+/ATPase caused by a decrement of intracellular Na^+. All these consequences result in a significant extracellular shift of intracellular K^+ in exchange for protons. On the contrary, organic acids can enters the cells; therefore, they do not have the same effects [2, 7].
3. The presence of comorbidities like diabetes mellitus associated with a low insulin secretion.
   It is well known that insulin promotes potassium entry into the cells by stimulating the activity of the Na^+/K^+/ATPase pump. In addition, the hyperosmolarity caused by the hyperglycaemic status leads to water movements from the cells to the extracellular space as a result intracellular potassium raise creating a gradient for K^+ to exit the cells [7, 12].
4. Pharmacological treatments with ACEi and ARB.
   Both these medications cause hyperkalemia by reducing renal perfusion and aldosterone secretion. It has been studied that the risk of developing severe and symptomatic hyperkalemia in CKD stage 3 or higher is low in those taking monotherapy RAAS inhibitors compared with dual RAAS inhibition, in fact KDIGO recommendations declare not to routinely prescribe the double blockage [6, 13].

In addition, in patients with impaired renal function, the presence of uremic toxin can decrease the transcription of mRNA for the a1 isoform of the Na^+/K^+/ATPase pump causing a reduction of K^+ cell uptake, thus leading to hyperkalemia [4, 6, 7] (Fig. 1).

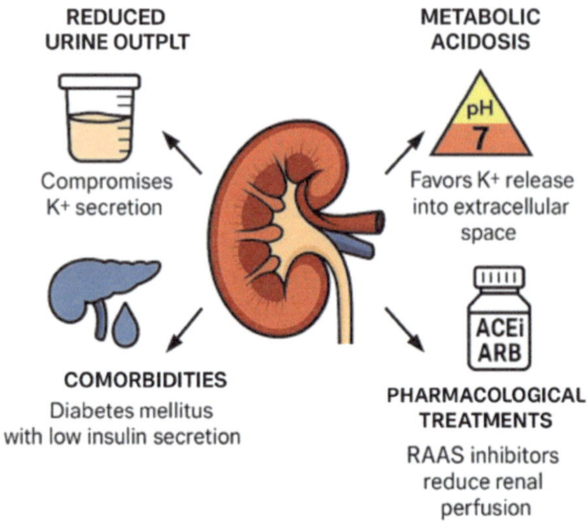

Fig. 1 Factors that play a crucial role in the pathophysiology of hyperkalemia

Complications of Hyperkalemia

Hyperkalemia is characterized by a serum or plasma potassium level exceeding the normal range, typically above 5.0 to 5.5 mmol/L. Mild hyperkalemia often does not show symptoms, but as potassium levels rise to 6.5 to 7 mmol/L, symptoms such as cardiac arrhythmias, cardiac arrest, muscle weakness, or paralysis may occur. However, the speed at which potassium levels change is more critical than the specific numerical value. Patients with chronic hyperkalemia may not show symptoms even at higher potassium levels, while those with rapid, acute changes in potassium may experience severe symptoms at lower levels [14].

Acute Hyperkalemia

Acute hyperkalemia is defined as a sudden increase in serum potassium concentration above the normal upper limit, typically ≥5.0 mmol/L, without prior evidence of chronic elevation. The rapid onset can lead to significant complications, necessitating immediate medical attention [15, 16].

Cardiovascular Complications [14]

The first test that should be ordered in a patient with suspected hyperkalemia is an ECG since the most lethal complication of hyperkalemia is cardiac condition abnormalities which can lead to dysrhythmias and death.

Elevated potassium causes ECG changes in a dose-dependent manner:

- $K = 5.5$ to 6.5 mEq/L ECG will show tall, peaked T-waves.
- $K = 6.5$ to 7.5 mEq/L ECG will show loss of P-waves.
- $K = 7$ to 8 ECG mEq/L will show widening of the QRS complex.
- $K = 8$ to 10 mEq/L will produce cardiac arrhythmias, sine wave pattern, and asystole.

It should be noted that the rate of rising serum potassium is a greater factor than the level. Patients with chronic hyperkalemia may have relatively normal EGCs even at high levels, and significant ECG changes may be present at much lower levels in patients with sudden spikes in serum potassium.

ECG features of hyperkalemia include:

- Small or absent P wave.
- Prolonged PR interval.
- Augmented R wave.
- Wide QRS.
- Peaked T-waves.

Neuromuscular Complications of Hyperkalemia: *Respiratory Failure*

Severe hyperkalemia can lead to respiratory failure due to diaphragmatic weakness. This is a medical emergency requiring immediate intervention [17].

Chronic Hyperkalemia

Chronic hyperkalemia can be defined as a biochemical condition characterized by persistently elevated serum potassium levels, with or without clinical symptoms. It typically requires pharmacological and/or non-pharmacological intervention [18].

The condition develops gradually over weeks to months and may present either persistently or in recurrent episodes. Despite its clinical relevance, according to the 2020 KDIGO *(Kidney Disease Improving Global Outcomes)* report, there is no consensus on the frequency, severity and duration of these episodes that describe chronicity [18, 19].

Chronic hyperkalemia is commonly associated with underlying chronic illnesses such as chronic kidney disease and heart failure. It is also frequently linked to the use of medications that impair potassium excretion, particularly those targeting the renin-angiotensin-aldosterone system (RAAS). While specific time frames can vary, chronic hyperkalemia is typically identified through repeated elevated potassium measurements over weeks to months [20].

1. *Renal Complications.*
   - *Reduced Renal Ammoniagenesis*: Hyperkalemia inhibits ammonium production in the proximal tubules, reducing the kidney's ability to excrete acid and thereby contributing to the development of metabolic acidosis [21].
   - *Decreased GFR*: Alters renal hemodynamic, lowering GFR and exacerbating underlying kidney disease [22].
2. *Gastrointestinal Complications.*
   - *Nausea, Vomiting, and Ileus*: Elevated potassium levels can reduce GI smooth muscle excitability, causing symptoms such as nausea, vomiting, abdominal distension, and even paralytic ileus [23] [24].
3. *Endocrine and Metabolic Complications.*
   - *Insulin Resistance*: Hyperkalemia can reduce insulin secretion, worsening glucose tolerance in diabetic individuals [25].
   - *Metabolic Acidosis*: Commonly observed due to impaired renal ammoniagenesis, especially in chronic renal impairment [26, 27].

Complications in Patients with Preexisting Risk Factors

Peripheral Neuropathy

Emerging evidence suggests hyperkalemia impairs neuronal excitability. In dialysis patients, median nerve conduction studies show axonal depolarization predialysis when serum potassium was ~5.4 mmol/L. Electrophysiological abnormalities were reversed by dialysis with low-dialysate potassium, suggesting hyperkalemia's role in uremic neuropathy [28, 29]. A single-blind RCT also found dietary potassium restriction improved peripheral nerve function in CKD patients [30].

Type IV Renal Tubular Acidosis (RTA)

The combination of hyperkalemia and impaired renal acid excretion defines type IV RTA [31].

Acute Flaccid Paralysis [32, 33]

Hyperkalemia-induced acute flaccid paralysis is a rare but serious condition. Patients typically present with rapidly progressive weakness, often starting in the lower limbs and ascending to involve the upper limbs.

Acute flaccid paralysis is a medical emergency that may be caused by severe hyperkalemia, especially in elderly patients with impaired renal function. It may constitute the dominant clinical presentation in patients with hyperkalemia. It may be caused by primary neuromuscular disorders, metabolic alterations, and iatrogenic effects.

Consequences of Hyperkalemia in Patients Receiving Dialysis

Patients on dialysis can be considered as a special group for two reasons: first, the prevalence of hyperkalemia (pre-dialysis serum [K^+] >5.5 mmol in ~20% of hemodialysis patients) and second, the prevalence of comorbidities that might potentiate any risk of cardiac arrhythmia and death (e.g., left ventricular hypertrophy) [34, 35].

In patients receiving maintenance hemo- and peritoneal dialysis, hyperkalemia has been associated with an increased risk of all-cause mortality, cardiac arrhythmia, and hospitalization [34–36]. In hemodialysis, the risks of hyperkalemia may be augmented during the long interdialytic gap. In an observational study of >50,000 hemodialysis patients, hyperkalemia (>5.5 mM pre-dialysis) was associated with an increased risk of hospitalization in the subsequent four days, and this risk was highest for K^+ measured before a three-day gap than for K^+ measured before a two-day gap [34].

Management of Hyperkalemia in CKD with New Potassium Binders

Hyperkalemia, defined as a serum potassium concentration > 5.0 mmol/L, is a common complication in patients with chronic kidney disease, particularly in advanced stages. It results from reduced renal excretion of potassium and is further exacerbated by the concurrent use of renin-angiotensin-aldosterone system inhibitors (RAASi), which are frequently prescribed to slow CKD progression and reduce cardiovascular risk. Recently, new potassium binders have been introduced, improving the management of hyperkalemia while allowing continuation of RAASi therapy and potentially preventing life-threatening events.

Potassium Binders: From Kayexalate to New Agents

Sodium polystyrene sulfonate (SPS), commercially known as Kayexalate, has been the mainstay treatment for hyperkalemia for decades. It can be administered orally or rectally and functions as a cation-exchange resin that promotes fecal elimination of potassium by exchanging sodium in the gut [37]. However, its clinical efficacy has been questioned, and its safety profile is limited by gastrointestinal side effects, including serious complications like intestinal necrosis [38].

Patiromer

Patiromer (Veltassa) is a non-absorbable cationic polymer that exchanges potassium for calcium in the colon, thereby reducing serum potassium through fecal excretion. It has a delayed onset of action (4–7 h), making it suitable for chronic rather than acute use. Studies have demonstrated its effectiveness in CKD patients receiving RAASi therapy, allowing continuation of treatment. Adverse effects include constipation, diarrhea, abdominal pain, and hypomagnesemia [39].

Sodium Zirconium Cyclosilicate

Sodium zirconium cyclosilicate (SZC) is a non-absorbable inorganic crystalline powder that selectively binds potassium throughout the gastrointestinal tract. It exchanges potassium and ammonium for sodium and hydrogen ions, with a favorable tolerability profile. Unlike Patiromer, it has a faster onset of action (1–6 h), making it suitable for subacute treatment. Adverse effects include edema—particularly at high doses—and gastrointestinal disturbances. SZC may temporarily raise gastric pH, and thus, pH-dependent drugs should be administered two hours before or after SZC intake [40].

Clinical Applications

New potassium binders are indicated for chronic management of hyperkalemia in patients with stage 3–5 CKD, particularly those receiving RAASi therapy. Typical daily doses are 8.4 g for Patiromer and 5–10 g for SZC, adjusted according to serum potassium levels (Table 1).

Table 1 Summary table of the initial and maintenance dosage of potassium binders

	Sodium zirconium cyclosilicate	Patiromer	Sodium polystyrene sulfonate
Initial dose	10 g orally 3 times/day for up to 48 h	8.4 g orally once daily	15 g orally 1–4 times/day
Maintenance dose	10 g once daily (range: 5 g every other day to 15 g once daily)	8.4–25.2 g orally once daily	15 g orally 1–4 times/day

Comparison Between SPS, Patiromer, and SZC

While Kayexalate has long been the standard therapy, newer binders present safer and more effective alternatives. These agents are associated with fewer gastrointestinal side effects and more predictable potassium control, enabling continued use of RAASi therapy [41].

Acute Hyperkalemia Management

Acute hyperkalemia is a potentially life-threatening condition, defined as a rapid elevation in serum potassium concentration, generally >5 mmol/L, with or without electrocardiographic (ECG) changes [42]. Due to its unpredictability and the immediate risk of ventricular arrhythmias, treatment must be initiated promptly [43].

The treatment strategy is structured into three fundamental phases:

1. *Stabilization of the Myocardial Cell Membrane*

The primary goal is to prevent the onset of fatal arrhythmias. The first-line agent is:

- *Calcium gluconate*: onset occurs within 1–3 min, with effects lasting 30–60 min. If ECG abnormalities persist after 5–10 min, the dose may be repeated [44].

Calcium does not lower serum potassium, but stabilizes the myocardial membrane potential, counteracting the depolarizing effects of extracellular K^+. Calcium chloride contains more ionized calcium than gluconate but is more irritating to peripheral veins and should preferably be administered via a central venous line [45].

2. *Intracellular Shift of Potassium*

This phase aims to temporarily lower serum potassium by driving potassium into the intracellular compartment:

- *Insulin (10–12 IU)* lowers K^+ levels by 0.5–1.5 mmol/L within 15–60 min. Insulin reduces potassium level by stimulating the Na^+/K^+-ATPase pump [46].
- *Salbutamol (β2-agonist)* decreases K^+ by ~0.5–1.0 mmol/L. Salbutamol has a synergic effect with insulin, and it cannot be used as monotherapy. It is contraindicated in patients with severe ischemic heart disease [47].
- *Sodium bicarbonate* is only recommended in the presence of metabolic acidosis (pH <7.2), since the effect with normal pH is modest [48].

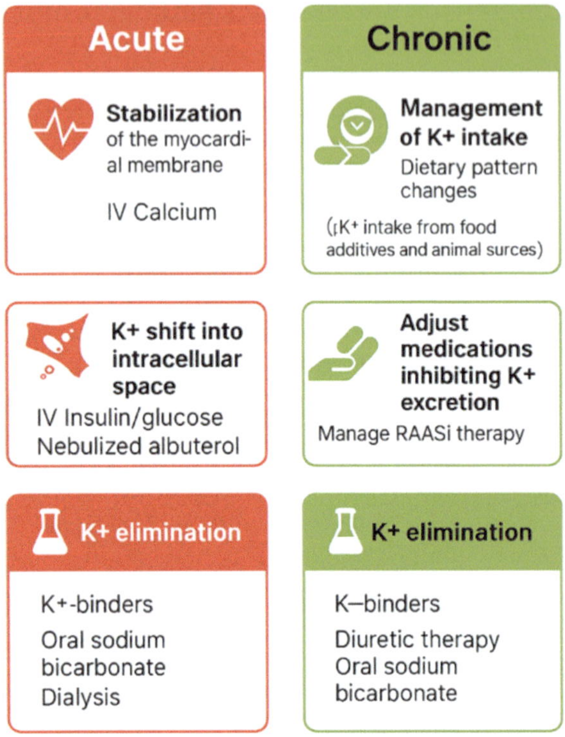

Fig. 2 Management of acute and chronic hyperkalemia

3. *Elimination of Potassium from the Body*

This step is essential for definitive potassium correction**:**

- *Loop diuretics*, but their efficacy varies in patients with renal impairment [49].
- *Oral Potassium Binders*:
- *Hemodialysis* is considered the most effective intervention when:
  - Conservative measures fail.
  - Advanced CKD or anuria is present.
    Severe hyperkalemia >7.0 mmol/L with symptoms or ECG changes.

Dialysis can reduce serum potassium by approximately 1 mmol/L per hour of treatment [50] (Fig. 2).

References

1. Viera AJ, Wouk N. Potassium disorders: hypokalemia and hyperkalemia. Am Fam Physician. 2015;92(6):487–95.
2. Sarnowski A, Gama RM, Dawson A, Mason H, Banerjee D. Hyperkalemia in chronic kidney disease: links, risks and management. Int J Nephrol Renovasc Dis. 2022;15:215–28.

3. Stallings VA, Harrison M, Oria M, editors. Dietary reference intakes for sodium and potassium. Washington, DC: National Academies Press; 2019.
4. Palmer BF, Clegg DJ. Physiology and pathophysiology of potassium homeostasis: core curriculum 2019. Am J Kidney Dis. 2019;74(5):682–95.
5. Giebisch G. Renal potassium transport: mechanisms and regulation. Am J Phys. 1998;274(5):F817–33.
6. Zacchia M, Abategiovanni ML, Stratigis S, Capasso G. Potassium: from physiology to clinical implications. Kidney Dis (Basel). 2016;2(2):72–9.
7. Valdivielso JM, Balafa O, Ekart R, Ferro CJ, Mallamaci F, Mark PB, et al. Hyperkalemia in chronic kidney disease in the new era of kidney protection therapies. Drugs. 2021;81(13):1467–89.
8. Palmer BF. Regulation of potassium homeostasis. Clin J Am Soc Nephrol. 2015;10(6):1050–60.
9. Sarafidis PA, Blacklock R, Wood E, Rumjon A, Simmonds S, Fletcher-Rogers J, et al. Prevalence and factors associated with hyperkalemia in predialysis patients followed in a low-clearance clinic. Clin J Am Soc Nephrol. 2012;7(8):1234–41.
10. Betts KA, Woolley JM, Mu F, McDonald E, Tang W, Wu EQ. The prevalence of hyperkalemia in the United States. Curr Med Res Opin. 2018;34(6):971–8.
11. Gennari FJ, Segal AS. Hyperkalemia: an adaptive response in chronic renal insufficiency. Kidney Int. 2002;62(1):1–9.
12. Palmer BF, Clegg DJ. Electrolyte and acid–base disturbances in patients with diabetes mellitus. N Engl J Med. 2015;373(6):548–59.
13. Weir MR, Rolfe M. Potassium homeostasis and renin-angiotensin-aldosterone system inhibitors. Clin J Am Soc Nephrol. 2010;5(3):531–48.
14. Simon LV, Hashmi MF, Farrell MW. Hyperkalemia [Internet]. In: StatPearls [Internet]. Treasure Island: StatPearls Publishing; 2023. [cited 2025 June 16].
15. Long B, Brit, et al. Controversies in management of hyperkalemia. J Emerg Med. 2025;55(2):192–205.
16. Lindner G, Burdmann EA, Clase CM, et al. Acute hyperkalemia in the emergency department: a summary from a kidney disease: improving global outcomes conference. Eur J Emerg Med. 2020;27(5):329–37.
17. Freeman SJ, Fale AD. Muscular paralysis and ventilatory failure caused by hyperkalaemia. Br J Anaesth. 1993;70(2):226–7.
18. Rico-Fontalvo J, Rodríguez-González MJ, Yama EY, et al. Chronic hyperkalemia, diagnosis and management. Colombian consensus. Arch Cardiol Mex. 2023;93(Supl):1–12. English
19. Clase CM, Ashuntantang GE, et al. Potassium homeostasis and management of dyskalemia in kidney diseases: conclusions from a kidney disease: improving global outcomes (KDIGO) controversies conference. Kidney Int. 2020;97(1):42–61.
20. Weinstein J, Girard LP, Lepage S, Mackelvie RS, Tennankore K. Prevention and management of hyperkalemia in patients treated with renin–angiotensin–aldosterone system inhibitors. CMAJ. 2021;193(48):E1836–41.
21. Soleimani M, Rastegar A. Pathophysiology of renal tubular acidosis: core curriculum 2016. Am J Kidney Dis. 2016;68(3):488–98.
22. Kovesdy C. Management of hyperkalaemia in chronic kidney disease. Nat Rev Nephrol. 2014;10:653–62.
23. Royal Children's Hospital Melbourne. Hyperkalaemia clinical guideline; [cited 2025 June 17] Available from: https://www.rch.org.au/clinicalguide/guideline_index/hyperkalaemia/
24. Currò D. The modulation of potassium channels in the smooth muscle as a therapeutic strategy for disorders of the gastrointestinal tract. In: Donev R, editor. Advances in protein chemistry and structural biology, vol. 104. Academic; 2016. p. 263–305.
25. Kim HW, Lee DH, Lee SA, Koh G. A relationship between serum potassium concentration and insulin resistance in patients with type 2 diabetes mellitus. Int Urol Nephrol. 2015;47(6):991–9.
26. Yartsev A. Type 4 (hyperkalemic) renal tubular acidosis [Internet]. Deranged Physiology. 2015 [updated 2020 Jan 8; cited 2025 June 16].

27. Treatment of hyperkalemia and metabolic acidosis. In: Metabolic acidosi Clin Exp Nephrol 2009;13:243–244.
28. Kiernan MC, Walters RJ, Andersen KV, Taube D, Murray NM, Bostock H. Nerve excitability changes in chronic renal failure indicate membrane depolarization due to hyperkalaemia. Brain. 2002;125(Pt 6):1366–78.
29. Arnold R, Pussell BA, Howells J, Grinius V, Kiernan MC, Lin CS-Y, Krishnan AV. Evidence for a causal relationship between hyperkalaemia and axonal dysfunction in end-stage kidney disease. Clin Neurophysiol. 2014;125(1):179–85.
30. Arnold R, Pianta TJ, Pussell BA, Kirby A, O'Brien K, Sullivan K, et al. Randomized, controlled trial of the effect of dietary potassium restriction on nerve function in CKD. Clin J Am Soc Nephrol. 2017;12(10):1569–77.
31. Karet FE. Mechanisms in hyperkalemic renal tubular acidosis. J Am Soc Nephrol. 2009;20(2):251–4. https://doi.org/10.1681/ASN.2008020166.
32. D'Ercole M, Cipriani L, Picciotto D, Bianzina S, Russo E, Viazzi F, Esposito P. Hyperkalemia-induced acute flaccid paralysis: a case report. Unit of nephrology, dialysis and transplantation. San Martino: IRCCS Ospedale Policlinico; n.d.
33. Karmacharya P, Poudel DR, Pathak R, Rettew A, Alweis R. Acute hyperkalemia leading to flaccid paralysis: a review of hyperkalemic manifestations. J Community Hosp Intern Med Perspect. 2015;5(3):27993.
34. Brunelli SM, et al. Serum potassium and short-term clinical outcomes among hemodialysis patients: impact of the long interdialytic interval. Am J Kidney Dis. 2017;70(1):21–9.
35. Karaboyas A, et al. Dialysate potassium, serum potassium, mortality, and arrhythmia events in hemodialysis: results from the Dialysis Outcomes and Practice Patterns Study (DOPPS). Am J Kidney Dis. 2017;69(2):266–77.
36. Rhee CM. Serum potassium and the long interdialytic interval: minding the gap. Am J Kidney Dis. 2017;70(1):4–7.
37. Sterns RH, et al. Kidney Int. 2016;89(3):546–54. PMID: 26880475
38. Harel Z, et al. Am J Med. 2013;126(3):264.e9–264.e24.
39. Weir MR, et al. N Engl J Med. 2015;372(3):211–21. PMID: 25372087
40. Levien TL, Baker DE. Hosp Pharm. 2019;54(1):12–9. PMID: 30718929
41. Fonseca C, et al. Heart Fail Rev. 2025;30(2):271–86. PMID: 39604607
42. Palmer BF, Clegg DJ. Diagnosis and treatment of hyperkalemia. N Engl J Med. 2017;376(6):548–59. https://doi.org/10.1056/NEJMra1607181.
43. Weisberg LS. Management of severe hyperkalemia. Crit Care Med. 2008;36(12):3246–51.
44. Batterink J, et al. Calcium for treating hyperkalemia: a systematic review. PLoS One. 2020;15(6):e0234922.
45. Sterns RH, et al. Therapy of hyperkalemia. Am J Kidney Dis. 2010;56(3):570–6.
46. Allon M. Insulin-induced hypokalemia: mechanisms and implications. Kidney Int. 1990;37(5):1135–42.
47. Mahoney BA, et al. Treatment of hyperkalemia with a combination of insulin, glucose, and albuterol. Arch Intern Med. 1999;159(6):675–80.
48. Adrogue HJ, Madias NE. Changes in plasma potassium concentration during acute acid-base disturbances. Am J Med. 1981;71(3):456–67.
49. Gennari FJ. Hypokalemia. N Engl J Med. 1998;339(7):451–8.
50. Kraut JA, Madias NE. Treatment of disorders of potassium balance: emerging insights. Kidney Int. 2007;72(5):544–54.

Antihypertensive Treatment in Chronic Kidney Disease: Blood Pressure Targets

Marieta P. Theodorakopoulou and Pantelis Sarafidis

Introduction

Hypertension represents the most frequent comorbidity in patients with chronic kidney disease (CKD), with reported rates of approximately 80–90%. Its prevalence rises in parallel with disease progression toward advanced CKD and affects up to 95% of individuals with stage 4 or 5 prior to initiation of kidney replacement therapy [1, 2]. Elevated blood pressure (BP) is a strong and independent risk factor for both development of CKD and progression to kidney failure [3, 4]. Hypertensive kidney disease is recognized as the second leading identifiable cause of end-stage kidney disease (ESKD), following diabetic kidney disease [5, 6]. In addition, hypertension is also a typical consequence of many primary and secondary kidney diseases. Thus, elevated BP is by far the most common modifiable factor for CKD progression. Treatment-resistant hypertension, elevated nighttime BP, and masked hypertension are common in patients with CKD and are associated with lower estimated glomerular filtration rate (eGFR), higher levels of albuminuria, progression to ESKD [7–13], as well as other hypertension-mediated organ damage (HMOD) and adverse cardiovascular outcomes [11–13].

The major role of the kidneys in the pathogenesis of essential hypertension is well established. In CKD, several mechanisms that originate from the kidney and promote hypertension are often amplified. These include increased sodium sensitivity, sodium and fluid retention, overactivation of the renin-angiotensin-system (RAS) and the sympathetic-nervous-system (SNS), as well as impaired endothelium-dependent vasodilation [4, 14]. Additional CKD-related factors, such as mineral bone disorder leading to arterial stiffness, increased prevalence of sleep-apnea syndrome, and administration of agents like erythropoietin, glucocorticoids, or

M. P. Theodorakopoulou (✉) · P. Sarafidis
1st Department of Nephrology, Aristotle University of Thessaloniki, Hippokration Hospital, Thessaloniki, Greece

P. Sarafidis, R. Pontremoli (eds.), *Hypertension and Chronic Kidney Disease*, Updates in Hypertension and Cardiovascular Protection,
https://doi.org/10.1007/978-3-032-29564-4_11

calcineurin inhibitors may also contribute to BP elevation in patients with CKD [15, 16]. Given the central role of hypertension in the development, progression, and complications of CKD, defining optimal treatment BP targets remains a challenge in both research and clinical practice. This chapter discusses major trials that examined this issue, including the Modification of Diet in Renal Disease (MDRD), African American Study of Kidney Disease and Hypertension (AASK), and Systolic Blood Pressure Intervention Trial (SPRINT) trials, including their strengths and limitations together with recommendations from contemporary guideline documents in the field.

Clinical Studies Examining Optimal BP Targets in CKD

Existing evidence indicates that lowering BP with any first-line antihypertensive class confers comparable protection against major cardiovascular outcomes and all-cause mortality, in individuals both with and without CKD [17]. However, the optimal BP targets in CKD have remained a subject of controversy until the recent past [18, 19]. Previous observational data suggested an association between BP and the risk for ESKD, starting from an SBP level of >120 mmHg [3]. However, robust clinical trial data defining the optimal BP goal in CKD are lacking; ideally, such evidence would come from a randomized clinical trial (RCT) comparing different BP targets (i.e., SBP < 140 vs. <130 mmHg), including a CKD population with an appropriate mixture of eGFR and albuminuria levels and etiology, achieving corresponding BP levels during follow-up and being powered to investigate hard kidney outcomes, cardiovascular outcomes, and mortality.

The evidence regarding optimal BP targets in CKD derives mainly from two previous trials in non-diabetic individuals that randomized patients to different levels or ranges of mean BP (Table 1) and examined renal outcomes. In the MDRD study, 840 nondiabetic patients with GFR of 13–55 mL/min/1.73 m^2 were randomized to a usual-protein or a low-protein diet and to a standard- or an intensive-BP target (mean arterial pressure (MAP) <107 and < 113 mmHg for patients <=60 and > 60 years, vs. MAP<92 and < 98 mmHg for patients ≤60 and > 60 years, respectively) in a 2 × 2 factorial design. The mean follow-up was 2.2 years. The projected GFR decline within 3 years, and the risk for ESKD and death were not significantly different between groups of low vs. usual BP target (hazard ratio, HR 0.85; 95% confidence interval (CI) 0.60–1.22) [20]. However, subgroups analyses stratifying patients by baseline proteinuria levels showed that those with proteinuria >1 g/day in the low-target group had a decrease in protein excretion and a slower eGFR loss over time compared to patients in the usual target group [21].

The AASK trial followed a 3 × 2 factorial design and randomized 1094 black patients with hypertensive CKD (eGFR: 20–65 mL/min/1.73 m^2) to two arms of BP control (mean BP: 102–107 vs. ≤92 mm Hg) and to initial therapy with three antihypertensive drug classes (metoprolol 50–200 mg/day or ramipril 2.5–10 mg/day or amlodipine 5–10 mg/day) [22]. In the main trial, results were similar to MDRD; no significant differences between the two BP goals for any of the outcomes studied

Table 1 Main characteristics and outcomes of major clinical trials and their long-term observational analyses including CKD patients that compared a low to a usual BP target

Study ID	Population	Intervention and comparator	Follow-up	Main findings
AASK [22]	1094 African-Americans with hypertensive CKD (GFR, 20–65 mL/min/1.73 m^2, mean proteinuria 0.6 g/day); mean age 54.6 years	Usual BP goal (MAP 102–107) compared to a low BP goal (MAP ≤92 mmHg, corresponding to <125/75)	3.8 years (median)	No difference between groups in mean GFR slope (-2.21 ± 0.17 vs. -1.95 ± 0.17 mL/min/1.73 m^2 per year; $p = 0.24$), or the composite outcome of reduction in GFR by 50% or more (or ≥ 25 mL/min/1.73 m^2), ESKD, or death (risk reduction for intensive BP group 2%; 95%CI, −22% to 21%; $p = 0.85$)
AASK trial and cohort phase analysis [25]		Trial period and a subsequent cohort period in which the BP target was <130/80 mmHg	Total follow-up 8.8–12.2 years	No difference between groups in the risk of the composite outcome of doubling of serum creatinine, ESKD, or death (HR in low-BP group, 0.91; 95%CI, 0.77–1.08). Significant interaction with the baseline level of proteinuria ($p = 0.02$). For patients with UPCR > 0.22 mg/g, HR 0.73; 95%CI, 0.58–0.93; for patients with UPCR ≤0.22, HR, 1.18; 95%CI: 0.93–1.50

(continued)

Table 1 (continued)

Study ID	Population	Intervention and comparator	Follow-up	Main findings
MDRD [20]	Study A: 585 patients (GFR 25–55 mL/min/1.73 m^2); study B: 255 patients (GFR 13–24 mL/min/1.73 m^2); mean age 51.7 years	Usual BP goal [MAP, <107 mmHg for patients ≤60 years (roughly corresponding to <140/90) and <113 for patients ≥61 years] compared to a low goal [MAP <92 mmHg for patients ≤60 years (corresponding to <125/75) and < 98 for patients ≥61 years]	2.2 years (mean)	No difference between groups in the projected GFR decline in 3 years (10.7 vs. 11.5 mL/min/1.73 m^2), and the risk of ESKD and death (0.85, 95%CI:0.60–1.22 for low BP arm)
MDRD trial and cohort phase analysis [24]		MDRD trial period (1989–1993) and a cohort period (1993–2000) during which no specific target BP was recommended	10.7 years (median)	Low target BP was associated with reduced risk for ESKD (adjusted HR 0.68; 95%CI:0.57–0.82) and the composite of ESKD or death (HR 0.77; 95%CI:0.65–0.91), compared with usual target BP. The *p-value for interaction of target BP with proteinuria was 0.09 for ESKD and 0.08 for the composite outcome*
MDRD and AASK trial and cohort phases combined [26]	1907 patients (mean age of 53 years, median GFR of 40 mL/min/1.73 m^2 and median urine protein excretion of 0.12 g/day at baseline	Trial period and subsequent cohort periods of both trials	14.9 years (median)	Low target BP was independently associated with lower risk of ESKD (HR 0.88; 95% CI 0.78–0.99) and death (HR 0.85; 95% CI 0.75–0.97). For patients with UPCR >0.44 g/g risk of ESKD (HR 0.77; 95% CI 0.64–0.92) and death (HR 0.77; 95% CI 0.62–0.96). For patients with UPCR<0.44 g/g no significant effects were shown

(continued)

Table 1 (continued)

Study ID	Population	Intervention and comparator	Follow-up	Main findings
SPRINT sub-analysis in CKD patients [28]	2646 patients with eGFR 20–60 mL/min/1.73 m^2 (individuals with proteinuria >1 g/day or > 1 g/g excluded); mean age 71.9 years	Intensive (SBP <120 mmHg) compared to standard (SBP <140 mmHg) BP lowering treatment based on unattended automated office BP measurements	3.3 years (median)	No difference between groups in the risk of the primary outcome (MI, acute coronary syndrome not resulting in MI, stroke, acute decompensated HF or death from cardiovascular causes) (HR, 0.81;95% CI, 0.63–1.05), and the main kidney outcome (≥50% decrease in eGFR from baseline or ESKD) (HR, 0.90; 95% CI, 0.44 to 1.83); low target BP was associated with lower all-cause mortality (HR, 0.72; 95% CI, 0.53–0.99)

MDRD Modification of Diet in Renal Disease Study, *AASK* African-American Study on Kidney Disease, *BP* Blood Pressure, *HF* Heart Failure, *SPRINT* Systolic Blood Pressure Intervention Trial, *MAP* Mean Arterial Pressure, *MI* Myocardial Infarction, *SBP* Systolic Blood Pressure, *eGFR* Estimated Glomerular Filtration Rate, *HR* Hazard Ratio, *ESKD* End-stage Kidney Disease, *UPCR* Urine Protein-to-Creatinine Ratio, *CKD* Chronic Kidney Disease, *CI* Confidence Interval

(eGFR slope, composite of ≥50% or ≥ 25 mL/min/1.73 m^2 reduction in eGFR from baseline, ESKD or death) were noted. However, in a post hoc analysis, again, low BP was associated with kidney benefit in the small subgroup of patients with proteinuria >1 g/day [23].

Subsequent analyses of both studies combined the randomized trial periods with subsequent observational follow-up phases (Table 1). In MDRD long-term follow-up analysis, low-target BP was associated with overall reduced risk for ESKD and the composite of ESKD or death, but this was again mainly driven from better outcomes in patients with baseline proteinuria >1 g/day [24]. In the AASK long-term follow-up analysis, no between-group difference in the risk of the composite outcome of doubling of serum creatinine, ESKD, or death was observed. However, for patients with urine protein-to-creatinine ratio (UPCR) > 0.22 g/g, low BP was again associated with better kidney outcomes [25]. A recent analysis combining the trial and cohort periods of both these trials (adding up to 1907 patients and a median follow-up of 14.9 years) showed that low target BP was associated with lower risk for ESKD and mortality in the total population; again this effect was mainly driven by changes in patients with UPCR >0.44 g/g (UACR roughly >200 mg/g) [26].

The SPRINT randomized 9361 non-diabetic, hypertensive patients to intensive or standard treatment (target SBP <120 vs. <140 mmHg, respectively) based on automated office BP recordings [27]. This trial was prematurely terminated (median follow-up 3.26 years) as the rate of the primary outcome (acute coronary syndrome with or without myocardial infarction, stroke, acute decompensated heart failure or death from cardiovascular causes) was significantly lower in the intensive treatment compared with the standard treatment group (HR 0.75; 95% CI 0.64–0.89; P < 0.001). Importantly, the low BP target in this study produced a significant reduction in total mortality (HR 0.73; 95% CI 0.60–0.90; P¼0.003), despite the premature termination of the study. From the total population, 28% had CKD (eGFR 20–60 mL/min/1.73 m^2), but very few had albuminuria A2 or A3, as individuals with proteinuria >1 g/24 h or > 1 g/g were excluded. In the overall trial, kidney outcomes did not differ between groups. In a pre-specified sub-analysis of the SPRINT in 2646 patients with CKD [28], in whom achieved BP was 123.3 ± 0.4/66.9 ± 0.3 mm Hg in the intensive group (vs. 136.9 ± 0.4/73.8 ± 0.3 mm Hg in the standard group), no difference between groups in the primary outcome nor in the pre-specified kidney outcome was detected, but mortality rate was lower in the intensive BP arm. The primary renal outcome (decrease in eGFR ≥50% or ESKD) occurred in 15/1330 intensive group and 16/1316 standard group participants (HR 0.90; 95% CI 0.44–1.83). The above results must be cautiously interpreted, as the SPRINT trial was not designed or powered to study kidney outcomes, and as such resulted in an extremely small number of kidney events (15 vs. 16 in the two groups). Most importantly, as previously mentioned, the majority of SPRINT participants with CKD had normoalbuminuria (median UACR 13.3 mg/g). A low BP target is obviously not expected to confer renal benefits in the short follow-up of this group at low risk for renal disease progression, in accordance with the aforementioned findings of MDRD and AASK. Moreover, SPRINT employed a trial-specific automated office BP measurement protocol, but its implementation lacked uniformity across study sites. Variations existed in whether staff were present or absent during the rest period and/or measurement phase (no attendance, attendance during rest periods, readings' period, or both), a fact that directly influenced the observed differences in outcomes [29]. It is also well recognized that unattended systolic BP, which was applied in approximately 42% of SPRINT participants, can differ markedly from conventional office BP, with individual discrepancies ranging from 5 to 15 mmHg [9].

In patients with diabetic CKD, no randomized trial has directly defined the optimal BP target. Earlier studies, including the United Kingdom Prospective Diabetes Study (UKPDS) 38 [30] and the sub-analysis of diabetic patients of the Hypertension Optimal Treatment (HOT) [31] trials, provided some evidence regarding DBP target, since they randomized patients in different DBP levels. The Action to Control CardiOvascular risk in Diabetes (ACCORD)-BP trial randomized high-risk patients with type 2 diabetes to target SBP < 120 vs. <140 mmHg [32]; apart from no difference in the primary outcome, most possibly due to interactions with other arms of the factorial design and the unexpectedly low event rate [19], ACCORD-BP excluded individuals with serum creatinine >1.5 mg/dL; thus, it can offer very little insight to the optimal BP in patients with diabetic CKD. A post hoc analysis of the Reduction of Endpoints in NIDDM with the Angiotensin II Antagonist Losartan (RENAAL) study demonstrated that baseline SBP of 140–159 mmHg increased risk for ESKD or death by 38% compared to SBP < 130 mmHg [33]. A relevant post hoc analysis from the Irbesartan Diabetic Nephropathy Trial (IDNT) showed that SBP > 149 mmHg was associated with a 2.2-fold increase in the risk for the composite of doubling SCr or ESKD compared with SBP < 134 mmHg. Progressive lowering of SBP to 120 mmHg improved renal and overall survival, but below 120 mmHg, all-cause mortality increased [34].

Taken together, although evidence remains indirect, these findings suggest that BP targets shown to be beneficial in proteinuric non-diabetic CKD may be cautiously extrapolated to patients with proteinuric diabetic CKD, given the shared pathways of kidney injury. Post hoc analyses of major kidney outcome trials in DM [33, 34] showed benefits when SBP is reduced <130 mmHg, but not <120 mmHg. In a recent pooled analysis AASK, ACCORD, MDRD, and SPRINT trials, all-cause mortality showed a tendency to a reduction with intensive treatments (BP <130 mmHg) [35]. In another meta-analysis of 18 RCTs (n = 15,924 CKD patients), more intensive vs. less intensive BP control (SBP 132 mmHg vs. 140 mmHg) was associated with 14% lower risk of all-cause mortality [36]. In general, however, meta-analytic efforts in patients with or without diabetes suffer from various limitations, most commonly mixture of studies that compared two different BP targets with studies comparing active drug treatment with placebo/no treatment and resulting in different BP levels [19].

Current Recommendations on BP Targets in CKD

Over the past decade, major guideline documents have reported recommendations on BP targets for patients with CKD (Table 2). The 2021 KDIGO guidelines do not discuss the thresholds on which antihypertensive treatment should be instituted [37]. In addition, they recommend for an SBP target of <120 mmHg for patients with CKD [37], with the specific notion that this refers to standardized office BP readings and it should be applied only if this target is well tolerated [37, 38]. No reference on a DBP target is made in this guideline. This is mainly based on the SPRINT trial, and particularly a single, hypothesis-generating sub-analysis of the SPRINT trial, which included only a narrow range of the CKD population (non-diabetic, non-proteinuric CKD with eGFR 20–60 mL/min/1.73 m^2 without prior stroke) and had both the primary and the main kidney outcomes (with only few events) being not significantly different between groups, while also the methodology for BP measurement was not consistent, as mentioned above [29]. As such subsequent Guidelines in this issue give different recommendations [19, 39].

The 2023 ESH Guidelines extensively discuss the thresholds for starting antihypertensive treatment; it is recommended that in patients 18 to 79 years, the office threshold for initiation of drug treatment is 140 mmHg for SBP and/or 90 mmHg for DBP [Class of Recommendation, (CoR) I, Level of Evidence (LoE) A] [40]. The exception to this rule is adult patients with a history of CVD, predominantly coronary artery disease (CAD), in whom drug treatment should be initiated in the high-normal BP range (SBP ≥130 or DBP ≥80 mmHg) (CoR I, LoE A); the clinical nephrologists should not overlook that many CKD patients fall into the latter

Table 2 BP targets for CKD patients in current guidelines

Guidelines	Recommendation for antihypertensive medication treatment	Recommendation for BP target
2021 KDIGO	Not applicable	In all adults with high BP and CKD the treatment target to lower standardized office SBP <120 mmHg (2B) In adult kidney transplant recipients, standardized office BP should be lowered to <130/80 mmHg (not graded)
2023 ESH	In patients 18 to 79 years, the recommended office threshold for initiation of drug treatment is 140 mmHg for SBP and/or 90 mmHg for DBP, except for patients with a history of CVD, predominantly CAD, in whom drug treatment should be initiated in the high-normal BP range (SBP ≥130 or DBP ≥80 mmHg) (CoR I, LoE A)	In all patients with CKD the primary goal is to lower office BP to <140/90 mmHg (CoR I, LoE A) In most patients with CKD (especially, young patients, patients with an UACR ≥ 300 mg/g, high CV risk patients) office BP should be lowered to <130/80 mmHg if tolerated (CoR II, LoE B) In kidney transplant recipients with hypertension, office BP should be lowered to <130/80 mmHg (CoR II, LoE B) In patients with CKD, a BP target of <120/70 mmHg is not recommended (CoR III, LoE C)
2024 ESC	It is recommended that in hypertensive patients with confirmed BP ≥ 140/90 mmHg, irrespective of CVD risk, lifestyle measure and pharmacological BP-lowering treatment are initiated promptly to reduce CVD risk (CoR I, LoE A) In patients with diabetic or non-diabetic moderate-to-severe CKD and confirmed BP ≥ 130/80 mmHg, lifestyle optimization and BP-lowering medication are recommended to reduce CVD risk, provided such treatment is well tolerated (CoR I, LoE A)	In adults with moderate-to-severe CKD who are receiving BP-lowering drugs and who have eGFR >30 mL/min/1.73 m^2, it is recommended to target SBP to 120–129 mmHg, if tolerated Individualized BP targets are recommended for those with lower eGFR or renal transplantation (CoR I, LoE A)
2025 AHA/ACC	In all adults with hypertension, initiation of medications to lower BP is recommended when average SBP is ≥140/90 mmHg to reduce the risk of CVD events and total mortality (CoR I, LoE A) In adults with hypertension and CKD, initiation of medications to lower BP is recommended when average SBP ≥ 130 mmHg (CoR I, LoE A) and/or DBP ≥ 90 mmHg (CoR I, LoE C-LD) to reduce the risk of CVD events and total mortality	For adults with hypertension and CKD as identified by eGFR <60 mL/min/1.73 m^2 or albuminuria of UACR ≥30 mg/g, treatment should target an SBP goal of <130 mmHg to decrease all-cause mortality (CoR I, LoE A)

BP Blood Pressure, *CAD* Coronary Artery Disease, *CKD* Chronic Kidney Disease, *CoR* Class of Recommendation, *CV* Cardiovascular, *CVD* Cardiovascular Disease, *DBP* Diastolic Blood Pressure, *eGFR* Estimated Glomerular Filtration Rate, *LoE* Level of Evidence, *SBP* Systolic Blood Pressure, *UACR* Urine Albumin-to-Creatinine Ratio

category and should be treated accordingly. In patients ≥80 years, the recommended office SBP threshold for initiation of drug treatment is 160 mmHg (CoR I, LoE A), but a lower SBP threshold of 140–159 mmHg may be considered (CoR II, LoE B). With regard to BP targets, this document recommends that in all patients with CKD the primary goal is to lower office SBP to <140 mmHg and DBP <90 mmHg (CoR I, LoE A) and that in most CKD patients (young patients, patients with a urine ACR ≥300 mg/g, high CV risk patients) office BP may be lowered to <130/80 mmHg, if tolerated (CoR II, LoE B) [40]. According to this document, a recommendation to target office SBP < 120 mmHg in persons with CKD cannot be made (CoR III, LoE C) due to insufficient evidence and the potential to cause harm. The 2023 ESH Guidelines also suggest that equivalent targets for HBPM or ABPM are not established; however, at an office BP <130/80, home or mean 24-h values are likely to be similar or only modestly different from BP values. Of note, a similar target of <130/80 mmHg is recommended for patients that have undergone kidney transplantation. The 2023 ESH Guidelines acknowledge that these recommendations have a number of limitations: (i) none of the trials comparing different BP targets included patients with diabetes and CKD, thus current evidence cannot be readily extrapolated to this subpopulation; (ii) MDRD and AASK trials randomized participants to different mean BP levels, which cannot be readily extrapolated to SBP and DBP values; (iii) MDRD and AASK trials recruited patient populations of a relatively young age (mean age 51.7 and 54.6 years, respectively), and thus their findings cannot be readily extrapolated to older patients with CKD; and (iv) even for the long-term observational analyses, the benefits associated with lower BP targets were mainly apparent in individuals with proteinuria.

The 2024 ESC Guidelines include patients with moderate-to-severe CKD (eGFR<60 mL/min/1.73 m^2 or albuminuria at or over 30 mg/g creatinine), among the high-risk groups that may benefit from pharmacotherapeutic agent initiation at SBP ≥130 mm Hg and/or DBP ≥80 mm Hg, in contrast to patients that do not fall in this category and would benefit from treatment initiation at SBP ≥ 140 mm Hg and/or DBP ≥ 90 mm Hg [41]. These guidelines recommend the same treatment target (120–129/70–79 mmHg), if tolerated, for patients with hypertension and CKD with an eGFR >30 mL/min/1.73 m^2, as for the general hypertensive population (Table 2). For patients with lower eGFR, patients with ESKD and those with kidney transplantation and individualized approach without discussion on BP targets are recommended [41].

Finally, the recent 2025 AHA/ACC guideline recommends that in all adult patients with hypertension, the office threshold for initiation of medication to lower BP is 140 mmHg for SBP and/or 90 mmHg for DBP (CoR I, LoE A) [42]. For selected adults who have clinical CVD, previous stroke, diabetes, CKD, or increased 10-year predicted cardiovascular risk of ≥7.5% defined by PREVENT™ (Predicting Risk of CVD EVENTs), initiation of medication therapy to lower BP is recommended for BP levels ≥130/80 mmHg (CoR I, LoE A for SBP and LoE C-LD for DBP) [42]. With regard to target BP, the recommendation in this guideline is for a treatment goal SBP <130 mmHg [42].

Conclusions

Hypertension is the most common comorbidity in CKD, affecting up to 95% of patients with advanced stages and being both a cause and consequence of kidney dysfunction. It accelerates progression to kidney failure and increases cardiovascular risk. Existing evidence suggests that antihypertensive therapy reduces cardiovascular events and mortality, but to date the optimal treatment BP target in CKD remains debated. Clinical trials such as MDRD and AASK have shaped the current understanding, but they were inarguably limited by population selection, short follow-up, and underrepresentation of high-risk groups such as patients with diabetes (in all three) or significant albuminuria/proteinuria (in SPRINT). Consequently, guideline recommendations over the past decade were some what different whereas most recent documents agree on a BP target <130/80 mmHg for most patients with CKD.

References

1. Sarafidis PA, Li S, Chen S-C, Collins AJ, Brown WW, Klag MJ, et al. Hypertension awareness, treatment, and control in chronic kidney disease. Am J Med. 2008;121:332–40.
2. Sarafidis PA, Sharpe CC, Wood E, Blacklock R, Rumjon A, Al-Yassin A, et al. Prevalence, patterns of treatment, and control of hypertension in predialysis patients with chronic kidney disease. Nephron Clin Pract. 2012;120:c147–55.
3. Klag MJ, Whelton PK, Randall BL, Neaton JD, Brancati FL, Ford CE, et al. Blood pressure and end-stage renal disease in men. N Engl J Med. 1996;334:13–8.
4. Loutradis C, Sarafidis P. Hypertension in patients with advanced chronic kidney disease. In: Mancia G, Grassi G, Tsioufis K, Dominiczak A, Rosei EA, editors. Manual of hypertension of the European Society of Hypertension. Boca Raton: CRC Press; 2019. https://doi.org/10.1201/9780429199189.
5. Boenink R, Astley ME, Huijben JA, Stel VS, Kerschbaum J, Ots-Rosenberg M, et al. The ERA registry annual report 2019: summary and age comparisons. Clin Kidney J. 2022;15:452–72.
6. Johansen KL, Chertow GM, Gilbertson DT, Herzog CA, Ishani A, Israni AK, et al. US renal data system 2021 annual data report: epidemiology of kidney disease in the United States. Am J Kidney Dis. 2022;79:A8–A12.
7. Rossignol P, Massy ZA, Azizi M, Bakris G, Ritz E, Covic A, et al. The double challenge of resistant hypertension and chronic kidney disease. Lancet. 2015;386:1588–98.
8. Sarafidis PA, Georgianos PI, Zebekakis PE. Comparative epidemiology of resistant hypertension in chronic kidney disease and the general hypertensive population. Semin Nephrol. 2014;34:483–91.
9. Drawz PE, Agarwal A, Dwyer JP, Horwitz E, Lash J, Lenoir K, et al. Concordance Between Blood Pressure in the Systolic Blood Pressure Intervention Trial and in Routine Clinical Practice. JAMA Intern Med 2020;180:1655–63.
10. Ruiz-Hurtado G, Ruilope LM, de la Sierra A, Sarafidis P, de la Cruz JJ, Gorostidi M, et al. Association between high and very high albuminuria and nighttime blood pressure: influence of diabetes and chronic kidney disease. Diabetes Care. 2016;39:1729–37.
11. De Nicola L, Gabbai FB, Agarwal R, Chiodini P, Borrelli S, Bellizzi V, et al. Prevalence and prognostic role of resistant hypertension in chronic kidney disease patients. J Am Coll Cardiol. 2013;61:2461–7.
12. Minutolo R, Gabbai FB, Agarwal R, Chiodini P, Borrelli S, Bellizzi V, et al. Assessment of achieved clinic and ambulatory blood pressure recordings and outcomes during treatment in

hypertensive patients with CKD: a multicenter prospective cohort study. Am J Kidney Dis. 2014;64:744–52.
13. Borrelli S, Garofalo C, Gabbai FB, Chiodini P, Signoriello S, Paoletti E, et al. Dipping status, ambulatory blood pressure control, cardiovascular disease, and kidney disease progression: a multicenter cohort study of CKD. Am J Kidney Dis. 2023;81:15–24.e1.
14. Schmieder RE. Renal denervation: where do we stand and what is the relevance to the nephrologist? Nephrol Dial Transplant. 2022;37:638–44.
15. Phan O, Burnier M, Wuerzner G. Hypertension in chronic kidney disease – role of arterial calcification and impact on treatment. Eur Cardiol. 2014;9:115–9.
16. Sarafidis PA, Persu A, Agarwal R, Burnier M, de Leeuw P, Ferro C, et al. Hypertension in dialysis patients: a consensus document by the European renal and cardiovascular medicine (EURECA-m) working group of the European renal association – European Dialysis and Transplant Association (ERA-EDTA) and the hypertension and the kidney working group of the European Society of Hypertension (ESH). J Hypertens. 2017;35:657–76.
17. Blood Pressure Lowering Treatment Trialists' Collaboration, Ninomiya T, Perkovic V, Turnbull F, Neal B, Barzi F, et al. Blood pressure lowering and major cardiovascular events in people with and without chronic kidney disease: meta-analysis of randomised controlled trials. BMJ. 2013;347:f5680.
18. Sarafidis PA, Ruilope LM. Aggressive blood pressure reduction and renin-angiotensin system blockade in chronic kidney disease: time for re-evaluation? Kidney Int. 2014;85:536–46.
19. Sarafidis PA, Lazaridis AA, Ruiz-Hurtado G, Ruilope LM. Blood pressure reduction in diabetes: lessons from ACCORD, SPRINT and EMPA-REG OUTCOME. Nat Rev Endocrinol. 2017;13:365–74.
20. Klahr S, Levey AS, Beck GJ, Caggiula AW, Hunsicker L, Kusek JW, et al. The effects of dietary protein restriction and blood-pressure control on the progression of chronic renal disease. Modification of Diet in Renal Disease Study Group. N Engl J Med. 1994;330:877–84.
21. Peterson JC, Adler S, Burkart JM, Greene T, Hebert LA, Hunsicker LG, et al. Blood pressure control, proteinuria, and the progression of renal disease. The Modification of Diet in Renal Disease Study. Ann Intern Med. 1995;123:754–62.
22. Wright JT, Bakris G, Greene T, Agodoa LY, Appel LJ, Charleston J, et al. Effect of blood pressure lowering and antihypertensive drug class on progression of hypertensive kidney disease: results from the AASK trial. JAMA. 2002;288:2421–31.
23. Lea J, Greene T, Hebert L, Lipkowitz M, Massry S, Middleton J, et al. The relationship between magnitude of proteinuria reduction and risk of end-stage renal disease: results of the African American study of kidney disease and hypertension. Arch Intern Med. 2005;165:947–53.
24. Sarnak MJ, Greene T, Wang X, Beck G, Kusek JW, Collins AJ, et al. The effect of a lower target blood pressure on the progression of kidney disease: long-term follow-up of the modification of diet in renal disease study. Ann Intern Med. 2005;142:342–51.
25. Appel LJ, Wright JT, Greene T, Agodoa LY, Astor BC, Bakris GL, et al. Intensive blood-pressure control in hypertensive chronic kidney disease. N Engl J Med. 2010;363:918–29.
26. Ku E, Sarnak MJ, Toto R, McCulloch CE, Lin F, Smogorzewski M, et al. Effect of blood pressure control on long-term risk of end-stage renal disease and death among subgroups of patients with chronic kidney disease. J Am Heart Assoc. 2019;8:e012749.
27. SPRINT Research Group, Wright JT, Williamson JD, Whelton PK, Snyder JK, Sink KM, et al. A randomized trial of intensive versus standard blood-pressure control. N Engl J Med. 2015;373:2103–16.
28. Cheung AK, Rahman M, Reboussin DM, Craven TE, Greene T, Kimmel PL, et al. Effects of intensive BP control in CKD. J Am Soc Nephrol. 2017;28:2812–23.
29. Johnson KC, Whelton PK, Cushman WC, Cutler JA, Evans GW, Snyder JK, et al. Blood Pressure Measurement in SPRINT (Systolic Blood Pressure Intervention Trial). Hypertension 2018;71:848–57.
30. Tight blood pressure control and risk of macrovascular and microvascular complications in type 2 diabetes: UKPDS 38. UK Prospective Diabetes Study Group. BMJ. 1998;317:703–13.
31. Hansson L, Zanchetti A, Carruthers SG, Dahlöf B, Elmfeldt D, Julius S, et al. Effects of intensive blood-pressure lowering and low-dose aspirin in patients with hypertension: principal

results of the Hypertension Optimal Treatment (HOT) randomised trial. HOT Study Group Lancet. 1998;351:1755–62.
32. ACCORD Study Group, Cushman WC, Evans GW, Byington RP, Goff DC, Grimm RH, et al. Effects of intensive blood-pressure control in type 2 diabetes mellitus. N Engl J Med. 2010;362:1575–85.
33. Bakris GL, Weir MR, Shanifar S, Zhang Z, Douglas J, van Dijk DJ, et al. Effects of blood pressure level on progression of diabetic nephropathy: results from the RENAAL study. Arch Intern Med. 2003;163:1555–65.
34. Pohl MA, Blumenthal S, Cordonnier DJ, De Alvaro F, Deferrari G, Eisner G, et al. Independent and additive impact of blood pressure control and angiotensin II receptor blockade on renal outcomes in the irbesartan diabetic nephropathy trial: clinical implications and limitations. J Am Soc Nephrol. 2005;16:3027–37.
35. Aggarwal R, Petrie B, Bala W, Chiu N. Mortality outcomes with intensive blood pressure targets in chronic kidney disease patients. Hypertension. 2019;73:1275–82.
36. Malhotra R, Nguyen HA, Benavente O, Mete M, Howard BV, Mant J, et al. Association between more intensive vs less intensive blood pressure lowering and risk of mortality in chronic kidney disease stages 3 to 5: a systematic review and meta-analysis. JAMA Intern Med. 2017;177:1498–505.
37. Kidney Disease: Improving Global Outcomes (KDIGO) Blood Pressure Work Group. KDIGO 2021 Clinical Practice Guideline for the Management of Blood Pressure in Chronic Kidney Disease. Kidney Int. 2021;99:S1–S87.
38. Cheung AK, Whelton PK, Muntner P, Schutte AE, Moran AE, Williams B, et al. International consensus on standardized clinic blood pressure measurement – a call to action. Am J Med. 2023;136:438–445.e1.
39. Castillo-Rodriguez E, Fernandez-Fernandez B, Alegre-Bellassai R, Kanbay M, Ortiz A. The chaos of hypertension guidelines for chronic kidney disease patients. Clin Kidney J. 2019;12:771–7.
40. Mancia G, Kreutz R, Brunström M, Burnier M, Grassi G, Januszewicz A, et al. 2023 ESH Guidelines for the management of arterial hypertension The Task Force For the management of arterial hypertension of the European Society of Hypertension: endorsed by the International Society of Hypertension (ISH) and the European renal association (ERA). J Hypertens. 2023;41:1874–2071.
41. McEvoy JW, McCarthy CP, Bruno RM, Brouwers S, Canavan MD, Ceconi C, et al. 2024 ESC Guidelines for the management of elevated blood pressure and hypertension: developed by the task force on the management of elevated blood pressure and hypertension of the European Society of Cardiology (ESC) and endorsed by the European Society of Endocrinology (ESE) and the European stroke organisation (ESO). Eur Heart J 2024; 45:3912–4018.
42. Jones DW, Ferdinand KC, Taler SJ, Johnson HM, Shimbo D, Abdalla M, et al. AHA/ACC/AANP/AAPA/ABC/ACCP/ACPM/AGS/AMA/ASPC/NMA/PCNA/SGIM Guideline for the prevention, detection, evaluation and Management of high blood pressure in adults: a report of the American College of Cardiology/American Heart Association Joint Committee on Clinical Practice Guidelines. Hypertension. 2025;82:e212-e316. Erratum in: Hypertension. 2025;82:e350. Erratum in: Hypertension. 2026;83:e000262. Erratum in: Hypertension. 2026;83:e00264.

Antihypertensive Treatment in Chronic Kidney Disease: Current Algorithms

Marieta P. Theodorakopoulou and Pantelis Sarafidis

Introduction

Hypertension is the most frequent comorbidity in patients with chronic kidney disease (CKD), affecting approximately 80–90% of individuals overall and up to 95% of those with stage 4–5 disease prior to the initiation of kidney replacement therapy [1, 2]. Elevated blood pressure (BP) not only accelerates loss of kidney function and progression to kidney failure, but is also a leading cause of incident CKD, with hypertensive kidney disease ranking as the second most common identifiable cause of end-stage kidney disease (ESKD) after diabetic kidney disease [3, 4]. Despite this substantial burden, and although hypertension awareness and treatment rates in CKD are high, BP control remains poor with <15% of patients achieving office BP targets <130/80 mmHg [1, 5]. Thus, treatment-resistant hypertension is highly prevalent in this population and is associated with lower estimated glomerular filtration rate (eGFR), higher albuminuria, faster progression to kidney failure and cardiovascular events [5]. Moreover, 24-h BP control is even more problematic in CKD, with abnormal nocturnal dipping patterns and elevated nighttime BP being exceedingly common and independently predictive of adverse outcomes [6].

Achieving recommended BP targets in CKD almost always requires multiple antihypertensive agents [7]; in both older and recent major trials in CKD, participants used on average 3–4 antihypertensive drugs at baseline, but mean office BP was still above 130/80 mmHg [5, 8]. Despite clear evidence that BP reduction improves cardiovascular and renal outcomes, optimal sequencing of antihypertensive medications and effective management of resistant hypertension remain challenging in clinical practice.

M. P. Theodorakopoulou (✉) · P. Sarafidis
1st Department of Nephrology, Aristotle University of Thessaloniki, Hippokration Hospital, Thessaloniki, Greece

P. Sarafidis, R. Pontremoli (eds.), *Hypertension and Chronic Kidney Disease*, Updates in Hypertension and Cardiovascular Protection,
https://doi.org/10.1007/978-3-032-29564-4_12

This chapter provides a structured overview of current antihypertensive treatment strategies in CKD. We first summarize the evidence and practical use of major drug classes (renin-angiotensin system (RAS) blockers, calcium-channel blockers (CCBs), diuretics, and others). We also discuss additional agents with modest BP-lowering properties that provide substantial nephroprotective and cardioprotective benefits, despite not being approved as antihypertensive medications. Finally, we integrate contemporary recommendations from major guideline documents (KDIGO, ESH, ESC, AHA/ACC) into practical treatment algorithms, highlighting areas of agreement and differences in the management of hypertension in CKD.

Lifestyle Interventions

Lifestyle interventions are fundamental for both the prevention and management of hypertension across all patient populations, including those with CKD [7, 9–11]. Current recommendations emphasize a personalized approach that considers individual patient characteristics, comorbidities, and the broader clinical context when addressing hypertension and cardiovascular risk [7, 9–11]. The core components of lifestyle management include weight loss, healthy dietary pattern, daily physical activity and structured exercise, reduction of alcohol intake close to abstinence, smoking cessation and salt restriction (Table 1) [7, 9–11]. Dietary salt restriction to <5 g (~2 g sodium) daily is recommended for all hypertensive patients, and is emphasized for those with CKD, who are commonly salt-sensitive. Large-scale randomized clinical trials (RCTs) have demonstrated that restricted sodium intake was associated with lower blood pressure and improved cardiovascular outcomes in the general population [12, 13]. In CKD, reducing dietary sodium lowers blood pressure and also albuminuria levels [14]. Clinical studies have also demonstrated that restricting dietary sodium might enhance the effectiveness of diuretics and RAS blockers in CKD. A recent meta-analysis of cohorts and randomized studies suggested that lower dietary sodium intake reduces the risk of composite kidney outcomes [15]. In a subgroup analysis in patients with eGFR >30 mL/min/1.73 m^2, lower sodium intake was associated with a lower risk of cardiovascular events [15]. Dietary modification can be challenging for patients; nevertheless, given the evidence that dietary sodium restriction improves blood pressure and albuminuria, all recent guidelines recommend sodium restriction <2 g sodium per day (equivalent to <5 g sodium chloride) to people with CKD [7, 9–11]. Increased potassium consumption via dietary modification is recommended for adults with elevated BP, except for patients with advanced CKD [7]. Better RCT data on the safety of potassium-based salt substitutes would be valuable in CKD, due to risk of hyperkalemia.

Table 1 Antihypertensive medication recommendations and treatment algorithms for patients with CKD in current guidelines

Therapeutic area	2021 KDIGO	2023 ESH	2024 ESC	2025 AHA
Antihypertensive drug use in CKD	Starting an ACEI or ARB in all patients with high BP, CKD, and severely increased albuminuria (G1–G4, A3) without diabetes, as well as in all diabetics with high BP, CKD, and moderately-to-severely increased albuminuria (G1–G4, A2 and A3) is recommended (1B) Starting RAS blockers (ACEI or ARB) in patients with high BP, CKD, and moderately increased albuminuria (G1–G4, A2) without diabetes, is suggested (2C)	An ACEI or an ARB, titrated to the maximum tolerated doses is recommended for patients with CKD and moderate (UACR 30 to 300 mg/g) or severe (UACR >300 mg/g) albuminuria. (CoR I, LoE A) *Step 1* of treatment includes combination of an ACEI or ARB + CCB or $_{T/TL}$Diuretic if eGFR ≥30 mL/min/1.73 m^2, or combination of an ACEI or ARB + CCB or Loop Diuretic if eGFR <30 mL/min/1.73 m^{2a} *Step 2* of treatment includes combination of the 3 above drug classes to maximum tolerated doses *Step 3* of treatment includes addition of spironolactone if eGFR ≥30 mL/min/1.73m^2 and potassium within the normal range or chlortalidone if eGFR <30 mL/min/1.73 m^{2a}	ACEI or ARBs are more effective at reducing albuminuria than other BP-lowering agents and should be considered as part of the treatment strategy for patients with hypertension and microalbuminuria or proteinuria (CoR IIa, LoE B) Combination therapy should be initiated as a combination of a RAS inhibitor and a CCB or diuretic. In patients with eGFR <30 mL/min/1.73 m^2, an adequately up-titrated loop diuretic is necessary to define resistant hypertension. Chlorthalidone, typically added to a loop diuretic, also effectively lowers BP and reduces microalbuminuria in patients with resistant hypertension with stage 4 CKD. The combination of an ACEI and an ARB is not recommended.	For adults with hypertension and CKD as identified by eGFR<60 mL/min/1.73 m^2 with albuminuria of ≥30 mg/g, RAS blocker (either ACEI or ARB but not both) is recommended to decrease CVD and delay progression of kidney disease (CoR I, LoE B-R) Not graded recommendation (only in the text): Treatment with RAS blocker may be considered for those with lower level albuminuria (<30 mg/g) based on expert opinion, and is also appropriate for less-severe CKD (stage 1 or 2) when moderate or severe albuminuria is present.

(continued)

Table1 (continued)

Therapeutic area	2021 KDIGO	2023 ESH	2024 ESC	2025 AHA
Kidney and heart protection	–	SGLT-2 inhibitors are recommended for patients with diabetic and nondiabetic CKD, if eGFR is at least 20 mL/min/1.73m^2. (CoR I, LoE A)	In hypertensive patients with CKD and eGFR>20 mL/min/1.73 m^2, SGLT-2 inhibitors are recommended to improve outcomes in the context of their modest BP-lowering properties (CoR I, LoE A)	–
	–	The non-steroidal MRA finerenone is recommended in patients with CKD and albuminuria associated with type 2 DM, if eGFR is at least 25 mL/min/1.73m^2 and serum potassium <5.0 mmol/L. (CoR I, LoE A)	–	–
Potassium management	Hyperkalemia associated with use of RAS blockers can often be managed by measures to reduce the serum potassium levels rather than decreasing the dose or stopping RAS blockers. (Not graded)	In CKD patients with hyperkalemia a potassium binder can be used to maintain potassium <5.5 mmol/L) to allow continuation of treatment with a RAS-blocker or a MRA to continue. (CoR II, LoE B)		–

Resistant hypertension	Mineralocorticoid receptor antagonists are effective for management of refractory hypertension but may cause hyperkalemia or a reversible decline in kidney function, particularly among patients with low eGFR. (Not graded)	In patients with CKD stage 1–3 and true-resistant hypertension step 3 of treatment includes addition of spironolactone (preferred) or other MRA. β-blockers, alpha-1 blockers or centrally acting agents can be used alternatively. (CoR II, LoE B) In patients with CKD stage 4–5[a] and true-resistant hypertension, step 3 of treatment includes the addition of chlortalidone (preferred) or other thiazide/thiazide-like diuretic. β-blockers, alpha-1 blockers or centrally acting agents can be used alternatively. (CoR II, LoE B)	In patients with resistant hypertension and uncontrolled BP despite use of first-line BP lowering therapies, the addition of spironolactone to existing treatment should be considered (CoR IIa, LoE B) In patients with resistant hypertension in whom spironolactone is not effective or tolerated, treatment with eplerenone instead of spironolactone, or the addition of a β-blocker if not already indicated and, next, a centrally acting BP-lowering medication, an alpha-blocker, hydralazine, or a potassium-sparing diuretic should be considered (CoR IIa, LoE B) Steroidal MRAs are contraindicated in patients with an eGFR of <30 mL/min/1.73 m².	In adults with uncontrolled resistant hypertension despite optimal treatment with first-line antihypertensive therapy (i.e. a combination of ACEI or ARB plus CCB and TL diuretic (chlorthalidone or indapamide) and with eGFR ≥45 mL/min/1.73 m², addition of a MRA is recommended to control BP (CoR I, LoE B-R) In adults with uncontrolled resistant hypertension who cannot tolerate or have contraindications to MRA, the addition of one of the following agents or classes—amiloride, BBs, alpha-blockers, central sympatholytic drugs, dual endothelin receptor antagonists, or direct vasodilators-is reasonable to control BP (CoR IIa, LoE B-NR) Not graded recommendation (only in the text): Use of nonsteroidal MRA for treating resistant hypertension in patients with moderate to advanced CKD has not been tested in a clinical trial but may be considered in selected patients with close monitoring of serum potassium.

ACEI angiotensin-converting enzyme inhibitor, *ARB* angiotensin-receptor blocker, *CKD* chronic kidney disease, *CoR* Class of Recommendation, *CCB* calcium channel blocker, *CVD* cardiovascular disease, *DM* diabetes mellitus, *eGFR* estimated glomerular filtration rate, *LoE* Level of Evidence, *MRA* mineralocorticoid receptor antagonist, *RAS* renin-angiotensin system, *SGLT2i* sodium-glucose transporter 2 inhibitor, *T/TLDiuretic* thiazide or thiazide-like diuretic, *UACR* urine albumin-to-creatinine ratio

[a]Excludes patients with CKD G5 on dialysis

Use of Antihypertensive Agents in CKD

Except for the lifestyle measures mentioned above, achieving recommended BP targets in CKD usually requires use of antihypertensive medications in combination therapy, which should be a combination of a RAS blocker with a CCB or diuretic in these patients, as in the general population.

Renin-Angiotensin System Blockers

An angiotensin converting enzyme inhibitor (ACEI) or an angiotensin-2 receptor blocker (ARB) is the treatment of choice for patients with albuminuria, following seminal clinical trials in diabetic [16–19] and non-diabetic CKD [20–22], where these agents were found to reduce proteinuria, the rate of GFR decline, and the risk of doubling of serum creatinine or ESKD. In the Reduction of Endpoints in NIDDM with the Angiotensin II Antagonist Losartan (RENAAL) study, treatment with losartan resulted in a 35% reduction in the urinary albumin-to-creatinine ratio and a 16% lower risk of the primary composite endpoint of doubling of serum creatinine, progression to ESKD or death. The median rate of decline in estimated clearance was 4.4 and 5.2 mL/min/1.73 m^2/per year in the losartan and placebo group, respectively [17]. Similarly, in the Irbesartan Diabetic Nephropathy Trial (IDNT) study, after a mean follow-up of 2.6 years, irbesartan therapy led to a 33% reduction in proteinuria, compared with 6% in the amlodipine group and 10% in the placebo group. Irbesartan also produced a 20% risk reduction versus placebo and a 23% reduction versus amlodipine in the primary composite outcome of doubling of serum creatinine, ESKD or death. The mean rate of decline of creatinine clearance was −5.5, −6.8, and −6.5 mL/min/1.73 m^2 per year in the irbesartan, placebo and amlodipine groups, respectively [18]. Post hoc analyses of both trials established a strong relationship between baseline proteinuria, its reduction during treatment, and renal outcomes. In RENAAL, baseline proteinuria showed an almost linear association with the risk of the primary endpoint. Moreover, every 50% reduction in albuminuria within the first 6 months translated to a 36% lower risk of the primary endpoint and a 45% lower risk of progression to ESKD by study end [23]. Similarly, in IDNT, every twofold increase in baseline proteinuria doubled the risk of the primary outcome, while each 50% reduction in proteinuria after 1 year halved that risk, irrespective of treatment allocation [24]. These results clearly supported the value of proteinuria as an intermediate outcome in patients with overt diabetic nephropathy. It must be noted that there are currently no outcome data supporting differences in renoprotection between ACEIs and ARBs. This was exemplified in the Diabetics Exposed to Telmisartan And enalapril (DETAIL) study, which compared the effects of enalapril and telmisartan in 250 patients with type 2 diabetes, hypertension and urine albumin excretion (UAE) between 11 and 999 μg/min. and showed the two drugs having similar effects on GFR change, UAE, BP, and the rates of ESKD, cardiovascular events and all-cause mortality [19].

In nondiabetic CKD patients with proteinuria, the efficacy of ACEI was first demonstrated in the Ramipril Efficacy in Nephropathy (REIN-2) study. Patients with a mean serum creatinine level of 2.4 mg/dL and proteinuria exceeding 3 g/day were randomized to ramipril or placebo. Ramipril therapy led to significant reductions in proteinuria, rate of GFR decline, and the risk of serum creatinine doubling or progression to ESKD compared with placebo. Importantly, the renoprotective effect of ramipril remained significant even after adjustment for systolic and diastolic BP changes [21]. In the African American Study of Kidney Disease and Hypertension (AASK) trial, patients treated with ramipril had a 36% reduction in the composite endpoint of 50% reduction of eGFR, ESKD or death compared to amlodipine, and a 22% reduction compared to metoprolol [20]. In another study in 224 Chinese patients with serum creatinine levels 3.1–5.0 mg/dL (274.3–442.5 μmol/L) and persistent proteinuria [mean urine protein excretion of 1600 mg/day (1.6 g/day)], benazepril was associated with a 43% reduction in the risk of the primary endpoint (doubling of serum creatinine, ESKD, or death), a 23% decrease in the rate of decline in kidney function and 2.5 times greater reduction in proteinuria compared to placebo after 3.4 years, benefits that were not attributable to better BP control [22]. The ACEI or ARB monotherapy should be at maximum tolerated approved doses to achieve optimal nephroprotection.

However, dual combination of an ACEI with an ARB or combination of aliskiren with any of the two is not recommended, following the premature termination of two outcome trials due to increased risk of adverse events (mainly hyperkalemia-related) with combination therapy [25, 26]. The Aliskiren Trial in Type-2 Diabetes Using Cardiorenal Endpoints (ALTITUDE) study evaluated the efficacy and safety of dual RAS blockade with aliskiren in combination with an ACEI or ARB versus ACEI or ARB monotherapy in 8561 patients with type 2 diabetes. ALTITUDE was prematurely terminated at 69% of events after safety concerns. The components of the primary outcome did not differ between groups, with the exception of resuscitated cardiac arrest; the main differences between groups were the proportion of patients with hyperkalemia (11.2% vs 7.2%) and hypotension (12.1% vs 8.3%) ($p < 0.001$ for both) [25]. The Veterans Affairs Nephropathy in Diabetes (VA NEPHRON-D) study investigated the effects of combined RAS blockade with losartan and lisinopril versus losartan monotherapy in 1850 patients with diabetes, eGFR 30–90 mL/min/1.73 m^2, and urine albumin-to-creatinine ratio (UACR) >300 mg/day. The trial was terminated early after enrollment of 1448 participants and a median follow-up of 2.2 years due to excess adverse events. No difference in the primary endpoint of eGFR change, ESKD or death (hazard ratio (HR) with combination therapy 0.88; 95% confidence interval (CI): 0.70–1.12; $p = 0.30$), mortality or cardiovascular events were noted with combination therapy, whereas risk of hyperkalemia (6.3 vs 2.6 events per 100 person-years, $p < 0.001$) was increased [26].

With regard to normoalbuminuric patients with hypertension, ACEIs or ARBs are able to delay the progression to severely increased albuminuria; in a randomized, double-blind, multicenter, controlled trial in 4447 patients with type 2 diabetes and normoalbuminuria, olmesartan was associated with a delayed onset of microalbuminuria (microalbuminuria 8.2% in the olmesartan group vs 9.8% in the placebo group; HR, 0.77; 95% CI, 0.63–0.94) compared to placebo [27]. No evidence exists for better preservation of renal function with RAS blockers compared to other major antihypertensive classes in the normoalbuminuric population [28].

Importantly, the vasodilatory action of ACEIs and ARBs on the efferent arteriole leads to a reduction in intraglomerular pressure and consequently in renal perfusion pressure. As a result, it is both expected and physiologically normal for eGFR to decline by approximately 10–15% within the first weeks of therapy initiation (eGFR dip). A similar hemodynamic effect can be seen with large BP reductions offered by any antihypertensive agent. Therefore, close monitoring of eGFR and serum electrolytes within 4–8 weeks after starting or intensifying RAS blockade (depending on baseline renal function) is essential. Clinicians should recognize that a modest, transient fall in eGFR does not necessitate discontinuation. However, if the decline exceeds 30% or continues beyond the initial adjustment period, the RAS blocker should be withheld and the patient evaluated for the presence of renovascular disease.

A common concern during RAS blockade in CKD is hyperkalemia, whose incidence increases with declining kidney function [29]. Incident hyperkalemia is associated with increased mortality [30] and is the most frequent reason for dose reduction or interruption of ACEIs and ARBs in CKD patients [31, 32]. However, as dose reduction or interruption of RAS blockers has been associated with increased risk in different populations [32], this strategy is generally not advisable by the major existing guidelines (Table 1). Novel potassium binders (patiromer and sodium zirconium cyclosilicate) were shown to effectively normalize elevated serum potassium and chronically maintain normal levels in CKD patients treated with ACEIs, ARBs or spironolactone, with generally good tolerability [33, 34]. Thus, these agents can be used to maintain serum potassium <5.5 mmol/L in patients with CKD [35, 36] and their use is also supported by current guidelines.

Calcium Channel Blockers

Most patients with CKD will not have their BP controlled with ACEI or ARB monotherapy, and a CCB or a diuretic should be included in the regimen. Selection of one of the two would be based on patient characteristics [37, 38]; however, this is largely a theoretical question as most patients with CKD would require a combination of at least three antihypertensives.

The two different subtypes of CCBs, non-dihydropyridine (non-DHPCCB) and dihydropyridine (DHPCCB) CCBs, have been shown to have divergent effects on proteinuria. In patients with overt diabetic nephropathy, treatment with non-DHPCCBs (verapamil, diltiazem) led to greater reductions in proteinuria and slower decline in creatinine clearance compared with atenolol [39, 40]; moreover, the achieved reductions were similar to those with lisinopril [39], with also similar BP control in the various groups. In another cohort of patients with overt diabetic nephropathy and a follow-up of 21 months, a DHPCCB, nifedipine XL, was associated with no changes in proteinuria levels, whereas diltiazem resulted in reductions of about 60% [41].

The underlying mechanism for the aforementioned different effects on proteinuria involves the predominant afferent arteriole dilation produced by DHPCCB [42]. This relates to increased renal blood flow and creates the misleading impression of preserved kidney function; however, in reality, it increases intraglomerular pressure and albumin permeability, leading to poorer long-term kidney outcomes. Further evidence that DHPCCBs increase proteinuria when used in the absence of a RAS blocker in patients with proteinuric CKD comes from multicenter trials. In the IDNT trial, amlodipine was associated with a 6% increase in proteinuria versus baseline and a 23% higher incidence of the primary endpoint compared to irbesartan [18]. In the non-diabetic population of the AASK trial, treatment with amlodipine was associated with a 58% increase in proteinuria after 6 months, which corresponded to a higher incidence of the composite endpoint (≥50% decline in eGFR, onset of ESKD, or death) compared with ramipril therapy, where proteinuria decreased by 20% [20]. Similarly, data from the REIN-2 study also question the ability of DHPCCBs to help towards regression of kidney function deterioration in proteinuric kidney disease even by means of BP-lowering [43]. However, a detrimental effect of DHPCCBs in kidney disease progression is not apparent in patients without proteinuria and preserved eGFR, as noted in the Antihypertensive and Lipid-Lowering Treatment to Prevent Heart Attack Trial (ALLHAT) trial [28] or when these agents are used in combination with ACEI, as noted in the Avoiding Cardiovascular Events through COMbination Therapy in Patients LIving with Systolic Hypertension (ACCOMPLISH) trial [44]. Moreover, in the general hypertensive population, where the majority of patients do not have moderately or severely increased albuminuria, dihydropyridine CCBs were shown to have similar effects on renal outcomes with RAS blockers or diuretics [28]. Similarly, in a study of hypertensive patients of which 19% had moderately and 5% had severely increased albuminuria at baseline, a combination of a RAS blocker with a dihydropyridine CCB was superior in reducing kidney outcomes compared to a RAS blocker-thiazide combination [44].

Diuretics

Diuretics play a key role in the management of hypertension in CKD patients, as these individuals are commonly sodium-sensitive (particularly those with older age, coexisting diabetes and/or obesity) and have a high prevalence of resistant hypertension [38, 45]. Treatment with diuretics has been shown to effectively reduce proteinuria when added to RAS blockers in proteinuric CKD [14]; moreover, potential benefit of diuretics relates to helping preserve the antiproteinuric effects of ACEIs/ARBs, which are blunted with high-salt diets [46]. When GFR falls <30–40 mL/min/1.73 m^2, the efficacy of thiazide diuretics diminishes, as these agents fail to reach their tubular site of action due to competition for tubular secretion with other substances that accumulate in CKD [47]. If GFR falls below that level, thiazides should be replaced by chlorthalidone (which recently showed BP-lowering efficacy in CKD Stage 4) [48], metolazone, or a loop diuretic. Among loop diuretics, torasemide is generally preferred due to longer half-life and simpler dosing scheme; furosemide has a very short duration of action (3–6 h), so adequate dosing (i.e. 3 times daily) is necessary to achieve optimal BP control and natriuresis, and this may affect patient adherence [49].

Resistant Hypertension

Hypertension is defined as treatment resistant when appropriate lifestyle measures and treatment with optimal or best tolerated doses of three or more drugs (a thiazide/thiazide-like diuretic, a RAS blocker and a CCB) fail to lower office BP to <140/90 mmHg [7]. The inadequate BP control should be confirmed by uncontrolled 24-h BP (≥130/80 mmHg), and evidence of adherence to therapy and exclusion of secondary causes of hypertension are also required to define true resistant hypertension. In major hypertension guidelines [7, 10, 11], after the combination of an ACEI/ARB, a CCB and a diuretic, spironolactone is recommended as the fourth drug to achieve BP control in resistant hypertension. The evidence to support this derives from the Spironolactone versus Placebo, Bisoprolol, and Doxazosin to determine the optimal treatment for drug-resistant hypertension (PATHWAY-2) trial [50] and relevant meta-analyses [51]; however, patients with an eGFR <45 mL/min/1.73 m^2 or potassium >4.5 mmol/L were excluded from this study [50] and, thus, the efficacy and safety of spironolactone in such individuals are not established. Indirect evidence comes from the Spironolactone With Patiromer in the Treatment of Resistant Hypertension in Chronic Kidney Disease (AMBER) trial that used spironolactone with addition of placebo or patiromer in patients with treatment-resistant hypertension and eGFR 25–≤45 mL/min/1.73 m^2, in which BP was effectively reduced in both groups, but patients in the spironolactone group had incidence of hyperkalemia (serum potassium ≥ 5.5 mmol/L) around 65% [52]. Subsequently, the Benefits of Aldosterone Receptor Antagonism in Chronic Kidney Disease (BARACK-D) trial, examining the addition of spironolactone on standard therapy versus standard therapy alone in CKD stage 3b, reported discontinuation rates of 67% with spironolactone due to hyperkalaemia and eGFR decline and no difference in cardiovascular outcomes between groups [53]. Based on the above, the use of spironolactone as a fourth antihypertensive agent in patients with advanced CKD (stage G3b or higher) and treatment-resistant hypertension is not advised. For patients with CKD stage 4, chlorthalidone is considered an alternative, based on the recent Chlorthalidone in Chronic Kidney Disease (CLICK) randomized trial that included 160 patients with uncontrolled hypertension, showing that the addition of chlorthalidone (mean dose 23 mg daily) on top of previous antihypertensive treatment (including a loop diuretic) was associated with 10.5 mmHg reduction in 24-h SBP (Table 1) [48]. Aldosterone synthase inhibitors (ASIs) represent a novel drug class currently examined for kidney and cardiovascular diseases, including uncontrolled and resistant hypertension. Baxdrostat has recently been approved as the first-in-class selective ASI for the treatment of uncontrolled hypertension in combination with other antihypertensive medications. Approval by the US Food and Drug

Administration (FDA) was based on results from the phase III BaxHTN trial, which showed significant reductions in office SBP after 12 weeks with both the 1- and 2-mg doses compared with placebo (placebo-corrected reductions of −8.7 mmHg and −9.8 mmHg, respectively, $p < 0.001$). Baxdrostat was generally well tolerated; potassium >6.0 mmol/L was reported in 2.3% of patients with 1-mg, 3.0% with 2-mg and 0.4% with placebo [54]. In the phase 3 Bax24 trial including 217 patients with resistant hypertension and 24-h ABPM, baxdrostat significantly reduced 24-h SBP versus placebo at week 12 by a mean placebo-corrected reduction of −14.0 mmHg (95% CI −17.2 to −10.8) [55]. Similar to the general hypertensive population, the Study to Evaluate CIN 107 for the Treatment of Patients With Uncontrolled Hypertension and Chronic Kidney Disease (FigHTN) investigated the effects of baxdrostat in CKD patients with uncontrolled hypertension. Baxdrostat, at both low (0.5–1 mg) and high (2–4 mg) doses, was superior to placebo in reducing office systolic BP (placebo-corrected change in the pooled group −8.1 mmHg (95% CI; −13.4 to −2.8) [56]. Ongoing, large outcome-driven trials (NCT06268873, NCT06742723, NCT06531824) are awaited to define long-term renal and cardiovascular efficacy and safety of these agents and guide the positioning of ASIs within contemporary CKD management.

Other Antihypertensive Classes

With regard to additional antihypertensive agents, β-blockers, alpha-blockers, and central-acting agents can offer important help toward BP lowering, especially since sympathetic nervous system activity is commonly elevated in CKD [57]; however, their effects in CKD have not been tested in hard kidney outcome trials. For β-blockers in more detail, there is no direct evidence that conventional β-blockers provide additional renoprotective effects. As mentioned above, in overt diabetic nephropathy, non-DHPCCBs produced greater proteinuria reductions than atenolol [40]. In patients with type 2 diabetes in the UKPDS-39 study there were no significant differences between captopril and atenolol in the level of BP achieved, incidence of overt nephropathy, and doubling of creatinine, data suggesting that any renoprotective effect is due to BP lowering [58]. The Glycemic Effects in Diabetes Mellitus: Carvedilol-Metoprolol Comparison in Hypertensives (GEMINI) trial showed that carvedilol was associated with significant reductions in the risk of microalbuminuria development in hypertensive type 2 diabetic patients compared to metoprolol [59]. These findings, however, were not confirmed by a trial in proteinuric CKD. Therefore, β-blockers are suggested to be used in patients with CKD mainly for BP reduction [37]; of importance, β-blockers can be used at any step as guideline-directed medical therapy in respective indications or considered in several other conditions (i.e. coronary artery disease, heart failure, arrhythmias, etc.). From the other antihypertensive drug classes, α-blockers and central-acting agents can also be used as fourth line agents. Direct vasodilators, such as hydralazine or minoxidil, should be used cautiously because they may cause severe fluid retention and reflex sympathetic activation with tachycardia.

Device-Based BP-Lowering

Renal denervation reduces sympathetic nervous system activity and, thereby, BP by interrupting afferent and efferent sympathetic nerves in the adventitia and perivascular tissue of the renal arteries. The latest guidelines from different societies [7, 10, 11] consider renal denervation as an adjunctive therapy option for patients who have uncontrolled BP despite the use of antihypertensive medications; however, the selection of patients should be made with caution and include only patients with eGFR >40 mL/min/1.73 m^2, based on evidence from the existing randomized clinical trials [60–62].

Use of Agents That Offer Nephroprotection and Cardioprotection in CKD

In addition to BP control at the targets (see Chap. 11) and with the agents described above, significant help towards retardation of CKD progression and reduction of cardiovascular events and mortality in CKD patients can be offered by additional therapeutic classes that also have some BP-lowering effects, although not approved as antihypertensive agents.

Sodium-Glucose Co-Transporter-2 (SGLT-2) Inhibitors

Sodium-glucose co-transporter-2 (SGLT-2) inhibitors were first introduced as oral hypoglycemic agents that reduce plasma glucose levels by inhibiting kidney glucose reabsorption through the SGLT-2, located in the proximal convoluted tubule. Early clinical studies in diabetic patients suggested that these agents can offer modest office BP reductions of around 3–5/1–2 mmHg [63], that were later confirmed with ambulatory BP monitoring (ABPM) studies [64], while data from patients with advanced CKD (eGFR <30 mL/min/1.73 m^2) suggest even greater SBP reductions of up to 7 mmHg [65]. The main underlying mechanism is the mild natriuretic/diuretic effect occurring from both inhibition of proximal sodium reabsorption and osmotic diuresis [63], while reductions in sympathetic nervous system activity, arterial stiffness, endothelial dysfunction, and systemic vascular resistance have also been proposed [63, 66, 67]. In parallel to the above, these agents were shown to offer reductions in urine albumin excretion of 25–40%, depending on the baseline albuminuria levels [68].

In the cardiovascular outcome trials with SGLT-2 inhibitors in patients with type 2 diabetes (that also included large proportions of patients with CKD), large and homogeneous reductions of around 40% in composite kidney endpoints were observed [69–71]. Moreover, in kidney outcome trials (CREDENCE, DAPA-CKD, EMPA-KIDNEY), treatment with SGLT-2 inhibitors in diabetic and non-diabetic CKD showed significant reductions compared to placebo on composite kidney outcomes and individual endpoints such as doubling of SCr and progression to

ESKD. The mild BP reduction is suggested as a contributor to the nephroprotective effect of SGLT-2 inhibitors. In addition, in CREDENCE and DAPA-CKD, SGLT-2 inhibitors were also able to reduce the risk of some cardiovascular events and in DAPA-CKD the risk of mortality in patients with CKD [72], something that was not previously evident with RAS blockade or any other drug treatment in this population [73–76].

Nonsteroidal Mineralocorticoid Receptor Antagonists

In the past few years, the Efficacy and Safety of Finerenone in Subjects With Type 2 Diabetes Mellitus and Diabetic Kidney Disease (FIDELIO-DKD) and Efficacy and Safety of Finerenone in Subjects With Type 2 Diabetes Mellitus and the Clinical Diagnosis of Diabetic Kidney Disease (FIGARO-DKD) trials evaluated the efficacy of finerenone, a novel, non-steroidal mineralocorticoid receptor antagonist (MRA) in type-2 diabetes patients with CKD and moderately or severely increased albuminuria on top of ACEI or ARB treatment [77, 78]. In the FIDELIO-DKD trial, finerenone significantly reduced the risk of both the primary kidney composite outcome and the secondary cardiovascular composite outcome compared with placebo [77]. The mean difference in blood pressure between groups during follow-up was modest (2.7/1.0 mmHg favoring finerenone), and treatment effects were consistent across all baseline BP groups [79]; however, in the trial, free up- or down-titration of antihypertensive agents was allowed during the long follow-up, thus, BP differences between arms were small and the net antihypertensive effect of finerenone could not be determined [8]. With regard to safety, hyperkalemia leading to discontinuation of the trial regimen was 2.3% with finerenone and 0.9% with placebo, and no fatal hyperkalemia adverse events were reported [77]. In FIGARO-DKD, finerenone was associated with a 13% significant reduction in the risk of the primary cardiovascular outcome, with consistent beneficial effects on kidney outcomes and a similar tolerability profile [80]. In the FIDELITY on-treatment analysis combining the patient population of both trials, finerenone reduced mortality by 18% compared to placebo [81]. Recently, the Finerenone Non-Diabetic Chronic Kidney Disease (FIND-CKD) trial provided important evidence for finerenone in non-diabetic CKD. In 1584 patients with eGFR 25–90 mL/min/1.73 m^2 and UACR 200–3500 mg/g, finerenone led to a slower decrease in the eGFR slope over 32 months compared with placebo (mean annual rate of change –3.3 vs –4.0 mL/min/1.73 m^2, $p < 0.001$), while also reduced the risk of a composite kidney or cardiovascular outcome (HR 0.77; 95% CI, 0.60–0.99). Hyperkalaemia was the most common adverse event and occurred more frequently with finerenone (17.0% vs 13.3%), but treatment discontinuation due to hyperkalaemia was uncommon (1.5% vs 0.1% respectively) [82].

More detailed evidence regarding the blood pressure effects of finerenone derives from the earlier Safety and Efficacy of Different Oral Doses of BAY94-8862 in Subjects With Type 2 Diabetes Mellitus and the Clinical Diagnosis of Diabetic Nephropathy (ARTS-DN) phase 2b trial, which randomized 823 patients with type 2 diabetes and CKD with a median UACR of 192.8 mg/g and eGFR of 66.3 mL/min/1.73 m^2 to placebo or finerenone (1.25–20 mg once daily in the morning) for 90 days. At day 90, placebo-adjusted changes in 24-h systolic BP were −8.3 mmHg, −11.2 mmHg, and −9.9 mmHg for the 10 mg, 15 mg, and 20 mg doses, respectively [83], representing substantial reductions for this population. With regard to safety, hyperkalemia and subsequent discontinuation of study drug occurred in 1.8% of patients receiving finerenone 7.5 to 20 mg, but were not observed in the placebo or finerenone 10 mg groups, indicating that this agent is generally well tolerated.

Antihypertensive Medication Algorithms in Current Recommendations in CKD

Over the past few years, major guideline documents have reported recommendations on antihypertensive medications for patients with CKD (Table 1).

The 2021 KDIGO guidelines primarily focus on the selection of appropriate first-line agents [9]. In particular, an ACEI or ARB is recommended as the treatment of choice for patients with high BP, CKD and increased albuminuria. Hyperkalemia associated with use of RAS blockers should generally be addressed through measures aimed at lowering serum potassium levels, rather than by reducing the dose or discontinuing the RAS blocker (not graded recommendation). For resistant hypertension, KDIGO provides a non-graded recommendation supporting cautious use of steroidal MRAs, acknowledging their efficacy but also the risk of hyperkalemia or reversible declines in eGFR, particularly in advanced CKD.

The 2023 ESH Guidelines provide specific algorithms on antihypertensive agent selection for BP-lowering in patients with hypertension and CKD (Fig. 1) [7]. Because most CKD patients require at least two agents to reach target BP levels, the recommended initial combinations include a RAS blocker with either a CCB or a thiazide/thiazide-like diuretic when eGFR is ≥45 mL/min/1.73 m^2 (CKD G1–G3a). Below an eGFR of 30 mL/min/1.73 m^2 (CKD G4–G5), thiazide/thiazide-like agents should generally be replaced by loop diuretics. Treatment with an ACEI or an ARB remains the first choice for patients with CKD and albuminuria (CoR I, LoE A); the ACEI or ARB monotherapy should be at maximum tolerated approved doses to achieve optimal nephroprotection. Dual combination of an ACEI with an ARB or combination of aliskiren with any of the two is not recommended (CoR III, LoE A). In order to deal with the problem of hyperkalemia, novel potassium binders (patiromer and sodium zirconium cyclosilicate) are recommended to be used to maintain serum potassium <5.5 mmol/L in individuals with CKD in order to allow optimal treatment with a RAS blocker or an MRA to continue [35, 36] (CoR II, LoE B).

In the same Guideline [7], there is a detailed commentary on the role of diuretics in CKD patients with resistant hypertension [38, 45]; a specific algorithm for treatment is proposed depending on underlying renal function. According to this, the fourth line treatment in patients with resistant hypertension and eGFR ≥30 mL/min/1.73 m^2 should include the MRA spironolactone, based on the fact that patients

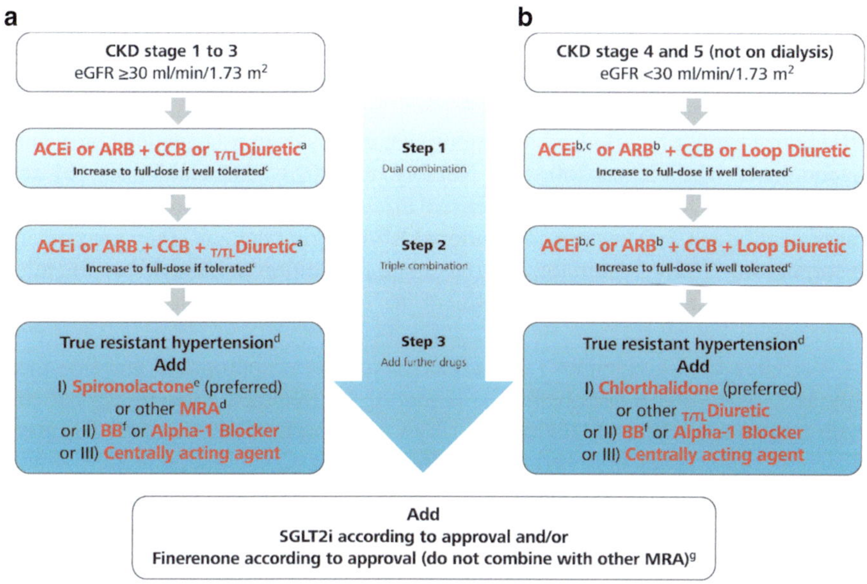

Fig. 1 BP-lowering therapy in patients with hypertension and chronic kidney disease (CKD). (**a**) Therapy for CKD G1-G3 (eGFR ≥30 mL/min/1.73 m^2). (**b**) Therapy for CKD G4-G5 (eGFR <30 mL/min/1.73 m^2) not on dialysis. (**a**) Transition from T/TL diuretic to loop diuretic should be individualized in patients with eGFR <45 mL/min/1.73 m^2. (**b**) Cautious start with low dose. (**c**) Check for dose adjustment according to renal impairment for drugs with relevant renal excretion rate. (**d**) When SBP is ≥140 mmHg or DBP is ≥90 mmHg provided that: maximum recommended and tolerated doses of a three-drug combination comprising a RAS blocker (either an ACEI or an ARB), a CCB and a T/TL diuretic have been used, adequate BP control has been confirmed by ABPM or by HBPM if ABPM is not feasible, various causes of pseudo-resistant hypertension (especially poor medication adherence) and secondary hypertension have been excluded. (**e**) Caution if eGFR <45 mL/min/1.73 m^2 or serum potassium >4.5 mmol/l. (**f**) Should be used at any step as guideline-directed medical therapy in respective indications or considered in several other conditions. (**g**) SGLT-2 inhibitors and Finerenone should be used according to their approval for CKD treatment. (From Mancia et al. [7], with permission). BP blood pressure, T/TL thiazide/thiazide-like, eGFR estimated glomerular filtration rate, SBP systolic blood pressure, DBP diastolic blood pressure, ACEI angiotensin-converting enzyme inhibitor, ARB angiotensin-receptor blocker, CCB calcium channel blocker, ABPM ambulatory blood pressure monitoring, HBPM home blood pressure monitoring, SGLT2is sodium-glucose co-transporter-2 inhibitors, MRA mineralocorticoid receptor antagonist

with an eGFR <45 mL/min/1.73 m^2 or potassium >4.5 mmol/L were excluded from the pivotal PATHWAY-2 trial [50]. Consequently, spironolactone should be used only when necessary, and with close potassium monitoring, in patients with CKD G3b and resistant hypertension, while it is not recommended in CKD G4 or higher. Instead, according to the recent evidence from the CLICK trial, the addition of chlortalidone is recommended as an effective and safer alternative for this patient group [7]. Other antihypertensive drug classes, β-blockers, alpha-blockers, and centrally acting agents can be useful for the management of hypertension, as they offer important help towards BP lowering in patients with CKD. Direct vasodilators, such as hydralazine or minoxidil, should be used parsimoniously because they may cause severe fluid retention and reflex sympathetic activation with tachycardia. For patients with eGFR >40 mL/min/1.73 m^2, endovascular renal denervation can be proposed as an adjunctive therapy to patients with resistant hypertension, in whom BP control cannot be achieved or serious side effects cannot be avoided with antihypertensive medications [60, 84]. Notably, the 2023 ESH Guidelines [7] also included for the first time a comprehensive discussion on nephroprotection and cardioprotection in CKD beyond conventional BP-lowering therapy. They recommend incorporating SGLT-2 inhibitors or finerenone in addition to lifestyle modification and standard antihypertensive treatment to enhance renal and cardiovascular outcomes.

The 2024 ESC Guidelines [11] similarly emphasize appropriate first-line therapy, recommending ACEIs or ARBs as part of the treatment strategy for patients with hypertension and microalbuminuria or proteinuria (CoR IIa, LoE B), given their superior efficacy in lowering albuminuria levels. Combination therapy should be started early, typically pairing a RAS blocker with a CCB or diuretic. In patients with eGFR <30 mL/min/1.73 m^2, an adequately titrated loop diuretic becomes necessary to classify hypertension as resistant. Chlorthalidone, typically added to a loop diuretic, also effectively lowers BP and reduces microalbuminuria in patients with resistant hypertension with stage 4 CKD. For resistant hypertension, spironolactone remains the preferred option (CoR IIa, LoE B). If spironolactone is ineffective or poorly tolerated, eplerenone, β-blockers, centrally acting agents, alpha-blockers, hydralazine, or potassium-sparing diuretics may be considered (CoR IIa, LoE B). Steroidal MRAs are contraindicated when eGFR <30 mL/min/1.73 m^2. The ESC also highlights the role of SGLT-2 inhibitors in hypertensive CKD patients with eGFR >20 mL/min/1.73 m^2 as a means of improving renal and cardiovascular outcomes (CoR I, LoE A).

Finally, the recent 2025 AHA/ACC guideline recommends [10] RAS blockers (either ACEI or ARB but not both) to decrease cardiovascular disease risk and delay progression of kidney disease (CoR I, LoE B-R). A non-graded recommendation notes that RAS blockers may also be considered in patients with low-grade albuminuria (<30 mg/g) or in early-stage CKD (G1–G2) when moderate or severe albuminuria is present.

For adults with resistant hypertension and eGFR ≥45 mL/min/1.73 m^2, despite optimal first-line triple therapy (ACEI/ARB + CCB + thiazide-like diuretic), the addition of an MRA is recommended (CoR I, LoE B-R). When MRAs are contraindicated or not tolerated, alternative add-on agents—including amiloride, β-blockers, alpha-blockers, central sympatholytics, dual endothelin receptor antagonists, or direct vasodilators—are considered reasonable (CoR IIa, LoE B-NR). A further non-graded recommendation suggests that non-steroidal MRAs may be considered for resistant hypertension in moderate-to-advanced CKD, although they have not yet been evaluated in dedicated outcome trials.

Conclusions

Despite the strong evidence that blood pressure reduction slows CKD progression and improves cardiovascular outcomes, achieving recommended BP targets in clinical practice remains difficult. Most patients require combination therapy with 3–4 antihypertensive agents; yet office BP frequently remains above 130/80 mmHg, and treatment-resistant hypertension is common and closely linked to adverse outcomes. Lifestyle interventions are fundamental for management of hypertension, but pharmacological therapy (centered on RAS blockade and complemented by CCBs and diuretics, as in the general population) remains the cornerstone of BP management in CKD. Agents with proven nephroprotective and cardioprotective benefits and modest BP reductions (SGLT-2 inhibitors and finerenone) further expand the therapeutic algorithms. Major existing guidelines are largely aligned in their overall recommendations, with small differences reflecting different emphasis on some topics (i.e. detailed algorithms on antihypertensive agent use), while others reflect evolution of important evidence in recent years. Baxdrostat can be an effective and safe treatment for uncontrolled hypertension in CKD and future guidelines are expected to incorporate its use accordingly.

References

1. Sarafidis PA, Li S, Chen S-C, Collins AJ, Brown WW, Klag MJ, et al. Hypertension awareness, treatment, and control in chronic kidney disease. Am J Med. 2008;121:332–40.
2. Sarafidis PA, Sharpe CC, Wood E, Blacklock R, Rumjon A, Al-Yassin A, et al. Prevalence, patterns of treatment, and control of hypertension in predialysis patients with chronic kidney disease. Nephron Clin Pract. 2012;120:c147–55.
3. Boenink R, Astley ME, Huijben JA, Stel VS, Kerschbaum J, Ots-Rosenberg M, et al. The ERA registry annual report 2019: summary and age comparisons. Clin Kidney J. 2022;15:452–72.
4. Johansen KL, Chertow GM, Gilbertson DT, Herzog CA, Ishani A, Israni AK, et al. US renal data system 2021 annual data report: epidemiology of kidney disease in the United States. Am J Kidney Dis. 2022;79:A8–A12.
5. Sarafidis PA, Georgianos PI, Zebekakis PE. Comparative epidemiology of resistant hypertension in chronic kidney disease and the general hypertensive population. Semin Nephrol. 2014;34:483–91.
6. Parati G, Pengo MF, Avolio A, Azizi M, Bothe TL, Burnier M, et al. Nocturnal blood pressure: pathophysiology, measurement and clinical implications. Position paper of the European Society of Hypertension. J Hypertens. 2025;43:1296–318.
7. Mancia G, Kreutz R, Brunström M, Burnier M, Grassi G, Januszewicz A, et al. 2023 ESH guidelines for the management of arterial hypertension the task force for the management of arterial hypertension of the European Society of Hypertension: endorsed by the International Society of Hypertension (ISH) and the European Renal Association (ERA). J Hypertens. 2023;41:1874–2071.
8. Ruilope LM, Agarwal R, Anker SD, Filippatos G, Pitt B, Rossing P, et al. Blood pressure and cardiorenal outcomes with Finerenone in chronic kidney disease in type 2 diabetes. Hypertension. 2022;79:2685–95.
9. Kidney Disease: Improving Global Outcomes (KDIGO) Blood Pressure Work Group. KDIGO 2021 Clinical practice guideline for the management of blood pressure in chronic kidney disease. Kidney Int. 2021;99:S1–S87.
10. Jones DW, Ferdinand KC, Taler SJ, Johnson HM, Shimbo D, Abdalla M, et al. AHA/ACC/AANP/AAPA/ABC/ACCP/ACPM/AGS/AMA/ASPC/NMA/PCNA/SGIM Guideline for the

prevention, detection, evaluation and Management of high blood pressure in adults: a report of the American College of Cardiology/American Heart Association Joint Committee on Clinical Practice Guidelines. Hypertension. 2025;82:e212-e316. Erratum in: Hypertension. 2025;82:e350. Erratum in: Hypertension. 2026;83:e000262. Erratum in: Hypertension. 2026;83:e00264.

11. McEvoy JW, McCarthy CP, Bruno RM, Brouwers S, Canavan MD, Ceconi C, et al. ESC guidelines for the management of elevated blood pressure and hypertension: developed by the task force on the management of elevated blood pressure and hypertension of the European Society of Cardiology (ESC) and endorsed by the European Society of Endocrinology (ESE) and the European stroke organisation (ESO). Eur Heart J. 2024;45:3912–4018.
12. Sacks FM, Svetkey LP, Vollmer WM, Appel LJ, Bray GA, Harsha D, et al. Effects on blood pressure of reduced dietary sodium and the dietary approaches to stop hypertension (DASH) diet. N Engl J Med. 2001;344:3–10.
13. Neal B, Wu Y, Feng X, Zhang R, Zhang Y, Shi J, et al. Effect of salt substitution on cardiovascular events and death. N Engl J Med. 2021;385:1067–77.
14. Vogt L, Waanders F, Boomsma F, de Zeeuw D, Navis G. Effects of dietary sodium and hydrochlorothiazide on the antiproteinuric efficacy of losartan. J Am Soc Nephrol. 2008;19:999–1007.
15. Shi H, Su X, Li C, Guo W, Wang L. Effect of a low-salt diet on chronic kidney disease outcomes: a systematic review and meta-analysis. BMJ Open. 2022;12(1):e050843.
16. Strippoli GFM, Craig M, Deeks JJ, Schena FP, Craig JC. Effects of angiotensin converting enzyme inhibitors and angiotensin II receptor antagonists on mortality and renal outcomes in diabetic nephropathy: systematic review. BMJ. 2004;329:828.
17. Brenner BM, Cooper ME, de Zeeuw D, Keane WF, Mitch WE, Parving HH, et al. Effects of losartan on renal and cardiovascular outcomes in patients with type 2 diabetes and nephropathy. N Engl J Med. 2001;345:861–9.
18. Lewis EJ, Hunsicker LG, Clarke WR, Berl T, Pohl MA, Lewis JB, et al. Renoprotective effect of the angiotensin-receptor antagonist irbesartan in patients with nephropathy due to type 2 diabetes. N Engl J Med. 2001;345:851–60.
19. Barnett AH, Bain SC, Bouter P, Karlberg B, Madsbad S, Jervell J, et al. Angiotensin-receptor blockade versus converting-enzyme inhibition in type 2 diabetes and nephropathy. N Engl J Med. 2004;351:1952–61.
20. Wright JT, Bakris G, Greene T, Agodoa LY, Appel LJ, Charleston J, et al. Effect of blood pressure lowering and antihypertensive drug class on progression of hypertensive kidney disease: results from the AASK trial. JAMA. 2002;288:2421–31.
21. Randomised placebo-controlled trial of effect of ramipril on decline in glomerular filtration rate and risk of terminal renal failure in proteinuric, non-diabetic nephropathy. The GISEN Group (Gruppo Italiano di Studi Epidemiologici in Nefrologia). Lancet. 1997;349:1857–63.
22. Hou FF, Zhang X, Zhang GH, Xie D, Chen PY, Zhang WR, et al. Efficacy and safety of benazepril for advanced chronic renal insufficiency. N Engl J Med. 2006;354:131–40.
23. de Zeeuw D, Remuzzi G, Parving H-H, Keane WF, Zhang Z, Shahinfar S, et al. Proteinuria, a target for renoprotection in patients with type 2 diabetic nephropathy: lessons from RENAAL. Kidney Int. 2004;65:2309–20.
24. Atkins RC, Briganti EM, Lewis JB, Hunsicker LG, Braden G, Champion de Crespigny PJ, et al. Proteinuria reduction and progression to renal failure in patients with type 2 diabetes mellitus and overt nephropathy. Am J Kidney Dis. 2005;45:281–7.
25. Parving H-H, Brenner BM, McMurray JJV, de Zeeuw D, Haffner SM, Solomon SD, et al. Cardiorenal end points in a trial of aliskiren for type 2 diabetes. N Engl J Med. 2012;367:2204–13.
26. Fried LF, Emanuele N, Zhang JH, Brophy M, Conner TA, Duckworth W, et al. Combined angiotensin inhibition for the treatment of diabetic nephropathy. N Engl J Med. 2013;369:1892–903.
27. Haller H, Ito S, Izzo JL, Januszewicz A, Katayama S, Menne J, et al. Olmesartan for the delay or prevention of microalbuminuria in type 2 diabetes. N Engl J Med. 2011;364:907–17.

28. Rahman M, Pressel S, Davis BR, Nwachuku C, Wright JT, Whelton PK, et al. Renal outcomes in high-risk hypertensive patients treated with an angiotensin-converting enzyme inhibitor or a calcium channel blocker vs a diuretic: a report from the antihypertensive and lipid-lowering treatment to prevent heart attack trial (ALLHAT). Arch Intern Med. 2005;165:936–46.
29. Sarafidis PA, Blacklock R, Wood E, Rumjon A, Simmonds S, Fletcher-Rogers J, et al. Prevalence and factors associated with hyperkalemia in predialysis patients followed in a low-clearance clinic. Clin J Am Soc Nephrol. 2012;7:1234–41.
30. Einhorn LM, Zhan M, Hsu VD, Walker LD, Moen MF, Seliger SL, et al. The frequency of hyperkalemia and its significance in chronic kidney disease. Arch Intern Med. 2009;169:1156–62.
31. Yildirim T, Arici M, Piskinpasa S, Aybal-Kutlugun A, Yilmaz R, Altun B, et al. Major barriers against renin-angiotensin-aldosterone system blocker use in chronic kidney disease stages 3–5 in clinical practice: a safety concern? Ren Fail. 2012;34:1095–9.
32. Epstein M, Reaven NL, Funk SE, McGaughey KJ, Oestreicher N, Knispel J. Evaluation of the treatment gap between clinical guidelines and the utilization of renin-angiotensin-aldosterone system inhibitors. Am J Manag Care. 2015;21:S212–20.
33. Bakris GL, Pitt B, Weir MR, Freeman MW, Mayo MR, Garza D, et al. Effect of patiromer on serum potassium level in patients with hyperkalemia and diabetic kidney disease: the AMETHYST-DN randomized clinical trial. JAMA. 2015;314:151–61.
34. Roger SD, Spinowitz BS, Lerma EV, Singh B, Packham DK, Al-Shurbaji A, et al. Efficacy and safety of sodium zirconium Cyclosilicate for treatment of hyperkalemia: an 11-month open-label extension of HARMONIZE. Am J Nephrol. 2019;50:473–80.
35. Sarafidis PA, Georgianos PI, Bakris GL. Advances in treatment of hyperkalemia in chronic kidney disease. Expert Opin Pharmacother. 2015;16:2205–15.
36. Valdivielso JM, Balafa O, Ekart R, Ferro CJ, Mallamaci F, Mark PB, et al. Hyperkalemia in chronic kidney disease in the new era of kidney protection therapies. Drugs. 2021;81:1467–89.
37. Sarafidis PA, Khosla N, Bakris GL. Antihypertensive therapy in the presence of proteinuria. Am J Kidney Dis. 2007;49:12–26.
38. Ott C, Schmieder RE. Diagnosis and treatment of arterial hypertension 2021. Kidney Int. 2022;101:36–46.
39. Bakris GL, Copley JB, Vicknair N, Sadler R, Leurgans S. Calcium channel blockers versus other antihypertensive therapies on progression of NIDDM associated nephropathy. Kidney Int. 1996;50:1641–50.
40. Bakris GL, Mangrum A, Copley JB, Vicknair N, Sadler R. Effect of calcium channel or beta-blockade on the progression of diabetic nephropathy in African Americans. Hypertension. 1997;29:744–50.
41. Smith AC, Toto R, Bakris GL. Differential effects of calcium channel blockers on size selectivity of proteinuria in diabetic glomerulopathy. Kidney Int. 1998;54:889–96.
42. Griffin KA, Picken MM, Bakris GL, Bidani AK. Class differences in the effects of calcium channel blockers in the rat remnant kidney model. Kidney Int. 1999;55:1849–60.
43. Ruggenenti P, Perna A, Loriga G, Ganeva M, Ene-Iordache B, Turturro M, et al. Blood-pressure control for renoprotection in patients with non-diabetic chronic renal disease (REIN-2): multicentre, randomised controlled trial. Lancet. 2005;365:939–46.
44. Bakris GL, Sarafidis PA, Weir MR, Dahlöf B, Pitt B, Jamerson K, et al. Renal outcomes with different fixed-dose combination therapies in patients with hypertension at high risk for cardiovascular events (ACCOMPLISH): a prespecified secondary analysis of a randomised controlled trial. Lancet. 2010;375:1173–81.
45. Sarafidis PA, Bakris GL. Resistant hypertension: an overview of evaluation and treatment. J Am Coll Cardiol. 2008;52:1749–57.
46. Slagman MCJ, Waanders F, Hemmelder MH, Woittiez A-J, Janssen WMT, Lambers Heerspink HJ, et al. Moderate dietary sodium restriction added to angiotensin converting enzyme inhibition compared with dual blockade in lowering proteinuria and blood pressure: randomised controlled trial. BMJ. 2011;343:d4366.
47. Sarafidis PA, Georgianos PI, Lasaridis AN. Diuretics in clinical practice. Part I: mechanisms of action, pharmacological effects and clinical indications of diuretic compounds. Expert Opin Drug Saf. 2010;9:243–57.

48. Agarwal R, Sinha AD, Cramer AE, Balmes-Fenwick M, Dickinson JH, Ouyang F, et al. Chlorthalidone for hypertension in advanced chronic kidney disease. N Engl J Med. 2021;385:2507–19.
49. Loutradis C, Sarafidis P. Hypertension in patients with advanced chronic kidney disease. In: Mancia G, Grassi G, Tsioufis K, Dominiczak A, Rosei EA, editors. Manual of hypertension of the European Society of Hypertension. Boca Raton: CRC Press; 2019. https://doi.org/10.1201/9780429199189.
50. Williams B, MacDonald TM, Morant S, Webb DJ, Sever P, McInnes G, et al. Spironolactone versus placebo, bisoprolol, and doxazosin to determine the optimal treatment for drug-resistant hypertension (PATHWAY-2): a randomised, double-blind, crossover trial. Lancet. 2015;386:2059–68.
51. Chen C, Zhu X-Y, Li D, Lin Q, Zhou K. Clinical efficacy and safety of spironolactone in patients with resistant hypertension: a systematic review and meta-analysis. Medicine (Baltimore). 2020;99:e21694.
52. Agarwal R, Rossignol P, Romero A, Garza D, Mayo MR, Warren S, et al. Patiromer versus placebo to enable spironolactone use in patients with resistant hypertension and chronic kidney disease (AMBER): a phase 2, randomised, double-blind, placebo-controlled trial. Lancet. 2019;394:1540–50.
53. Richard Hobbs FD, McManus RJ, Taylor CJ, et al. Low-dose spironolactone and cardiovascular outcomes in moderate stage chronic kidney disease: a randomized controlled trial. Nat Med. 2024;30:3634–45.
54. Flack JM, Azizi M, Brown JM, et al. Efficacy and safety of baxdrostat in uncontrolled and resistant hypertension. N Engl J Med. 2025;393:1363–74.
55. Azizi M, Brown JM, Dwyer JP, et al. Effect of baxdrostat on ambulatory blood pressure in patients with resistant hypertension (Bax24): a phase 3, randomised, double-blind, placebo-controlled trial. Lancet. 407:988–99.
56. Dwyer JP, Maklad N, Vedin O, et al. Efficacy and safety of baxdrostat in participants with CKD and uncontrolled hypertension: a randomized, double-blind, placebo-controlled trial. J Am Soc Nephrol. 2026;37:299–311.
57. Bakris GL, Hart P, Ritz E. Beta blockers in the management of chronic kidney disease. Kidney Int. 2006;70:1905–13.
58. UK Prospective Diabetes Study Group. Efficacy of atenolol and captopril in reducing risk of macrovascular and microvascular complications in type 2 diabetes: UKPDS 39. UK Prospective Diabetes Study Group. BMJ. 1998;317:713–20.
59. Bakris GL, Fonseca V, Katholi RE, McGill JB, Messerli FH, Phillips RA, et al. Metabolic effects of carvedilol vs metoprolol in patients with type 2 diabetes mellitus and hypertension: a randomized controlled trial. JAMA. 2004;292:2227–36.
60. Azizi M, Sanghvi K, Saxena M, Gosse P, Reilly JP, Levy T, et al. Ultrasound renal denervation for hypertension resistant to a triple medication pill (RADIANCE-HTN TRIO): a randomised, multicentre, single-blind, sham-controlled trial. Lancet. 2021;397:2476–86.
61. Azizi M, Schmieder RE, Mahfoud F, Weber MA, Daemen J, Davies J, et al. Endovascular ultrasound renal denervation to treat hypertension (RADIANCE-HTN SOLO): a multicentre, international, single-blind, randomised, sham-controlled trial. Lancet. 2018;391:2335–45.
62. Böhm M, Kario K, Kandzari DE, Mahfoud F, Weber MA, Schmieder RE, et al. Efficacy of catheter-based renal denervation in the absence of antihypertensive medications (SPYRAL HTN-OFF MED pivotal): a multicentre, randomised, sham-controlled trial. Lancet. 2020;395:1444–51.
63. Imprialos KP, Sarafidis PA, Karagiannis AI. Sodium-glucose cotransporter-2 inhibitors and blood pressure decrease: a valuable effect of a novel antidiabetic class? J Hypertens. 2015;33:2185–97.
64. Papadopoulou E, Loutradis C, Tzatzagou G, Kotsa K, Zografou I, Minopoulou I, et al. Dapagliflozin decreases ambulatory central blood pressure and pulse wave velocity in patients with type 2 diabetes: a randomized, double-blind, placebo-controlled clinical trial. J Hypertens. 2021;39:749–58.

65. Cherney DZI, Cooper ME, Tikkanen I, Pfarr E, Johansen OE, Woerle HJ, et al. Pooled analysis of phase III trials indicate contrasting influences of renal function on blood pressure, body weight, and HbA1c reductions with empagliflozin. Kidney Int. 2018;93:231–44.
66. Jordan J, Tank J, Heusser K, Heise T, Wanner C, Heer M, et al. The effect of empagliflozin on muscle sympathetic nerve activity in patients with type II diabetes mellitus. J Am Soc Hypertens. 2017;11:604–12.
67. Chilton R, Tikkanen I, Cannon CP, Crowe S, Woerle HJ, Broedl UC, et al. Effects of empagliflozin on blood pressure and markers of arterial stiffness and vascular resistance in patients with type 2 diabetes. Diabetes Obes Metab. 2015;17:1180–93.
68. Piperidou A, Sarafidis P, Boutou A, Thomopoulos C, Loutradis C, Alexandrou ME, et al. The effect of SGLT-2 inhibitors on albuminuria and proteinuria in diabetes mellitus: a systematic review and meta-analysis of randomized controlled trials. J Hypertens. 2019;37:1334–43.
69. Zinman B, Wanner C, Lachin JM, Fitchett D, Bluhmki E, Hantel S, et al. Empagliflozin, cardiovascular outcomes, and mortality in type 2 diabetes. N Engl J Med. 2015;373:2117–28.
70. Neal B, Perkovic V, Mahaffey KW, de Zeeuw D, Fulcher G, Erondu N, et al. Canagliflozin and cardiovascular and renal events in type 2 diabetes. N Engl J Med. 2017;377:644–57.
71. Wiviott SD, Raz I, Bonaca MP, Mosenzon O, Kato ET, Cahn A, et al. Dapagliflozin and cardiovascular outcomes in type 2 diabetes. N Engl J Med. 2019;380:347–57.
72. Sarafidis P, Ortiz A, Ferro CJ, Halimi J-M, Kreutz R, Mallamaci F, et al. Sodium–glucose co-transporter-2 inhibitors for patients with diabetic and nondiabetic chronic kidney disease: a new era has already begun. J Hypertens. 2021;39:1090–7.
73. Sarafidis PA, Stafylas PC, Kanaki AI, Lasaridis AN. Effects of renin-angiotensin system blockers on renal outcomes and all-cause mortality in patients with diabetic nephropathy: an updated meta-analysis. Am J Hypertens. 2008;21:922–9.
74. Sharma P, Blackburn RC, Parke CL, McCullough K, Marks A, Black C. Angiotensin-converting enzyme inhibitors and angiotensin receptor blockers for adults with early (stage 1 to 3) non-diabetic chronic kidney disease. Cochrane Database Syst Rev. 2011;7:CD007751.
75. Lin Y-C, Lin J-W, Wu M-S, Chen K-C, Peng C-C, Kang Y-N. Effects of calcium channel blockers comparing to angiotensin-converting enzyme inhibitors and angiotensin receptor blockers in patients with hypertension and chronic kidney disease stage 3 to 5 and dialysis: a systematic review and meta-analysis. PLoS One. 2017;12:e0188975.
76. Sarafidis P, Papadopoulos CE, Kamperidis V, Giannakoulas G, Doumas M. Cardiovascular protection with sodium-glucose Cotransporter-2 inhibitors and mineralocorticoid receptor antagonists in chronic kidney disease: a milestone achieved. Hypertension. 2021;77:1442–55.
77. Bakris GL, Agarwal R, Anker SD, Pitt B, Ruilope LM, Rossing P, et al. Effect of Finerenone on chronic kidney disease outcomes in type 2 diabetes. N Engl J Med. 2020;383:2219–29.
78. Pitt B, Filippatos G, Agarwal R, Anker SD, Bakris GL, Rossing P, et al. Cardiovascular events with Finerenone in kidney disease and type 2 diabetes. N Engl J Med. 2021;385:2252–63.
79. Ruilope LM, Agarwal R, Anker SD, Filippatos G, Pitt B, Rossing P, et al; FIDELIO-DKD Investigators. Blood Pressure and Cardiorenal Outcomes With Finerenone in Chronic Kidney Disease in Type 2 Diabetes. Hypertension. 2022;79:2685–95.
80. Ruilope LM, Agarwal R, Anker SD, Bakris GL, Filippatos G, Nowack C, et al. Design and baseline characteristics of the Finerenone in reducing cardiovascular mortality and morbidity in diabetic kidney disease trial. Am J Nephrol. 2019;50:345–56.
81. Filippatos G, Anker SD, August P, Coats AJS, Januzzi JL, Mankovsky B, et al. Finerenone and effects on mortality in chronic kidney disease and type 2 diabetes: a FIDELITY analysis. Eur Heart J Cardiovasc Pharmacother. 2023;9:183.
82. Heerspink HJL, Neuen BL, Agarwal R, et al. Finerenone in persons with chronic kidney disease without diabetes. N Engl J Med. 2026. https://doi.org/10.1056/NEJMoa2604625.
83. Agarwal R, Ruilope LM, Ruiz-Hurtado G, Haller H, Schmieder RE, Anker SD, et al. Effect of finerenone on ambulatory blood pressure in chronic kidney disease in type 2 diabetes. J Hypertens. 2023;41:295–302.
84. Barbato E, Azizi M, Schmieder RE, Lauder L, Böhm M, Brouwers S, et al. Renal denervation in the management of hypertension in adults. A clinical consensus statement of the ESC Council on hypertension and the European Association of Percutaneous Cardiovascular Interventions (EAPCI). Eur Heart J. 2023;44:1313–30.

Adherence to Antihypertensive Medications in Chronic Kidney Disease

Aikaterini Damianaki and Michel Burnier

Abbreviations

ACC/AHA	American College of Cardiology/American Heart Association
ADA	American Diabetes Association
ADPKD	Autosomal dominant polycystic kidney disease
BP	Blood pressure
CAT	Chemical adherence testing
CCB	Calcium channel blocker
CDC	Center of disease control and prevention
CKD	Chronic kidney disease
CKD-aP	Chronic kidney disease—associated pruritus
CV	Cardiovascular
CVD	Cardiovascular diseases
eGFR	Estimated glomerular filtration rate
ESA	Erythropoietin stimulating agents
ESC	European Society of Cardiology
ESH	European Society of Hypertension
ESKD	End-stage kidney disease
GLP-1 RA	Glucagon-like peptide-1 receptor agonists
KDIGO	Kidney Disease Improving Outcomes

A. Damianaki
Service of Nephrology and Hypertension, Department of Medicine, University Hospital, Lausanne, Switzerland

M. Burnier (✉)
Faculty of Biology and Medicine, University of Lausanne, Lausanne, Switzerland
e-mail: michel.burnier@unil.ch; michel.burnier@netplus.ch

P. Sarafidis, R. Pontremoli (eds.), *Hypertension and Chronic Kidney Disease*, Updates in Hypertension and Cardiovascular Protection,
https://doi.org/10.1007/978-3-032-29564-4_13

MEMS	Medication event monitoring system
NHANES	National Health and Nutrition Examination Survey
nsMRA	Nonsteroidal mineralocorticoid receptor antagonists
PDC	Proportion of days covered
RAS	Renin-angiotensin system
SGLT2i	Sodium–glucose cotransporter 2 inhibitors
SHPTH	Secondary hyperparathyroidism
SLE	Systemic lupus erythematosus

Introduction

Chronic kidney disease (CKD) affects an estimated 850 million people globally, with a median prevalence of 9.5% (Interquartile range 5.9–11.7%) [1, 2]. However, these figures are likely underestimated due to limited screening and diagnostic programs in many regions, contributing to widespread unawareness of the disease—particularly in its earlier stages [3, 4]. Importantly, many affected people die prematurely due either to CKD-associated complications such as hypertension, diabetes and the resulting cardiovascular diseases (CVD) or to insufficient access to essential life-saving treatments such as dialysis and transplantation [5, 6]. Worldwide, CKD accounted for 1.2 million deaths in 2017, but projections suggest this number could rise to 2.2 million by 2040 under optimistic assumptions, and up to 4.0 million in the worst-case scenario [7]. Another important consideration is that the economic burden of CKD is disproportionately high compared to other diseases with similar prevalence [8]. Healthcare costs rise substantially with each advancing stage of CKD, but the greatest financial strain stems from the treatment of patients with end-stage kidney disease (ESKD), due to the high cost of dialysis and transplantation.

Simultaneously, several major CKD risk factors—such as hypertension, diabetes, and obesity- are continuing to rise globally along with the increasing and aging population, which further contributes to the CKD burden due to the natural decline in renal function with age. According to the Center of Disease Control (CDC) Chronic Kidney Disease in the United States 2023 report, CKD coexists in at least one in five individuals with hypertension and one in three individuals with diabetes [9]. Notably, developing countries are witnessing a rapid increase in CKD prevalence, largely due to the growing burden of diabetes and hypertension associated with urbanization and environmental issues, unhealthy lifestyles, and limited preventive care.

Definition of Adherence and Methods of Assessment

Medication adherence is generally defined as the extent to which a patient's medication-taking behavior aligns with the therapeutic plans proposed by healthcare providers in the context of a shared-decision process [10]. Adherence has three principal components: *initiation*, which is the time from prescription to the first dosing of the medication; *implementation*, which reflects how accurately the patient follows the prescribed dosing regimen on a daily basis and accounts for missed doses, delays, or prolonged interruptions such as "drug holidays" (typically defined as ≥3 consecutive days without intake); and *discontinuation*, which marks the point at which the patient stops medications. The latter enables the definition of persistence. While an 80% adherence threshold is often cited as the minimum required to achieve therapeutic benefits, this cut-off is largely arbitrary and not supported by evidence, and may not apply uniformly across drug classes or disease states [11].

Various methods exist to assess adherence, though each one comes with limitations. They are commonly divided into three categories: subjective (e.g., patient interviews and questionnaires), indirect (e.g., pill counts, electronic databases, electronic monitoring systems), and direct methods (measurement of drug/metabolite levels and directly observed treatment) [12–14]. Table 1 summarizes the strengths and limitations of each method [14]. Assessing adherence in clinical and research settings is challenging in people with CKD, who often face complex multidrug regimens. Electronic monitoring systems such as the Medication Event Monitoring System (MEMS) represent an objective assessment method, enabling them to track execution by recording the date and time when the medication container is opened. It is the only method providing a long-term dosing history. However, its use in CKD patients may be limited by the high number of prescribed medications, which complicates the monitoring (although it is not always necessary to monitor all prescribed medications simultaneously). Of course, electronic monitoring does not confirm drug ingestion. Yet, any non-opening of the pillbox is very likely associated with a non-ingestion [15]. Today, biochemical testing in urine and blood is promoted as the new standard of adherence monitoring. The chemical adherence testing (CAT) can provide objective adherence data, particularly for drugs with measurable serum levels [16]. This approach ascertains drug intake, but it also has its own limitations, the most important being that patients have better adherence before and after medical terms. In CKD patients, the interpretation of results may become complicated because of the CKD-related variations in pharmacodynamics and pharmacokinetics [17]. These limitations underscore the need for multifaceted adherence assessments and tailored interventions to support consistent, high-quality medication use in CKD care.

Table 1 Strengths and limitations of different methods to assess drug adherence

Method	Accuracy	Resistance to manipulation	Cost and/or workload	Clinical use
Assessment by clinician	🟥🟥	🟥🟥	🟩🟩🟩🟩🟩🟩	🟩🟩🟩🟩🟩🟩
Questionnaire	🟥🟥	🟥🟥	🟩🟩🟩🟩🟩🟩	🟩🟩🟩🟩🟩🟩
Pill count	🟧🟧🟧🟧	🟧🟧🟧🟧	🟧🟧🟧🟧	🟧🟧🟧🟧
Refill data	🟧🟧🟧🟧	🟧🟧🟧🟧	🟧🟧🟧🟧	🟧🟧🟧🟧
Witnessed drug intake	🟩🟩🟩🟩🟩🟩	🟧🟧🟧🟧	🟥🟥	🟥🟥
Electronic monitoring	🟩🟩🟩🟩🟩🟩	🟩🟩🟩🟩🟩🟩	🟥🟥	🟧🟧🟧🟧
Drug assay	🟩🟩🟩🟩🟩🟩	🟧🟧🟧🟧	🟥🟥	🟧🟧🟧🟧

"Resistance to manipulation" reflects the robustness to manipulation by the patient, with poor robustness resulting in misleading information on true adherence. Scores on characteristics are shown as follows: red bars – weak score; orange bars – average score; green bars – excellent score.

From Ref. [13], with permission

Adherence to Clinical Recommendations and Guidelines

With the global trends pointing to an escalating CKD burden that demands urgent attention, clinical practice guidelines offer a clear framework for physicians to prevent and manage the disease [18–20]. These guidelines published by nephrologists as well as by experts in other areas (hypertension, diabetes, …) are regularly updated and completed, driven by robust evidence emerging from high-quality clinical trials, ensuring that treatment strategies remain effective and aligned with the lasted scientific achievements. However, data have shown that adherence to specific CKD recommendations to retard the disease progression is far from being optimal in clinical practice with large variations among countries [21]. For example, the use of inhibitors of the renin-angiotensin system (RAS)—a cornerstone of CKD management for over three decades—has improved consistently over the years; yet, persistence rates remain low [22, 23]. A similar trend is being observed with new drugs recently added to the armamentarium of CKD such as sodium–glucose cotransporter 2 inhibitors (SGLT2is), glucagon-like peptide-1 receptor agonists (GLP-1 RAs) and nonsteroidal mineralocorticoid receptor antagonists (nsMRAs) [24–26].

Clinical Inertia and Polypharmacy: Two Major Barriers in CKD Patients

A key factor contributing to the therapeutic gap observed in most chronic diseases is clinical inertia, defined as the failure to initiate or to intensify treatment when clinically indicated [27, 28]. In CKD, this often manifests as a failure to prescribe or increase the dose of RAS inhibitors or an underuse of newer nephro- and cardioprotective agents, even in eligible patients. This inertia may stem from a range of factors, including clinicians' as well as patients' concerns about side effects (hyperkalemia, a drop in eGFR), assumptions about patient non-adherence, limited familiarity with newer agents, and the constraints imposed by heavy clinical overloads and brief appointment durations [27, 29]. In some countries, the administrative burden of obtaining pre-authorizations, although beneficial in reducing the use of inappropriate or expensive medications, may also play a negative role because it is time-consuming [30]. For primary care physicians—who manage most people with early-stage CKD—keeping up with evolving guideline recommendations from various authorities (guidelines from the Kidney Disease Improving Outcomes (KDIGO), the American Diabetes Association (ADA), the European Society of Hypertension (ESH), the European Society of Cardiology (ESC), etc.) can be challenging, particularly as updates are frequent and sometimes with differences. The perception that guidelines focus more on *what to do* rather than *how to do* further complicates their implementation in everyday practice [29, 31]. Additionally, performing ongoing monitoring for CKD patients—whose care is frequently fragmented due to multimorbidity and the involvement of multiple specialists—adds another layer of complexity, often leading providers to hesitate when acting outside their perceived scope [28, 32].

Patient-related barriers also contribute to clinical inertia because of polypharmacy, limited health literacy, poor language and communication skills, lack of self-management and involvement in decision making (empowerment) [26]. As for polypharmacy—commonly defined as the use of five medications or more daily—a recent systematic review and meta-analysis of 127 studies has reported a pooled mean number of prescribed medications of 9.7 in more than 80% of people with CKD, with the highest figures in dialysis patients and kidney transplant recipients [33]. Hence, inappropriate prescribing, multiple medication changes and polypharmacy remain persistent challenges in CKD [34]. Of note, polypharmacy has been associated with poor medication adherence, as well as with a more rapid decline of GFR, a lower quality of life, more adverse drug reactions and a higher all-cause mortality [33]. In a cohort of 5217 patients with moderate CKD, 8 of 10 participants were exposed to polypharmacy, and 2 of 10 were taking more than 10 different substances per day [35]. Similar findings were reported in the CKD-REIN cohort study, where polypharmacy prevalence reached 72%, and more than half of the patients received at least one inappropriate prescription relative to their level of kidney function [36]. A US survey of dialysis patients reported a median intake of 19 pills per day, with approximately one-quarter of patients taking over 25 medications daily. Likewise, a more recent study among Japanese dialysis patients reported an average of 16.4 (±8.34) oral medications per day on dialysis days and 16.3 (±8.55) on non-dialysis days [37]. Unfortunately, even in the hypothetical scenario where clinical inertia is fully addressed, and physicians consistently follow guideline-recommended treatments, polypharmacy will remain largely unavoidable. People with CKD typically require complex medication regimens to manage not only blood pressure (BP) but also glycemic control, lipid levels, anemia, and several CKD-related comorbidities. As expected, such a therapeutic complexity and high pill burden can further undermine adherence and persistence, as the sheer volume and variety of medications contribute to confusion, fatigue, and reduced patient engagement in long-term treatment care.

Treatment Management of CKD and Adherence

The effective management of CKD requires addressing several kidney-specific conditions including: (i) the cause of CKD, whenever possible, (ii) risk factors contributing to renal function deterioration (e.g. hypertension, diabetes, dyslipidemia) and (iii) common CKD complications (e.g. anemia, hyperphosphatemia, hyperkalemia) as CKD progresses. This can be achieved through multidrug prescriptions and the implementation of lifestyle measures.

Disease-Specific Treatments

The foundation of CKD management often begins with addressing the cause of the renal disease, particularly in patients with glomerular or autoimmune kidney diseases. Immunosuppressive therapies, corticosteroids, and other disease-modifying agents may be indicated, and these treatments often require long-term use—ranging from several months to years—as part of induction and maintenance therapy. These important medications add to the overall medication burden and adherence challenges. In a study by Cunha et al., hydroxychloroquine levels were monitored to identify non-adherent patients with lupus nephritis, and the authors reported that at least 15.6% had very low levels; other authors have reported that up to 44% of systemic lupus erythematosus (SLE) patients were not taking their most important medications as prescribed [38–40]. In other primary renal diseases, such as autosomal dominant polycystic kidney disease (ADPKD), clinical trial data suggest relatively high adherence and persistence with long-term therapy. Tolvaptan, a selective vasopressin V2-receptor antagonist approved to slow cyst growth and preserve kidney function in ADPKD, has demonstrated encouraging adherence in clinical settings. In the TEMPO3:4 trial, the 3-year discontinuation rate of tolvaptan was 23% while the REPRISE trial reported that 84.6% of patients completed the study one year after introduction [41, 42]. However, real-world data are less favorable. Persistence rates for tolvaptan at 12, 24, and 36 months were estimated to be 70.8% (95% CI: 48.2–93.4), 46.5% (23.2–66.9), and 38.7% (16.4–60.8), respectively [43].

Management of Risk Factors

Managing common risk factors such as hypertension and diabetes is essential to slow CKD progression and to reduce the CV risk of people with CKD.

Hypertension

Hypertension and CKD are closely linked as hypertension can be a cause and a consequence of kidney diseases. Hypertension is highly prevalent across all stages of CKD. As hypertension is both a driver of kidney function decline and a key CV risk factor, reaching optimal BP control is essential in CKD. However, impaired renal function makes BP control more challenging. In general, the achievement of defined BP targets necessitates the prescription of several antihypertensive agents associated with lifestyle modifications [44, 45].

This is the reason why BP control remains largely insufficient among people with CKD. Older studies consistently reported suboptimal control, with only 13.2% achieving a BP <130/80 mmHg in the KEEP study, 35% meeting targets in a Veterans Administration cohort, and over 60% exceeding this threshold in the REGARDS study [46–48]. More recent data from the National Health and Nutrition Examination Survey (NHANES) confirm these figures, showing that less than half of individuals with CKD had a BP at goal according to the 2017 American College of Cardiology/American Heart Association (ACC/AHA) guideline (<130/80 mmHg) [49]. Recent data have suggested that BP control in CKD is also low in European countries, with 30% of patients having uncontrolled BP [50].

In this context, it is not surprising that low adherence to prescribed antihypertensive medications is highly prevalent. The pooled prevalence of non-adherence to antihypertensive medications in people with CKD not on kidney replacement therapy was found to be 33% (95% confidence interval 25–40%) [51]. Advanced CKD stages have been associated with medication non-adherence in most studies, although some authors have found an improved self-reported adherence to BP medications as kidney function declines probably reflecting a progressive engagement of patients and their physicians due in part to the fear of progressing towards ESKD [46, 47, 52–55].

In dialysis patients, assessing BP control is particularly challenging due to the lack of standardized BP targets and variability in timing of BP measurements. Adherence to antihypertensive medications is challenging in this population, too. A recent systematic review reported that nonadherence to antihypertensive medications among chronic hemodialysis patients ranged between 12.5 and 97.5% (mean 38.2%) [56]. This very large range reflects substantial heterogeneity due to differences in definitions and assessment methods. When considering the methods, mean nonadherence rates were 24.3% by patient self-report and 38.5% using more objective measures.

According to its definition, true resistant hypertension can be diagnosed only once out-of-office BP measurements have been obtained and proper medication adherence has been confirmed [57]. This is based on the observation that poor adherence is a frequent cause of apparent resistant hypertension [58]. Indeed, several studies have suggested that low adherence to the prescribed medications can affect up to 50% of patients with resistant hypertension [59]. Since the prevalence of apparent resistant hypertension is high among CKD patients—with estimates reaching up to 42% [60]—management of adherence should be a key objective in individuals with CKD and uncontrolled hypertension or apparent resistant hypertension [59].

Type 2 Diabetes

Type 2 diabetes represents the most common cause of CKD, with a mean prevalence of 38% across all CKD stages, based on data from 547,422 patients [33]. Diabetes significantly increases the risk of CKD progression and CV events, making glycemic control another central goal of therapy. Management typically involves complex regimens, including oral hypoglycemic agents, insulin, and now newer agents such as SGLT2is and GLP-1 RAs, which have been shown to provide significant renal and CV benefits [61–64]. Whereas older hypoglycemic agents have little if any effect on BP, SGLT2is have been shown to lower BP when prescribed on top of RAS blockers or diuretics [65]. However, how much these BP-lowering properties contribute to the beneficial effects of SGLT2i on CKD progression and CV morbidity and mortality remains a matter of debate [66]. The same is true for GLP-1 RAs, which have been found to lower systolic BP by about 2–5 mmHg [67, 68]. Whether this slight reduction of BP contributes to the renal and CV benefits of this new class of agents remains uncertain.

Reflecting their growing importance, these agents have been rapidly incorporated into recent clinical practice guidelines for CKD associated with type 2 diabetes, including KDIGO, ESH, ESC and ADA recommendations [18–20]. However, some concerns have been raised regarding their long-term persistence due essentially to their cost and their impact on the pill burden.

Despite their proven efficacy, with long-term projections suggesting that their combination can reduce relative risk for major CV events by 35% and slow CKD progression by 58% compared to RAS inhibitors alone in CKD patients with type 2 diabetes, the real-world adoption of these therapies for CKD management is very slow, particularly in low-income countries. Indeed, data point out that among people with a diagnosis of CKD, the average proportion of individuals receiving appropriate therapy with SGLT2is to delay CKD progression is less than 10% (after 90 days) [26].

Large-scale observational data tend to confirm that even in populations with established CKD or CVD, these therapies remain under-prescribed. In national estimates from the U.S. (2017–2020), fewer than 6% of eligible adults with type 2 diabetes and eGFR ≥30 mL/min/1.73 m^2 were receiving an SGLT2i, with GLP-1 RA use trailing slightly behind [69]. A similar pattern of underuse was observed in a cohort of over 300,000 people with diabetes and known CVD, with less than 4% receiving either class [70]. Data from the UK and Australia, while showing slightly higher usage, still reflect substantial treatment gaps, particularly in disadvantaged regions and among patients with CV comorbidities, who arguably have the most to gain. In the UK, adoption remained limited in 2019, with SGLT2i use in people with CVD at 9.8% vs. 13.8% in those without CVD, and GLP-1 RA use at only 4.3% and 4.9%, respectively [71]. Australian data from New South Wales show somewhat higher adoption (29.7% for SGLT2is, 8.3% for GLP-1 RAs in metformin users), though disparities persist by geography and socioeconomic status [72]. Similar trends were found in the U.S. Veterans Affairs system, where only 11.2% of patients with type 2 diabetes and atherosclerotic CVD received SGLT2i and 8.0% were prescribed GLP-1 RA in 2020 [73]. A comparative study across the U.S., Sweden, and Israel further highlighted that adoption was inconsistent, and not clearly aligned with comorbidity profiles such as atherosclerotic CVD or CKD [74]. Encouragingly, a more recent analysis from the TriNetX U.S. dataset showed a rise in combined use of these agents from 9.2% in 2018 to 27.1% in 2022 among people with type 2 diabetes and atherosclerotic CVD, but the overall adoption still lags behind clinical guidelines [75]. With the accumulation of new results further demonstrating their cardiac and renal benefits, the penetration of these new drugs will probably increase substantially soon. Among approximately 113,000 patients with CKD and diabetes from Europe, Japan, and U.S., only about 50% of patients were receiving SGLT2i treatments during the period 2012–2021, highlighting substantial room for improvement [76]. Analysis from the same data showed that GLP-1 RA use steadily increased across multinational cohorts and persistence with treatment was higher (between 52% and 78%) [77].

Regarding patients' adherence, in a recent analysis of U.S. claims data, only 44% of White and 37% of Black patients with diabetic kidney disease remained persistent with SGLT2i therapy for at least one year, highlighting a substantial drop-off in use over time [78]. Interestingly, adherence rates (defined as proportion of days covered (PDC) ≥80%) were higher among White patients (85%) than among Black patients (78%). In Sweden, data from the National registry have reported that among 73,895 new users of GLP-1 RA, the cumulative incidence of treatment discontinuation was 23.6% at 1 year and 38.5% at 3 years. However, among patients who discontinued, treatment reinitiation was frequent, respectively 41.1% at 1 year and 57.4% at 3 years after discontinuation. Among 113,207 new users of SGLT2is, the cumulative incidence of treatment discontinuation was 27.9% at 1 year and 45.9% at 3 years, with a cumulative incidence of reinitiation of 40.4% at 1 year and 55.7% at 3 years after discontinuation [79].

Nonsteroidal mineralocorticoid receptor antagonists (nsMRA) have also demonstrated significant benefits in slowing CKD progression and reducing CV events in type 2 diabetes [66, 80–83]. In the two large clinical trials conducted with finerenone [84, 85], the impact of nsMRA on BP was very modest, suggesting no contribution of BP changes on the renal and cardiac benefits of this class of agents. However, in both these trials, free up-titration or down-titration of antihypertensive agents was allowed over a long follow-up period and, thus, the true effect of finerenone on BP could not be assessed. Nevertheless, other nsMRA than finerenone have been shown to lower BP [86, 87]. So far, information on adherence to finerenone has remained limited. A subgroup analysis of the FIDELITY suggested that Hispanic patients exhibit lower adherence rates, but overall adherence was more than 80% [80].

Management of Common Complications

The management of CKD also includes treating several other CKD-associated complications as illustrated in Fig. 1. These include metabolic acidosis, secondary hyperparathyroidism, anemia, iron deficiency, pruritus and electrolyte imbalances (sodium, potassium, magnesium). Some of these treatments are characterized by a very high pill burden, which may interfere with the adherence and persistence of other medications. Among those drug classes, phosphate binders are particularly notable for their high pill burden, accounting for about one-half of the daily pill burden in advanced CKD and dialysis patients [88–90]. Therefore, it is not surprising that adherence to these agents in an already overmedicated population is notably poor with a reported non-adherence rate as high as 93% [56, 91]. Other common factors leading to the high discontinuation rates of these medications are patients' perception that they are less important, side effects (predominantly gastrointestinal), need for administration with meals and the difficulty to swallow due to their size, texture and taste [92].

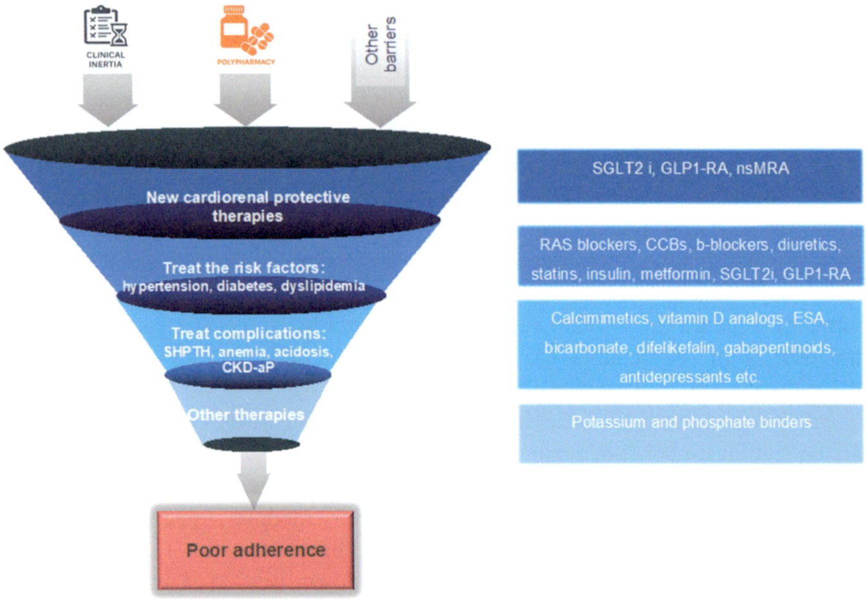

Fig. 1 CKD-associated complications and their impact on adherence. *CCBs* calcium channel blockers, *CKD-aP* chronic kidney disease–associated pruritus, *ESA* erythropoietin-stimulating agents, *GLP-1 RA* glucagon-like peptide-1 receptor agonist, *nsMRA* nonsteroidal mineralocorticoid receptor antagonist, *SGLT2i* sodium–glucose cotransporter 2 inhibitor, *SHPTH* secondary hyperparathyroidism

Strategies to Improve Medication Adherence and Clinical Inertia

Addressing the challenges of medication nonadherence and clinical inertia in CKD requires a coordinated, multi-level approach that spans policy, healthcare systems, providers, and patients. As nephrologists, we should ensure that our patients not only receive effective therapies but also that they are well equipped and empowered to use them consistently.

Starting with ensuring that CKD is recognized as a national health priority is fundamental, with appropriate investment in infrastructure, disease monitoring, and equitable access to essential diagnostic tools and therapies [24, 26]. Health systems must embed CKD management into the primary care framework, supported by quality standards, streamlined clinical pathways, and simplified treatment protocols to reduce complexity and improve continuity of care. In this respect, the European Kidney Health Alliance has recently adopted a resolution on kidney health recognizing kidney disease as a global public health issue in Europe, thereby supporting the WHO initiative which promoted kidney health as a priority among noncommunicable diseases [93].

Key to overcoming clinical inertia is empowering all members of the healthcare team. For example, expanding the roles of pharmacists has shown promise in improving adherence through structured interventions. This was demonstrated in the PANDIA-IRS study, where community pharmacist engagement led to improved medication persistence in diabetic kidney disease [94]. Similarly, improved BP was achieved in CKD stage 2–4 patients by engaging community pharmacists in a multidisciplinary team [95]. In a recent meta-analysis, interventions led by pharmacists reduced BP and improved hypertension outcomes in CKD, whereas mixed effects were found regarding medication adherence [96].

Deprescribing initiatives, such as those in Canada, have introduced structured approaches to minimize unnecessary medications and reduce treatment burden in patients with complex regimens [97]. Managing hypertension and diabetes while reducing cardiorenal risk in overmedicated CKD patients increasingly calls for strategies that simplify treatment while maintaining effectiveness. Therefore, single-pill combinations to manage hypertension as well as diabetes and lipid disorders are effective, practical solutions enabling a reduction in the pill burden. Thus, the use of single-pill combinations in hypertension has been found to improve drug adherence and persistence, leading to better BP control and a significant reduction in CV morbidity and mortality [98–100]. Reinforcement of dietary interventions and regular reassessment of therapy are some of the essential components of individualized care. Additional ways to support long-term adherence include improving patient information and knowledge, addressing medication-related costs, encouraging the use of well-regulated generics, and supporting policies that facilitate access to essential therapies.

Patient-centered strategies and technological innovations must also be part of the solution. Advances in digital health—such as mobile apps, smart pill organizers, remote monitoring, and telehealth—offer practical tools to support adherence and patient-provider communication. However, the current evidence for the use of eHealth interventions in CKD is of low quality, with uncertain effects due to methodological limitations and heterogeneity of eHealth modalities and intervention types [101]. Digital health technologies show potential in supporting medication adherence, but the current evidence is limited, as most studies involve small samples, short follow-up periods, and address only a narrow range of adherence challenges [102]. Whereas tailored education, collaborative goal setting, and development of personalized action plans can empower individuals with CKD to take an active role in their care, fostering better self-management, there is currently only weak or no evidence on the impact of self-activation on medication adherence in CKD [103].

Conflict of Interest Authors declare no conflict of interest for this publication.

Financial Support None.

References

1. Jager KJ, Kovesdy C, Langham R, Rosenberg M, Jha V, Zoccali C. A single number for advocacy and communication-worldwide more than 850 million individuals have kidney diseases. Nephrol Dial Transplant. 2019;34(11):1803–5. https://doi.org/10.1093/ndt/gfz174.
2. Bello AK, Okpechi IG, Levin A, Ye F, Damster S, Arruebo S, et al. An update on the global disparities in kidney disease burden and care across world countries and regions. Lancet Glob Health. 2024;12(3):e382–e95. https://doi.org/10.1016/S2214-109X(23)00570-3.
3. Tuot DS, Plantinga L. Approaches to raise awareness of CKD among patients and the general population. Nat Rev Nephrol. 2025;21(3):147–8. https://doi.org/10.1038/s41581-025-00928-3.
4. Tangri N, Moriyama T, Schneider MP, Virgitti JB, De Nicola L, Arnold M, et al. Prevalence of undiagnosed stage 3 chronic kidney disease in France, Germany, Italy, Japan and the USA: results from the multinational observational REVEAL-CKD study. BMJ Open. 2023;13(5):e067386. https://doi.org/10.1136/bmjopen-2022-067386.
5. Francis A, Harhay MN, Ong ACM, Tummalapalli SL, Ortiz A, Fogo AB, et al. Chronic kidney disease and the global public health agenda: an international consensus. Nat Rev Nephrol. 2024;20(7):473–85. https://doi.org/10.1038/s41581-024-00820-6.
6. Chronic Kidney Disease Prognosis C, Matsushita K, van der Velde M, Astor BC, Woodward M, Levey AS, et al. Association of estimated glomerular filtration rate and albuminuria with all-cause and cardiovascular mortality in general population cohorts: a collaborative meta-analysis. Lancet. 2010;375(9731):2073–81. https://doi.org/10.1016/S0140-6736(10)60674-5.
7. Foreman KJ, Marquez N, Dolgert A, Fukutaki K, Fullman N, McGaughey M, et al. Forecasting life expectancy, years of life lost, and all-cause and cause-specific mortality for 250 causes of death: reference and alternative scenarios for 2016-40 for 195 countries and territories. Lancet. 2018;392(10159):2052–90. https://doi.org/10.1016/s0140-6736(18)31694-5.
8. Golestaneh L, Alvarez PJ, Reaven NL, Funk SE, McGaughey KJ, Romero A, et al. All-cause costs increase exponentially with increased chronic kidney disease stage. Am J Manag Care. 2017;23(10 Suppl):S163–s72.
9. https://www.niddk.nih.gov/health-information/health-statistics/kidney-disease. Accessed.
10. Vrijens B, De Geest S, Hughes DA, Przemyslaw K, Demonceau J, Ruppar T, et al. A new taxonomy for describing and defining adherence to medications. Br J Clin Pharmacol. 2012;73(5):691–705. https://doi.org/10.1111/j.1365-2125.2012.04167.x.
11. Burnier M. Is there a threshold for medication adherence? Lessons learnt from electronic monitoring of drug adherence. Front Pharmacol. 2018;9:1540. https://doi.org/10.3389/fphar.2018.01540.
12. Burnier M. Medication adherence and persistence as the cornerstone of effective antihypertensive therapy*. Am J Hypertens. 2006;19(11):1190–6. https://doi.org/10.1016/j.amjhyper.2006.04.006.
13. Burnier M, Egan BM. Adherence in hypertension. Circ Res. 2019;124(7):1124–40. https://doi.org/10.1161/circresaha.118.313220.
14. Robberechts T, Stoenoiu MS, Burnier M, Persu A. Optimizing drug adherence in hypertension: more than a mind game. Kardiol Pol. 2024;82(3):259–66. https://doi.org/10.33963/v.phj.99493.
15. Burnier M, Pruijm M, Wuerzner G, Santschi V. Drug adherence in chronic kidney diseases and dialysis. Nephrol Dial Transplant. 2015;30(1):39–44. https://doi.org/10.1093/ndt/gfu015.
16. Lane D, Lawson A, Burns A, Azizi M, Burnier M, Jones DJL, et al. Nonadherence in hypertension: how to develop and implement chemical adherence testing. Hypertension. 2022;79(1):12–23. https://doi.org/10.1161/HYPERTENSIONAHA.121.17596.

17. Vondracek SF, Teitelbaum I, Kiser TH. Principles of kidney pharmacotherapy for the nephrologist: core curriculum 2021. Am J Kidney Dis. 2021;78(3):442–58. https://doi.org/10.1053/j.ajkd.2021.02.342.
18. KDIGO. 2024 clinical practice guideline for the evaluation and Management of Chronic Kidney Disease. Kidney Int. 2024;105(4s):S117–314. https://doi.org/10.1016/j.kint.2023.10.018.
19. KDIGO. 2022 clinical practice guideline for diabetes Management in Chronic Kidney Disease. Kidney Int. 2022;102(5s):S1–s127. https://doi.org/10.1016/j.kint.2022.06.008.
20. Chronic Kidney Disease and Risk Management: Standards of Care in Diabetes-2024. Diabetes Care. 2024;47(Suppl 1):S219–30. https://doi.org/10.2337/dc24-S011.
21. Stengel B, Muenz D, Tu C, Speyer E, Alencar de Pinho N, Combe C, et al. Adherence to the kidney disease: improving global outcomes CKD guideline in nephrology practice across countries. Kidney Int Rep. 2021;6(2):437–48. https://doi.org/10.1016/j.ekir.2020.11.039.
22. Nicholas SB, Daratha KB, Alicic RZ, Jones CR, Kornowske LM, Neumiller JJ, et al. Prescription of guideline-directed medical therapies in patients with diabetes and chronic kidney disease from the CURE-CKD Registry, 2019–2020. Diabetes Obes Metab. 2023;25(10):2970–9. https://doi.org/10.1111/dom.15194.
23. Murphy DP, Drawz PE, Foley RN. Trends in angiotensin-converting enzyme inhibitor and angiotensin II receptor blocker use among those with impaired kidney function in the United States. J Am Soc Nephrol. 2019;30(7):1314–21. https://doi.org/10.1681/asn.2018100971.
24. Nee R, Yuan CM, Narva AS, Yan G, Norris KC. Overcoming barriers to implementing new guideline-directed therapies for chronic kidney disease. Nephrol Dial Transplant. 2022;38(3):532–41. https://doi.org/10.1093/ndt/gfac283.
25. Kim D, Perkovic V, Kotwal S. Barriers to care: new medications and CKD. Kidney Int Rep. 2024;9(3):504–7. https://doi.org/10.1016/j.ekir.2023.12.012.
26. Luyckx VA, Tuttle KR, Abdellatif D, Correa-Rotter R, Fung WWS, Haris A, et al. Mind the gap in kidney care: translating what we know into what we do. Kidney Res Clin Pract. 2025;44(1):6–19. https://doi.org/10.23876/j.krcp.24.100.
27. Phillips LS, Branch WT Jr, Cook CB, Doyle JP, El-Kebbi IM, Gallina DL, et al. Clinical inertia. Ann Intern Med. 2001;135(9):825–34.
28. Burnier M. Poor physician adherence to clinical guidelines in hypertension-time for physicians to face clinical inertia. JAMA Netw Open. 2024;7(8):e2426830. https://doi.org/10.1001/jamanetworkopen.2024.26830.
29. Sperati CJ, Soman S, Agrawal V, Liu Y, Abdel-Kader K, Diamantidis CJ, et al. Primary care physicians' perceptions of barriers and facilitators to management of chronic kidney disease: a mixed methods study. PLoS One. 2019;14(8):e0221325. https://doi.org/10.1371/journal.pone.0221325.
30. Ismail WW, Witry MJ, Urmie JM. The association between cost sharing, prior authorization, and specialty drug utilization: a systematic review. J Manag Care Spec Pharm. 2023;29(5):449–63. https://doi.org/10.18553/jmcp.2023.29.5.449.
31. Wright EE, Nicholas SB. Making treatment guideline recommendations in chronic kidney disease and type 2 diabetes more accessible to primary care providers in the United States. Postgrad Med. 2024;136(4):347–57. https://doi.org/10.1080/00325481.2024.2350924.
32. Lu Y, Arowojolu O, Qiu X, Liu Y, Curry L, Krumholz HM. Barriers to optimal clinician guideline adherence in the Management of Markedly Elevated Blood Pressure: a qualitative content analysis of electronic health records. medRxiv. 2024; https://doi.org/10.1101/2024.01.12.24301223.
33. Oosting IJ, Colombijn JMT, Kaasenbrood L, Liabeuf S, Laville SM, Hooft L, et al. Polypharmacy in patients with CKD: a systematic review and meta-analysis. Kidney360. 2024;5(6):841–50. https://doi.org/10.34067/kid.0000000000000447.
34. Marienne J, Laville SM, Caillard P, Batteux B, Gras-Champel V, Masmoudi K, et al. Evaluation of changes over time in the drug burden and medication regimen complexity in ESRD patients before and after renal transplantation. Kidney Int Rep. 2021;6(1):128–37. https://doi.org/10.1016/j.ekir.2020.10.011.

35. Schmidt IM, Hübner S, Nadal J, Titze S, Schmid M, Bärthlein B, et al. Patterns of medication use and the burden of polypharmacy in patients with chronic kidney disease: the German Chronic Kidney Disease Study. Clin Kidney J. 2019;12(5):663–72. https://doi.org/10.1093/ckj/sfz046.
36. Laville SM, Metzger M, Stengel B, Jacquelinet C, Combe C, Fouque D, et al. Evaluation of the adequacy of drug prescriptions in patients with chronic kidney disease: results from the CKD-REIN cohort. Br J Clin Pharmacol. 2018;84(12):2811–23. https://doi.org/10.1111/bcp.13738.
37. Iwashita Y, Ohya M, Kunimoto S, Iwashita Y, Mima T, Negi S, et al. A survey of drug burden in patients undergoing maintenance hemodialysis in Japan. Intern Med. 2018;57(20):2937–44. https://doi.org/10.2169/internalmedicine.0108-17.
38. Cunha C, Alexander S, Ashby D, Lee J, Chusney G, Cairns TD, et al. Hydroxycloroquine blood concentration in lupus nephritis: a determinant of disease outcome? Nephrol Dial Transplant. 2018;33(9):1604–10. https://doi.org/10.1093/ndt/gfx318.
39. Durcan L, Clarke WA, Magder LS, Petri M. Hydroxychloroquine blood levels in systemic lupus erythematosus: clarifying dosing controversies and improving adherence. J Rheumatol. 2015;42(11):2092–7. https://doi.org/10.3899/jrheum.150379.
40. Costedoat-Chalumeau N, Houssiau FA. Improving medication adherence in patients with lupus nephritis. Kidney Int. 2021;99(2):285–7. https://doi.org/10.1016/j.kint.2020.10.037.
41. Torres VE, Chapman AB, Devuyst O, Gansevoort RT, Grantham JJ, Higashihara E, et al. Tolvaptan in patients with autosomal dominant polycystic kidney disease. N Engl J Med. 2012;367(25):2407–18.
42. Torres VE, Chapman AB, Devuyst O, Gansevoort RT, Perrone RD, Koch G, et al. Tolvaptan in later-stage autosomal dominant polycystic kidney disease. N Engl J Med. 2017;377(20):1930–42.
43. Saito R, Yamamoto H, Ichihara N, Kumamaru H, Nishimura S, Shimada K, et al. Persistence of tolvaptan medication for autosomal dominant polycystic kidney disease: a retrospective cohort study using Shizuoka Kokuho Database. Medicine. 2022;101(40):e30923. https://doi.org/10.1097/md.0000000000030923.
44. Ku E, Lee BJ, Wei J, Weir MR. Hypertension in CKD: core curriculum 2019. Am J Kidney Dis. 2019;74(1):120–31. https://doi.org/10.1053/j.ajkd.2018.12.044.
45. Burnier M, Damianaki A. Hypertension as cardiovascular risk factor in chronic kidney disease. Circ Res. 2023;132(8):1050–63. https://doi.org/10.1161/circresaha.122.321762.
46. Schmitt KE, Edie CF, Laflam P, Simbartl LA, Thakar CV. Adherence to antihypertensive agents and blood pressure control in chronic kidney disease. Am J Nephrol. 2010;32(6):541–8. https://doi.org/10.1159/000321688.
47. Muntner P, Judd SE, Krousel-Wood M, McClellan WM, Safford MM. Low medication adherence and hypertension control among adults with CKD: data from the REGARDS (Reasons for Geographic and Racial Differences in Stroke) Study. Am J Kidney Dis. 2010;56(3):447–57. https://doi.org/10.1053/j.ajkd.2010.02.348.
48. Sarafidis PA, Li S, Chen SC, Collins AJ, Brown WW, Klag MJ, et al. Hypertension awareness, treatment, and control in chronic kidney disease. Am J Med. 2008;121(4):332–40. https://doi.org/10.1016/j.amjmed.2007.11.025.
49. Akbari S, Ten Eyck P, Wendt L, Yamada M, Boucher R, Beddhu S, et al. Trends of blood pressure control in chronic kidney disease among US adults: findings from NHANES 2011 to 2020. J Am Heart Assoc. 2024;13(20):e034568. https://doi.org/10.1161/jaha.124.034568.
50. Halimi JM, Sarafidis P, Azizi M, Bilo G, Burkard T, Bursztyn M, et al. Management of patients with hypertension and chronic kidney disease referred to Hypertension Excellence Centres among 27 countries. On behalf of the European Society of Hypertension Working Group on Hypertension and the Kidney. Blood Press. 2024;33(1):2368800. https://doi.org/10.1080/08037051.2024.2368800.
51. Tesfaye WH, Erku D, Mekonnen A, Tefera YG, Castelino R, Sud K, et al. Medication non-adherence in chronic kidney disease: a mixed-methods review and synthesis using

the theoretical domains framework and the behavioural change wheel. J Nephrol. 2021;34(4):1091–125. https://doi.org/10.1007/s40620-020-00895-x.
52. Curtin RB, Walters BA, Schatell D, Pennell P, Wise M, Klicko K. Self-efficacy and self-management behaviors in patients with chronic kidney disease. Adv Chronic Kidney Dis. 2008;15(2):191–205. https://doi.org/10.1053/j.ackd.2008.01.006.
53. Cedillo-Couvert EA, Ricardo AC, Chen J, Cohan J, Fischer MJ, Krousel-Wood M, et al. Self-reported medication adherence and CKD progression. Kidney Int Rep. 2018;3(3):645–51. https://doi.org/10.1016/j.ekir.2018.01.007.
54. Magacho EJ, Ribeiro LC, Chaoubah A, Bastos MG. Adherence to drug therapy in kidney disease. Braz J Med Biol Res. 2011;44(3):258–62. https://doi.org/10.1590/s0100-879x2011007500013.
55. Wang SL, Chiu YW, Kung LF, Chen TH, Hsiao SM, Hsiao PN, et al. Patient assessment of chronic kidney disease self-care using the chronic kidney disease self-care scale in Taiwan. Nephrology (Carlton). 2019;24(6):615–21. https://doi.org/10.1111/nep.13475.
56. Ghimire S, Castelino RL, Lioufas NM, Peterson GM, Zaidi ST. Nonadherence to medication therapy in haemodialysis patients: a systematic review. PLoS One. 2015;10(12):e0144119. https://doi.org/10.1371/journal.pone.0144119.
57. Acelajado MC, Hughes ZH, Oparil S, Calhoun DA. Treatment of resistant and refractory hypertension. Circ Res. 2019;124(7):1061–70. https://doi.org/10.1161/circresaha.118.312156.
58. Burnier M, Wuerzner G, Struijker-Boudier H, Urquhart J. Measuring, analyzing, and managing drug adherence in resistant hypertension. Hypertension. 2013;62(2):218–25. https://doi.org/10.1161/HYPERTENSIONAHA.113.00687.
59. Burnier M. Managing 'resistance': is adherence a target for treatment? Curr Opin Nephrol Hypertens. 2014;23(5):439–43. https://doi.org/10.1097/mnh.0000000000000045.
60. Rossignol P, Massy ZA, Azizi M, Bakris G, Ritz E, Covic A, et al. The double challenge of resistant hypertension and chronic kidney disease. Lancet. 2015;386(10003):1588–98. https://doi.org/10.1016/S0140-6736(15)00418-3.
61. Perkovic V, Jardine MJ, Neal B, Bompoint S, Heerspink HJL, Charytan DM, et al. Canagliflozin and renal outcomes in type 2 diabetes and nephropathy. N Engl J Med. 2019;380(24):2295–306. https://doi.org/10.1056/NEJMoa1811744.
62. Heerspink HJL, Stefánsson BV, Correa-Rotter R, Chertow GM, Greene T, Hou FF, et al. Dapagliflozin in patients with chronic kidney disease. N Engl J Med. 2020;383(15):1436–46. https://doi.org/10.1056/NEJMoa2024816.
63. Herrington WG, Staplin N, Wanner C, Green JB, Hauske SJ, Emberson JR, et al. Empagliflozin in patients with chronic kidney disease. N Engl J Med. 2023;388(2):117–27. https://doi.org/10.1056/NEJMoa2204233.
64. Perkovic V, Tuttle KR, Rossing P, Mahaffey KW, Mann JFE, Bakris G, et al. Effects of semaglutide on chronic kidney disease in patients with type 2 diabetes. N Engl J Med. 2024;391(2):109–21. https://doi.org/10.1056/NEJMoa2403347.
65. Mancia G, Cannon CP, Tikkanen I, Zeller C, Ley L, Woerle HJ, et al. Impact of empagliflozin on blood pressure in patients with type 2 diabetes mellitus and hypertension by background anti-hypertensive medication. Hypertension. 2016;68(6):1355–64. https://doi.org/10.1161/hypertensionaha.116.07703.
66. Damianaki A, Polychronopoulou E, Wuerzner G, Burnier M. New aspects in the management of hypertension in patients with chronic kidney disease not on renal replacement therapy. High Blood Press Cardiovasc Prev. 2022;29(2):125–35. https://doi.org/10.1007/s40292-021-00495-1.
67. Goud A, Zhong J, Peters M, Brook RD, Rajagopalan S. GLP-1 agonists and blood pressure: a review of the evidence. Curr Hypertens Rep. 2016;18(2):16. https://doi.org/10.1007/s11906-015-0621-6.
68. Wang B, Zhong J, Lin H, Zhao Z, Yan Z, He H, et al. Blood pressure-lowering effects of GLP-1 receptor agonists exenatide and liraglutide: a meta-analysis of clinical trials. Diabetes Obes Metab. 2013;15(8):737–49. https://doi.org/10.1111/dom.12085.

69. Limonte CP, Hall YN, Trikudanathan S, Tuttle KR, Hirsch IB, de Boer IH, et al. Prevalence of SGLT2i and GLP1RA use among US adults with type 2 diabetes. J Diabetes Complicat. 2022;36(6):108204. https://doi.org/10.1016/j.jdiacomp.2022.108204.
70. Nelson AJ, O'Brien EC, Kaltenbach LA, Green JB, Lopes RD, Morse CG, et al. Use of lipid-, blood pressure–, and glucose-lowering pharmacotherapy in patients with type 2 diabetes and atherosclerotic cardiovascular disease. JAMA Netw Open. 2022;5(2):e2148030-e. https://doi.org/10.1001/jamanetworkopen.2021.48030.
71. Farmer RE, Beard I, Raza SI, Gollop ND, Patel N, Tebboth A, et al. Prescribing in type 2 diabetes patients with and without cardiovascular disease history: a descriptive analysis in the UK CPRD. Clin Ther. 2021;43(2):320–35. https://doi.org/10.1016/j.clinthera.2020.12.015.
72. de Oliveira Costa J, Lin J, Milder TY, Greenfield JR, Day RO, Stocker SL, et al. Geographic variation in sodium-glucose cotransporter 2 inhibitor and glucagon-like peptide-1 receptor agonist use in people with type 2 diabetes in New South Wales, Australia. Diabetes Obes Metab. 2024;26(7):2787–95. https://doi.org/10.1111/dom.15597.
73. Mahtta D, Ramsey DJ, Lee MT, Chen L, Al Rifai M, Akeroyd JM, et al. Utilization rates of SGLT2 inhibitors and GLP-1 receptor agonists and their facility-level variation among patients with atherosclerotic cardiovascular disease and type 2 diabetes: insights from the Department of Veterans Affairs. Diabetes Care. 2022;45(2):372–80. https://doi.org/10.2337/dc21-1815.
74. Lyu B, Sang Y, Selvin E, Chang AR, Alexander GC, Cohen CM, et al. Pharmacologic treatment of type 2 diabetes in the U.S., Sweden, and Israel. Diabetes Care. 2022;45(12):2926–34. https://doi.org/10.2337/dc22-1253.
75. King A, Tan X, Dhopeshwarkar N, Bohn R, Dea K, Leonard CE, et al. Recent trends in GLP-1 RA and SGLT2i use among people with type 2 diabetes and atherosclerotic cardiovascular disease in the USA. BMJ Open Diabetes Res Care. 2024;12(5) https://doi.org/10.1136/bmjdrc-2024-004431.
76. Johannes CB, Ziemiecki R, Pladevall-Vila M, Ebert N, Kovesdy CP, Thomsen RW, et al. Clinical profile and treatment adherence in patients with type 2 diabetes and chronic kidney disease who initiate an SGLT2 inhibitor: a multi-cohort study. Diabetes Ther. 2025;16(2):205–26. https://doi.org/10.1007/s13300-024-01671-x.
77. Pladevall-Vila M, Ziemiecki R, Johannes CB, Khan AM, Mines D, Ebert N, et al. Clinical profile and treatment patterns in individuals with type 2 diabetes and chronic kidney disease who initiate a GLP-1 receptor agonist: a multinational cohort study. Diabetes Ther. 2025;16(5):931–54. https://doi.org/10.1007/s13300-025-01717-8.
78. Kuranz S. EPH55 adherence and persistence with SGLT-2 inhibitors among White and black diabetic kidney disease patients: real-world evidence from a large US Claims Database. Value Health. 2023;26(6):S174. https://doi.org/10.1016/j.jval.2023.03.937.
79. Lim CE, Pasternak B, Eliasson B, Ueda P. Treatment discontinuation among users of GLP-1 receptor agonists and SGLT2 inhibitors in a national population of individuals with type 2 diabetes. Diabetologia. 2025; https://doi.org/10.1007/s00125-025-06439-x.
80. Rosas SE, Ruilope LM, Anker SD, Pitt B, Rossing P, Bonfanti AAC, et al. Finerenone in Hispanic patients with CKD and type 2 diabetes: a post hoc FIDELITY analysis. Kidney Med. 2023;5(10):100704. https://doi.org/10.1016/j.xkme.2023.100704.
81. Filippatos G, Anker SD, Pitt B, Rossing P, Joseph A, Kolkhof P, et al. Finerenone and heart failure outcomes by kidney function/albuminuria in chronic kidney disease and diabetes. JACC Heart Fail. 2022;10(11):860–70. https://doi.org/10.1016/j.jchf.2022.07.013.
82. Agarwal R, Filippatos G, Pitt B, Anker SD, Rossing P, Joseph A, et al. Cardiovascular and kidney outcomes with finerenone in patients with type 2 diabetes and chronic kidney disease: the FIDELITY pooled analysis. Eur Heart J. 2022;43(6):474–84. https://doi.org/10.1093/eurheartj/ehab777.
83. Sarafidis P, Iatridi F, Ferro C, Alexandrou M-E, Fernandez-Fernandez B, Kanbay M, et al. Mineralocorticoid receptor antagonist use in chronic kidney disease with type 2 diabetes: a clinical practice document by the European Renal Best Practice (ERBP)

Board of the European Renal Association (ERA). Clin Kidney J. 2023;16(11):1885–907. https://doi.org/10.1093/ckj/sfad139.
84. Filippatos G, Anker SD, Agarwal R, Pitt B, Ruilope LM, Rossing P, et al. Finerenone and cardiovascular outcomes in patients with chronic kidney disease and type 2 diabetes. Circulation. 2021;143(6):540–52. https://doi.org/10.1161/circulationaha.120.051898.
85. Bakris GL, Agarwal R, Anker SD, Pitt B, Ruilope LM, Rossing P, et al. Effect of finerenone on chronic kidney disease outcomes in type 2 diabetes. N Engl J Med. 2020;383(23):2219–29. https://doi.org/10.1056/NEJMoa2025845.
86. Lerma E, White WB, Bakris G. Effectiveness of nonsteroidal mineralocorticoid receptor antagonists in patients with diabetic kidney disease. Postgrad Med. 2023;135(3):224–33. https://doi.org/10.1080/00325481.2022.2060598.
87. Kario K, Ohbayashi H, Hashimoto M, Itabashi N, Kato M, Uchiyama K, et al. Home blood pressure-lowering effect of a non-steroidal mineralocorticoid receptor blocker, esaxerenone, versus trichlormethiazide for uncontrolled hypertension: the EXCITE-HT randomized controlled study. Hypertens Res. 2024;47(9):2435–46. https://doi.org/10.1038/s41440-024-01762-z.
88. Chiu YW, Teitelbaum I, Misra M, de Leon EM, Adzize T, Mehrotra R. Pill burden, adherence, hyperphosphatemia, and quality of life in maintenance dialysis patients. Clin J Am Soc Nephrol. 2009;4(6):1089–96. https://doi.org/10.2215/cjn.00290109.
89. Nagano N, Ito K, Ono T, Ariyoshi Y, Masima S, Kobayashi H, et al. Prescription characteristics of phosphate binders in a high pill burden for hemodialysis patients. Renal Replace Ther. 2021;7(1):5. https://doi.org/10.1186/s41100-021-00322-2.
90. Parker K, Bull-Engelstad I, Aasebø W, von der Lippe N, Reier-Nilsen M, Os I, et al. Medication regimen complexity and medication adherence in elderly patients with chronic kidney disease. Hemodial Int. 2019;23(3):333–42. https://doi.org/10.1111/hdi.12739.
91. Mohammed MA, Moles RJ, Chen TF. Medication-related burden and patients' lived experience with medicine: a systematic review and metasynthesis of qualitative studies. BMJ Open. 2016;6(2):e010035. https://doi.org/10.1136/bmjopen-2015-010035.
92. Mechta Nielsen T, Frøjk Juhl M, Feldt-Rasmussen B, Thomsen T. Adherence to medication in patients with chronic kidney disease: a systematic review of qualitative research. Clin Kidney J. 2018;11(4):513–27. https://doi.org/10.1093/ckj/sfx140.
93. Vanholder R, Bé A, De Barbieri I, Gallego D, Fontana M, Faure M, et al. Combating the rising tide of kidney advocacy in Europe: the seminal role of the European Kidney Health Alliance (EKHA). Clin Kidney J. 2025;18(3):sfaf005. https://doi.org/10.1093/ckj/sfaf005.
94. Bandiera C, Dotta-Celio J, Locatelli I, Nobre D, Wuerzner G, Pruijm M, et al. The differential impact of a 6-versus 12-month pharmacist-led interprofessional medication adherence program on medication adherence in patients with diabetic kidney disease: the randomized PANDIA-IRIS study. Front Pharmacol. 2024;15:1294436. https://doi.org/10.3389/fphar.2024.1294436.
95. Santschi V, Lord A, Berbiche D, Lamarre D, Corneille L, Prud'homme L, et al. Impact of collaborative and multidisciplinary care on management of hypertension in chronic kidney disease outpatients. J Pharm Health Serv Res. 2011;2 https://doi.org/10.1111/j.1759-8893.2011.00038.x.
96. Ardavani A, Curtis F, Hopwood E, Highton P, Katapa P, Khunti K, et al. Effect of pharmacist interventions in chronic kidney disease: a meta-analysis. Nephrol Dial Transplant. 2024;40(5):884–907. https://doi.org/10.1093/ndt/gfae221.
97. Lefebvre MJ, Ng PCK, Desjarlais A, McCann D, Waldvogel B, Tonelli M, et al. Development and validation of nine deprescribing algorithms for patients on hemodialysis to decrease polypharmacy. Can J Kidney Health Dis. 2020;7:2054358120968674. https://doi.org/10.1177/2054358120968674.
98. Parati G, Kjeldsen S, Coca A, Cushman WC, Wang J. Adherence to single-pill versus free-equivalent combination therapy in hypertension: a systematic review and meta-analysis. Hypertension. 2021;77(2):692–705. https://doi.org/10.1161/HYPERTENSIONAHA.120.15781.

99. Schmieder RE, Wassmann S, Predel HG, Weisser B, Blettenberg J, Gillessen A, et al. Improved persistence to medication, decreased cardiovascular events and reduced all-cause mortality in hypertensive patients with use of single-pill combinations: results from the START-Study. Hypertension. 2023;80(5):1127–35. https://doi.org/10.1161/HYPERTENSIONAHA.122.20810.
100. Simonyi G, Burnier M, Narkiewicz K, Rokszin G, Abonyi-Toth Z, Kovacs G, et al. Effect of single-pill versus free equivalent combinations on persistence and major adverse cardiovascular events in hypertension: a real-world analysis. J Hypertens. 2025;43(3):405–12. https://doi.org/10.1097/HJH.0000000000003916.
101. Stevenson JK, Campbell ZC, Webster AC, Chow CK, Tong A, Craig JC, et al. eHealth interventions for people with chronic kidney disease. Cochrane Database Syst Rev. 2019;8(8):Cd012379. https://doi.org/10.1002/14651858.CD012379.pub2.
102. O'Hara DV, Yi TW, Lee VW, Jardine M, Dawson J. Digital health technologies to support medication adherence in chronic kidney disease. Nephrology (Carlton). 2022;27(12):917–24. https://doi.org/10.1111/nep.14113.
103. Lunardi LE, Hill K, Xu Q, Le Leu R, Bennett PN. The effectiveness of patient activation interventions in adults with chronic kidney disease: a systematic review and meta-analysis. Worldviews Evid-Based Nurs. 2023;20(3):238–58. https://doi.org/10.1111/wvn.12634.

Resistant Hypertension in Chronic Kidney Disease

Francesca Mallamaci and Giovanni Tripepi

Resistant Hypertension (RH) is defined as blood pressure above target (≥140/90 mmHg, or ≥130/80 mmHg in high cardiovascular risk patients) despite treatment with three antihypertensive agents of different classes, including a diuretic, at maximally tolerated doses, or as blood pressure controlled but requiring at least four drugs [1]. This definition, now widely endorsed in the major Guidelines, underscores the complexity and heterogeneity inherent in this condition. The epidemiological burden of RH is both substantial and alarming [2]: its prevalence is estimated at 19% among hypertensive patients in Europe and 13% in the USA, figures that translate into millions of individuals at risk for adverse cardiovascular and renal outcomes. The public health implications are profound, as RH is not merely a marker of poor blood pressure control but a sign of increased morbidity and mortality, particularly from stroke, myocardial infarction, heart failure, and progressive renal dysfunction [2–5]. Thus, the identification, comprehensive evaluation, and effective management of RH must be regarded as priorities in contemporary clinical practice and public health policy.

A nuanced understanding of the etiological landscape of RH is essential for its rational management. Secondary forms of hypertension must be excluded or identified, as they frequently underlie apparent resistance to therapy. Among these, chronic kidney disease (CKD) emerges as the most prevalent and clinically significant cause, followed by less common but important entities such as primary aldosteronism, renovascular disease, and rare endocrine disorders like pheochromocytoma [2]. The relationship between CKD and RH is bidirectional and synergistic: CKD

F. Mallamaci
Associazione Ipertensione, Nefrologia Trapianto (IPNET), Reggio Calabria, Italy

G. Tripepi (✉)
Institute of Clinical Physiology of the National Research Council (IFC-CNR), Reggio Calabria, Italy
e-mail: giovanniluigi.tripepi@cnr.it

P. Sarafidis, R. Pontremoli (eds.), *Hypertension and Chronic Kidney Disease*, Updates in Hypertension and Cardiovascular Protection,
https://doi.org/10.1007/978-3-032-29564-4_14

both predisposes to and is exacerbated by poorly controlled blood pressure, creating a vicious cycle of progressive organ damage. Notably, sleep apnea—particularly obstructive sleep apnea (OSA)—has gained recognition as a dominant and often underappreciated contributor to RH [6], especially in patients with CKD. In well-characterized cohorts of resistant hypertensive patients, the prevalence of sleep apnea has been documented to approach 60%, a figure that is many times the prevalence of other secondary causes such as renal parenchymal disease, which typically accounts for only 10–13% of cases [6]. Indeed, sleep apnea is estimated to be six to twelve times more frequent than other etiologies of resistance to antihypertensive therapy, highlighting the necessity of systematic screening for this condition in all patients with difficult-to-control blood pressure.

The pathophysiological mechanisms underpinning RH are multifactorial and complex, involving both hemodynamic and neurohumoral perturbations [2]. In patients with CKD, sodium retention and volume overload are central features, driven by impaired renal excretory capacity. Sodium retention manifests not only as peripheral edema, such as ankle swelling, but also as more insidious systemic and regional fluid accumulation. Magnetic resonance imaging studies have revealed that in CKD patients, particularly when supine during sleep, the anatomical spaces of the upper airway—including the uvula and pharynx—become further constricted due to interstitial edema. This anatomical narrowing is a key precipitant of nocturnal snoring and obstructive sleep apnea, which, in turn, leads to recurrent episodes of hypoxia [7]. Importantly, RH in the context of CKD is not merely a surrogate marker of disease severity; it is an independent and powerful risk factor for adverse cardiovascular and renal events, as demonstrated in longitudinal cohort studies [8]. Patients with both CKD and RH experience higher rates of myocardial infarction, stroke, heart failure, and accelerated progression to end-stage renal disease, underscoring the imperative for aggressive therapeutic intervention [8]. The therapeutic approach to RH is necessarily multifaceted, combining pharmacological and non-pharmacological strategies [2]. The traditional stepwise escalation of antihypertensive therapy begins with the optimization of diuretic regimens, often incorporating mineralocorticoid receptor antagonists such as spironolactone or eplerenone, particularly in the setting of normal or low serum potassium. Additional agents—including angiotensin-converting enzyme inhibitors, angiotensin receptor blockers, calcium channel blockers, and drugs targeting the sympathetic nervous system—are sequentially added as needed. However, pharmacotherapy alone is frequently insufficient, necessitating rigorous attention to lifestyle modifications. Among these, dietary sodium restriction is of paramount importance. A randomized crossover study [9] in resistant hypertensive patients demonstrated that a low-salt diet can significantly enhance the efficacy of antihypertensive medications, although complete blood pressure normalization remains elusive in many cases. The persistent inadequacy of blood pressure control, despite maximal medical and lifestyle interventions, has spurred the search for novel therapeutic modalities.

Historically, the recognition of sympathetic nervous system hyperactivity as a central driver of refractory hypertension [10] led to the exploration of surgical sympathectomy in the mid-twentieth century. While effective in lowering blood pressure, this invasive procedure was ultimately abandoned due to its considerable morbidity. In recent years, attention has shifted to less invasive techniques, most notably catheter-based renal denervation. The rationale for this approach derives from the observation that afferent and efferent renal nerves play a critical role in modulating systemic sympathetic tone. Initial enthusiasm for renal denervation was tempered by the results of randomized controlled trials [11], including those synthesized in a recent Cochrane review, which found that the procedure had inconclusive effects on the gold standard of blood pressure assessment—24-h ambulatory blood pressure monitoring—and did not significantly reduce the risk of major cardiovascular events such as myocardial infarction, ischemic stroke, or unstable angina. Nevertheless, ongoing technological refinements and the development of new devices and protocols have yielded promising results in more recent studies, particularly in selected patient populations. Notably, in CKD patients, longitudinal analyses suggest that renal denervation may confer renoprotective benefits independent of its effects on blood pressure, as evidenced by stabilization of glomerular filtration rate over extended follow-up periods, even in the absence of substantial reductions in systolic blood pressure [12]. These findings are hypothesis-generating and warrant further investigation in larger, well-designed clinical trials.

The challenge of RH is further magnified in patients with end-stage renal disease (ESRD) undergoing hemodialysis. In this population, sympathetic hyperactivity attains levels rarely observed outside of conditions such as pheochromocytoma or advanced heart failure. Seminal studies have demonstrated that sympathetic nerve activity is approximately doubled in dialysis patients compared to healthy controls [13], and that surgical removal of native kidneys (bilateral nephrectomy) results in a marked reduction in both sympathetic tone and blood pressure. The afferent nerves from the diseased kidneys are pivotal in sustaining this heightened sympathetic state. Epidemiological studies reveal that hypertension is nearly ubiquitous among hemodialysis patients, with 84% being hypertensive or on antihypertensive therapy. Of these, approximately 18–42% meet criteria for treatment RH [14], defined as uncontrolled blood pressure despite the use of three or more antihypertensive agents, or controlled blood pressure on four or more drugs. Intriguingly, only about one-third of these patients exhibit clear evidence of fluid overload, indicating that mechanisms beyond volume expansion—such as persistent sympathetic activation—contribute substantially to treatment resistance.

Effective volume management remains a cornerstone of hypertension control in the dialysis population. Randomized trials, such as the Frequent Hemodialysis Network study, have demonstrated that more frequent and gentle dialysis sessions can achieve significant reductions in systolic blood pressure—by as much as 12 mmHg—compared to conventional thrice-weekly regimens [15]. This benefit is likely multifactorial, reflecting not only improved volume status but also amelioration of sleep apnea, as intensive nocturnal dialysis has been shown to dramatically reduce the frequency of apneic episodes. Nonetheless, a subset of patients remains hypertensive despite optimal volume control and maximal pharmacotherapy. In such cases, the potential role of renal denervation remains still highly debated in CKD patients, and to this promising technique is dedicated a special chapter in this book. Bilateral nephrectomy, while effective in selected cases, is a drastic intervention reserved for the most refractory and high-risk patients.

In conclusion, RH represents a complex, multifactorial, and clinically significant entity that demands a sophisticated and individualized approach. The interplay between renal dysfunction, sympathetic nervous system activation, and comorbid conditions such as sleep apnea creates a therapeutic landscape that is both challenging and evolving. While traditional pharmacological and lifestyle interventions remain foundational, emerging therapies targeting the sympathetic nervous system offer hope for improved outcomes in carefully selected patients. Ongoing research is essential to elucidate the optimal strategies for diagnosis, risk stratification, and management, with the ultimate goal of reducing the substantial burden of cardiovascular and renal disease attributable to RH.

References

1. Mancia G, Kreutz R, Brunstrom M, et al. 2023 ESH guidelines for the management of arterial hypertension. The task force for the management of arterial hypertension of the European Society of Hypertension: endorsed by the International Society of Hypertension (ISH) and the European Renal Association (ERA). J Hypertens. 2023;41:1874–2071.
2. Buso G, Agabiti-Rosei C, Lemoli M, Corvini F, Muiesan ML. The global burden of resistant hypertension and potential treatment options. Eur Cardiol. 2024;19:e07.
3. Sim JJ, Bhandari SK, Shi J, Reynolds K, Calhoun DA, Kalantar-Zadeh K, Jacobsen SJ. Comparative risk of renal, cardiovascular, and mortality outcomes in controlled, uncontrolled resistant, and nonresistant hypertension. Kidney Int. 2015;88:622–32.
4. Cuspidi C, Macca G, Sampieri L, et al. High prevalence of cardiac and extracardiac target organ damage in refractory hypertension. J Hypertens. 2001;19:2063–70.
5. Muiesan ML, Salvetti M, Rizzoni D, et al. Resistant hypertension and target organ damage. Hypertens Res. 2013;36:485–91.
6. Pedrosa RP, Drager LF, Gonzaga CC, et al. Obstructive sleep apnea: the most common secondary cause of hypertension associated with resistant hypertension. Hypertension. 2011;58:811–7.
7. Hartfield PJ, Janczy J, Sharma A, Newsome HA, Sparapani RA, Rhee JS, Woodson BT, Garcia GJM. Anatomical determinants of upper airway collapsibility in obstructive sleep apnea: a systematic review and meta-analysis. Sleep Med Rev. 2023;68:101741.
8. Fay KS, Cohen DL. Resistant hypertension in people with CKD: a review. Am J Kidney Dis. 2021;77:110–21.
9. Pimenta E, Gaddam KK, Oparil S, Aban I, Husain S, Dell'Italia LJ, Calhoun DA. Effects of dietary sodium reduction on blood pressure in subjects with resistant hypertension: results from a randomized trial. Hypertension. 2009;54:475–81.
10. Dudenbostel T, Acelajado MC, Pisoni R, et al. Refractory hypertension: evidence of heightened sympathetic activity as a cause of antihypertensive treatment failure. Hypertension. 2015;66:126–33.
11. Bakris GL, Townsend RR, Liu M, Cohen SA, D'Agostino R, Flack JM, Kandzari DE, Katzen BT, Leon MB, Mauri L, Negoita M, O'Neill WW, Oparil S, Rocha-Singh K, Bhatt DL, SYMPLICITY HTN-3 Investigators. Impact of renal denervation on 24-hour ambulatory blood pressure: results from SYMPLICITY HTN-3. J Am Coll Cardiol. 2014;64:1071–8.
12. Sanders MF, Reitsma JB, Morpey M, Gremmels H, Bots ML, Pisano A, Bolignano D, Zoccali C, Blankestijn PJ. Renal safety of catheter-based renal denervation: systematic review and meta-analysis. Nephrol Dial Transplant. 2017;32:1440–7.

13. Converse RL Jr, Jacobsen TN, Toto RD, Jost CM, Cosentino F, Fouad-Tarazi F, Victor RG. Sympathetic overactivity in patients with chronic renal failure. N Engl J Med. 1992;327:1912–8.
14. Georgianos PI, Agarwal R. Resistant hypertension in dialysis: epidemiology, diagnosis, and management. J Am Soc Nephrol. 2024;35:505–14.
15. Kotanko P, Garg AX, Depner T, Pierratos A, Chan CT, Levin NW, Greene T, Larive B, Beck GJ, Gassman J, Kliger AS, Stokes JB, FHN Trial Group. Effects of frequent hemodialysis on blood pressure: results from the randomized frequent hemodialysis network trials. Hemodial Int. 2015;19:386–401.

Sodium–Glucose Cotransporter-2 Inhibitors for Renoprotection and Cardioprotection in CKD

Marieta P. Theodorakopoulou and Fotini Iatridi

Introduction

Chronic kidney disease (CKD) is a major global health issue; approximately 850 million individuals worldwide have CKD, of whom about four million receive kidney replacement therapy [1]. Diabetic kidney disease (DKD) is the leading cause of CKD globally [2, 3]. CKD is associated with increased morbidity as well as higher cardiovascular and all-cause mortality [4]. Both low estimated glomerular filtration rate (eGFR) and albuminuria are independently associated with an increased risk of cardiovascular events and death [5, 6]. Following the above, CKD is one of the fastest growing causes of death and is projected to become the fifth global cause of mortality by 2040 [7]. Importantly, with worsening kidney function, the predominant cardiovascular phenotype shifts from atherosclerotic and thromboembolic disease toward heart failure and sudden cardiac death [8]. In a large U.S. cohort of over 15,000 adults, 10-year cardiovascular mortality was 3.4% in those without diabetes or CKD, 6.7% in those with diabetes alone, and 9.9% in those with CKD alone. Notably, patients with both diabetes and CKD had a cumulative mortality of 19.6% [9].

For nearly two decades, management of CKD relied on lifestyle interventions, blood pressure, glycemic and lipid control, and renin–angiotensin system (RAS) blockade with angiotensin-converting enzyme inhibitors (ACEI) or angiotensin-2 receptor blockers (ARB) [10–12]. However, despite these measures, substantial residual renal risk persisted [13], and RAS blockade did not reduce cardiovascular events or mortality in DKD outcome trials [14]. Until recently, progress in preventing kidney failure due to diabetes remained limited, despite the availability of multiple glucose-lowering agents. Over the past decade, however,

M. P. Theodorakopoulou (✉) · F. Iatridi
1st Department of Nephrology, Aristotle University of Thessaloniki, Hippokration Hospital, Thessaloniki, Greece

P. Sarafidis, R. Pontremoli (eds.), *Hypertension and Chronic Kidney Disease*, Updates in Hypertension and Cardiovascular Protection,
https://doi.org/10.1007/978-3-032-29564-4_15

cardiovascular and renal outcome trials have demonstrated that sodium–glucose cotransporter-2 (SGLT-2) inhibitors markedly delay CKD progression and reduce cardiovascular risk in patients with diabetes [15, 16]. More recently, major renal outcome trials have confirmed that SGLT-2 inhibitors also provide effective and safe renoprotection in patients with CKD irrespective of diabetes status [13, 16].

Main Effects and Mode of Action of SGLT-2 Inhibitors

The class of SGLT-2 inhibitors includes several agents (dapagliflozin, canagliflozin, empagliflozin, ipragliflozin, luseogliflozin, tofogliflozin, and ertugliflozin) (Fig. 1). Their primary mechanism involves inhibiting glucose reabsorption through SGLT-2 transporters in the S1 segment of the proximal convoluted tubule, which normally accounts for about 90% of filtered glucose uptake [17]. This action lowers plasma glucose while simultaneously inducing glycosuria-related calorie loss, typically resulting in weight reduction of 3–5 kg [17]. Beyond glucose lowering, SGLT-2 inhibition modestly reduces sodium reabsorption in the proximal tubule, producing mild natriuresis and diuresis that are further amplified by osmotic diuresis due to glucosuria [18]. These hemodynamic effects translate into consistent, though modest, blood pressure (BP) reductions. Early studies in diabetes with preserved renal function demonstrated systolic/diastolic BP (SBP/DBP) decreases of approximately 3–5/1–2 mmHg [19]. Studies using ambulatory BP monitoring confirmed these reductions in patients with type-2 diabetes mellitus (T2D) and hypertension [20, 21], while data from patients with advanced CKD (eGFR <30 mL/min/1.73 m^2) suggest even greater SBP reductions of up to 7 mmHg. The possible mechanisms contributing to the BP reduction observed with SGLT-2 inhibitors include this diuretic effect along with reductions in sympathetic nervous system activity, arterial stiffness, endothelial dysfunction, and systemic vascular resistance [19, 22, 23].

SGLT-2 Inhibitors for Renoprotection in CKD

Renoprotective Effects of SGLT-2 Inhibitors Observed in Cardiovascular Outcome Trials in Type 2 Diabetes

Studies that examined the effects of SGLT-2 inhibitors on glycemic control and also included urine albumin excretion as a secondary outcome demonstrated an average 25% reduction in albuminuria compared with placebo or other hypoglycemic agents, with even greater reductions of up to 40% in patients with moderate or severe baseline albuminuria [24]. The cardiovascular and kidney benefits of SGLT-2 inhibitors on hard outcomes were first identified in cardiovascular outcome trials (CVOTs) mandated by the U.S. Food and Drug Administration to establish cardiovascular safety in T2D. While their primary endpoints focused on major adverse cardiovascular events (MACE), each also included prespecified renal outcomes.

Chemical structure	Name	Recommended dosage
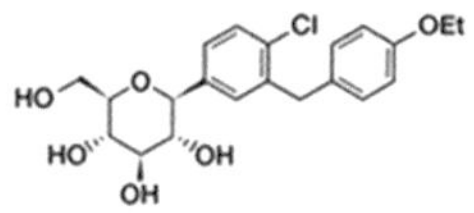	Dapagliflozin	5, 10mg
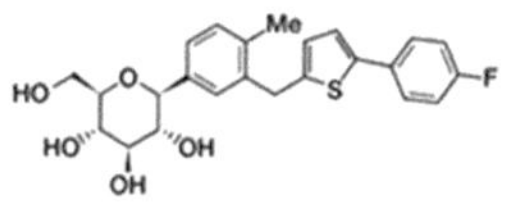	Canagliflozin	100, 300mg
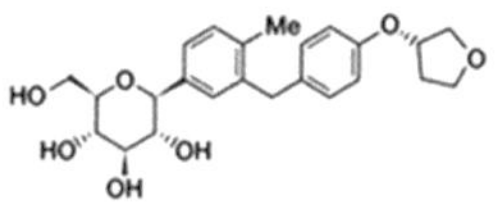	Empagliflozin	10, 25mg
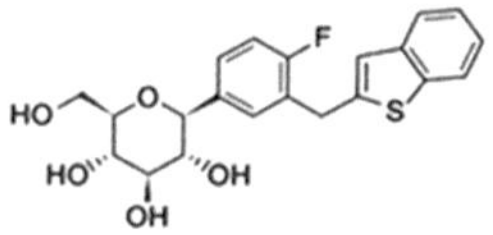	Ipragliflozin	25, 50mg
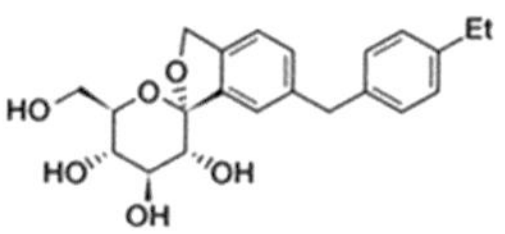	Tofogliflozin	20mg
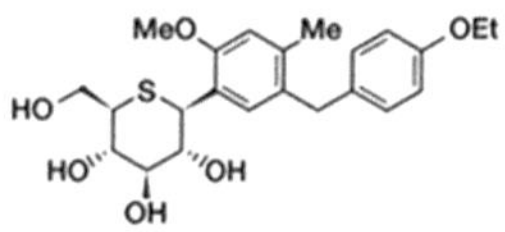	Luseogliflozin	2.5, 5mg
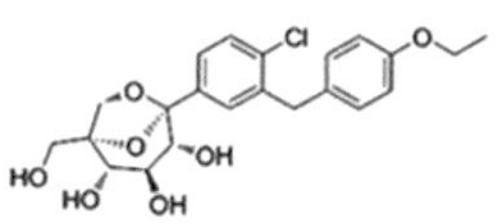	Ertugliflozin	5, 15mg
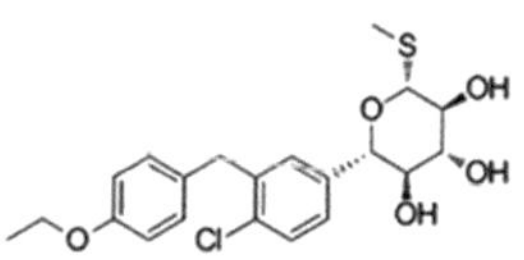	Sotagliflozin	200, 400mg

Fig. 1 Chemical structure and recommended dosage of the different SGLT-2 inhibitors

Table 1 Main clinical trials demonstrating reno- and cardioprotection in patients with type-2 diabetes receiving SGLT-2 inhibitors

Trial (year)	SGLT-2 inhibitor (dose)	Patient population	Number of patients	Mean eGFR (mL/min/1.73 m²)	Median follow-up	Cardiovascular outcome (HR, 95% CI)	Kidney outcome (HR, 95% CI)
EMPA-REG OUTCOME (2015) [25]	Empagliflozin (10 or 25 mg)	T2D with established CVD	7020	74 ± 21	3.1 years	MACE 0.86 (0.74–0.99); CV death or HHF 0.66 (0.55–0.79); CV death 0.62 (0.49–0.77)	Incident or worsening nephropathy 0.61 (0.55–0.69); Doubling of serum creatinine 0.56 (0.39–0.79); KRT initiation 0.45 (0.21–0.97)
CANVAS (2017) [26]	Canagliflozin (100 or 300 mg)	T2D with high CVD risk	10,142	76.5 ± 20.5	2.6 years	MACE 0.86 (0.75–0.97); HF 0.67 (0.52–0.87)	Progression of albuminuria 0.73 (0.67–0.79); Sustained ≥40% eGFR decline, KRT or renal death 0.60 (0.47–0.77)
DECLARE–TIMI 58 (2018) [27]	Dapagliflozin (10 mg)	T2D with at least 1 CV risk factor	17,160	85.2 ± 16	4.2 years	MACE 0.93 (0.84–1.03); CV death or HHF 0.83 (0.73–0.95)	≥40% eGFR reduction, ESKD ≥90 days, (dialysis, sustained eGFR <15 mL/min/1.73 m², or kidney transplantation), or renal/CV death 0.76 (0.67–0.87)
VERTIS CV (2019) [28]	Ertugliflozin (5 or 15 mg)	T2D with established CVD	8246	76.1 ± 20.9 (75.7 ± 20.8 in the placebo group)	3.5 years	HHF 0.88 (0.75–1.03); CV death or HHF 0.97 (0.85–1.11)	Doubling of serum creatinine, KRT or renal death 0.81 (0.63–1.04)

CV cardiovascular, *CVD* cardiovascular disease, *CI* confidence interval, *CKD* chronic kidney disease, *eGFR* estimated glomerular filtration rate, *ESKD* end-stage kidney disease, *HF* heart failure, *HHF* hospitalization for heart failure, *HR* hazard ratio, *MACE* major adverse cardiovascular events, *KRT* kidney replacement therapy, *SGLT-2i* sodium-glucose co-transporter 2 inhibitors, *T2D* type 2 diabetes mellitus

Table 1 summarizes the major CVOTs as well as the renal outcome trials with SGLT-2 inhibitors.

In the Empagliflozin Cardiovascular Outcome Event Trial in Type 2 Diabetes Mellitus Patients (EMPA-REG OUTCOME) trial 7028 patients with T2D (80% on ACEi/ARB therapy) were randomized to empagliflozin (10 or 25 mg) or placebo and followed for a mean of 3.1 years [25]. Among study participants, 1819 had an eGFR<60 mL/min/1.73 m^2 and about half of those presented moderately high or high albuminuria. In the analysis of renal outcomes [29], empagliflozin showed large reductions in the pre-specified composite outcome of progression to macroalbuminuria, doubling of SCr, initiation of renal replacement therapy or renal death (hazard ratio, HR 0.61; 95% confidence interval (CI) 0.53–0.70). In addition, empagliflozin also reduced the post hoc renal composite of doubling of SCr, initiation of renal replacement therapy or renal death (HR 0.54; 95% CI 0.40–0.75). Of note, significant between-group differences were observed in the individual analyses of all the above components. Further, hyperkalemia or acute kidney failure episodes were lower or similar in the empagliflozin vs placebo groups, irrespective of baseline kidney function [29].

The Canagliflozin Cardiovascular Assessment Study (CANVAS) program consisted of two double-blind, randomized trials (CANVAS and CANVAS-R) [30]. In CANVAS, participants were randomly assigned to receive 300 mg canagliflozin, 100 mg canagliflozin or placebo [26]. In CANVAS-R, participants were randomized to canagliflozin 100 mg or placebo (optional uptitration to 300 mg). At baseline, 20.1% of participants had eGFR <60 mL/min/1.73 m^2 [31]. In a prespecified explanatory analysis of the two studies, canagliflozin showed a significant decrease in the primary composite renal endpoint (40% reduction in eGFR levels, need for renal replacement therapy, or renal death) by 40% compared to placebo (HR 0.60; 95% CI 0.47–0.77) [32]. The effect of canagliflozin was consistent across all eGFR categories (baseline eGFR ≥90, 60–<90, 45–<60, and <45 mL/min/1.73 m^2) (*p* heterogeneity = 0.28 and >0.50, respectively) [32]. Another analysis of the CANVAS study showed a comparable reduction in the outcome of doubling of SCr, end-stage kidney disease (ESKD) and renal death in the intervention arm versus placebo (HR 0.53; 95% CI 0.33–0.84) [33].

The Multicenter Trial to Evaluate the Effect of Dapagliflozin on the Incidence of Cardiovascular Events Thrombolysis In Myocardial Infarction 58 (DECLARE-TIMI 58) randomized 17,160 patients with T2D (including 10,186 without atherosclerotic cardiovascular disease) to dapagliflozin or placebo [27]. Importantly, the study excluded individuals with an eGFR lower than 60 mL/min/1.73 m^2. The composite outcome of ≥40% decrease in eGFR to <60 mL/min/1.73 m^2, ESKD, or cardiovascular or renal death was decreased with dapagliflozin (HR 0.76; 95% CI 0.67–0.87). The main renal composite outcome of ≥40% decrease in eGFR to <60 mL/min/1.73 m^2, ESKD, or renal death was also decreased (HR 0.53; 95% CI 0.43–0.66). In separate analyses, the risk of "≥40% decrease in eGFR to <60 mL/min/1.73 m^2" was almost halved in the intervention arm (HR 0.54; 95% CI 0.43–0.67); ESKD occurred in 0.1% of patients treated with dapagliflozin vs 0.2% of those treated with placebo (HR 0.31; 95% CI 0.13–0.79) (Table 1) [27].

Renoprotective Effects of SGLT-2 Inhibitors Observed in Renal Outcome Trials in Diabetic and Non-Diabetic CKD

The Canagliflozin and Renal Events in Diabetes with Established Nephropathy Clinical Evaluation (CREDENCE) study was the first trial evaluating the effect of an SGLT-2 inhibitor on major renal outcomes in CKD [33]. This study randomized 4401 patients with T2D, eGFR 30 to <90 mL/min/1.73 m^2 and urine albumin to creatinine ratio (UACR) 300–5000 mg/g, already on maximum tolerated dose of an ACEI or ARB to canagliflozin or placebo. The primary outcome was ESKD defined as dialysis, transplantation, or sustained eGFR <15 mL/min/1.73 m^2; doubling of serum creatinine; or death from renal or cardiovascular causes. The mean age of study participants was 63 years, and 33.9% of the patients were women. The mean eGFR was 56.2 mL/min/1.73 m^2, and the median UACR was 927 mg/g. The study was prematurely terminated for efficacy (median follow-up 2.62 versus a projected duration of 5.5 years). The relative risk of the primary outcome was 30% lower with canagliflozin, with event rates of 43.2 and 61.2 per 1000 patient-years, respectively (HR 0.70; 95% CI 0.59–0.82). The relative risk of the renal-specific composite of ESKD, doubling of SCr, or death from renal causes was lower by 34% (HR 0.66; 95% CI 0.53–0.81), while ESKD itself was lower by 32% (HR 0.68; 95% CI 0.54–0.86) with canagliflozin treatment [33]. Furthermore, the geometric mean of UACR was 31% lower with canagliflozin, while the eGFR slope was typical of an acute eGFR dip with canagliflozin during the first 3 weeks (-3.72 ± 0.25 vs. -0.55 ± 0.25 mL/min/1.73 m^2), followed by slower eGFR decline thereafter (-1.85 ± 0.13 vs. -4.59 ± 0.14 mL/min/1.73 m^2 for canagliflozin versus placebo).

The Study to Evaluate the Effect of Dapagliflozin on Renal Outcomes and Cardiovascular Mortality in Patients With Chronic Kidney Disease (DAPA-CKD) assessed dapagliflozin versus placebo on top of maximally tolerated ACEi or ARB therapy in patients with eGFR 25–75 mL/min/1.73 m^2 and UACR 200–5000 mg/g [34]. The primary endpoint was a composite of ≥50% sustained decline in eGFR, ESKD, or cardiovascular/renal death. The study population consisted of 4304 patients with mean eGFR 43.1 mL/min/1.73 m^2 and median UACR of 949 mg/g. Two-thirds (67.5%) had T2D, while in 396 participants, CKD was attributed to non-diabetic causes (Table 2). The trial was also stopped early after a median follow-up of 2.4 years because of efficacy. The primary outcome occurred in 9.2% of dapagliflozin-treated patients versus 14.5% in the placebo group (HR 0.61; 95% CI 0.51–0.72). For the renal component of the composite endpoint (≥50% sustained eGFR decline, ESKD, or renal death), dapagliflozin provided significant protection (HR 0.56; 95% CI 0.45–0.68), with consistent benefit across all individual renal outcomes. Treatment also reduced geometric mean UACR by 29.3% (95% CI −33.1 to −25.2; $p < 0.0001$) [37]. As expected, an initial eGFR dip was observed within the first 2 weeks (-3.97 ± 0.15 vs -0.82 ± 0.15 mL/min/1.73 m^2), followed by a slower annual decline compared with placebo (-1.67 ± 0.11 vs -3.59 ± 0.11 mL/min/1.73 m^2).

The Study of Heart and Kidney Protection With Empagliflozin (EMPA-KIDNEY) [36] has largely reproduced the DAPA-CKD results for empagliflozin in a more

Table 2 Main clinical trials demonstrating reno- and cardioprotection in patients with CKD receiving SGLT-2 inhibitors

Trial (year)	SGLT-2 inhibitor (dose)	Patient population	Number of patients	Mean eGFR (mL/min/1.73 m²)	Median follow-up	Cardiovascular outcome (HR, 95% CI)	Kidney outcome (HR, 95% CI)
CREDENCE (2019) [33]	Canagliflozin (100 mg)	T2D with CKD	4401	56.2 ± 18.2	2.6 years	MACE 0.80 (0.67–0.95); HHF or CV death 0.69 (0.57–0.83)	Doubling of serum creatinine, ESKD or renal/CV death) 0.70 (0.59–0.82)
DAPA-CKD (2020) [34]	Dapagliflozin (10 mg)	CKD with/without T2D	4304	43.1 ± 12.4	2.4 years	CV death or HHF 0.71 (0.55–0.92)	≥50% eGFR decline, ESKD, or renal/CV death 0.61 (0.51–0.72) Sustained ≥50% eGFR decline, ESKD, or renal death 0.72 (0.64–0.82)
SCORED (2020) [35]	Sotagliflozin (200–400 mg)	CKD and CV risk	10.584	Median 44.4 (37.0–51.3) [44.7 (37.0–51.5) in the placebo group]	16 months	Total CV deaths, HHF or urgent visits for HF 0.74 (0.63–0.88)	Sustained ≥50% eGFR decline, long-term dialysis, renal transplantation, or a sustained eGFR <15 mL/min/1.73 m² 0.71 (0.46–1.08)
EMPA-KIDNEY (2022) [36]	Empagliflozin (10 mg)	CKD with/without T2D	6609	37.5 ± 14.8	2 years	CV death or HHF 0.84 (0.67–1.07)	Progression of kidney disease (sustained eGFR <10 mL/min/1.73 m², ESKD, or sustained ≥40% eGFR decline) or CV death 0.72 (0.64–0.82)

CV cardiovascular, *CVD* cardiovascular disease, *CI* confidence interval, *CKD* chronic kidney disease, *eGFR* estimated glomerular filtration rate, *ESKD* end-stage kidney disease, *HF* heart failure, *HFpEF* heart failure with preserved ejection fraction, *HFrEF* heart failure with reduced ejection fraction, *HHF* hospitalization for heart failure, *HR* hazard ratio, *MACE* major adverse cardiovascular events, *KRT* kidney replacement therapy, *SGLT-2i* sodium-glucose co-transporter 2 inhibitors, *T2D* type 2 diabetes mellitus

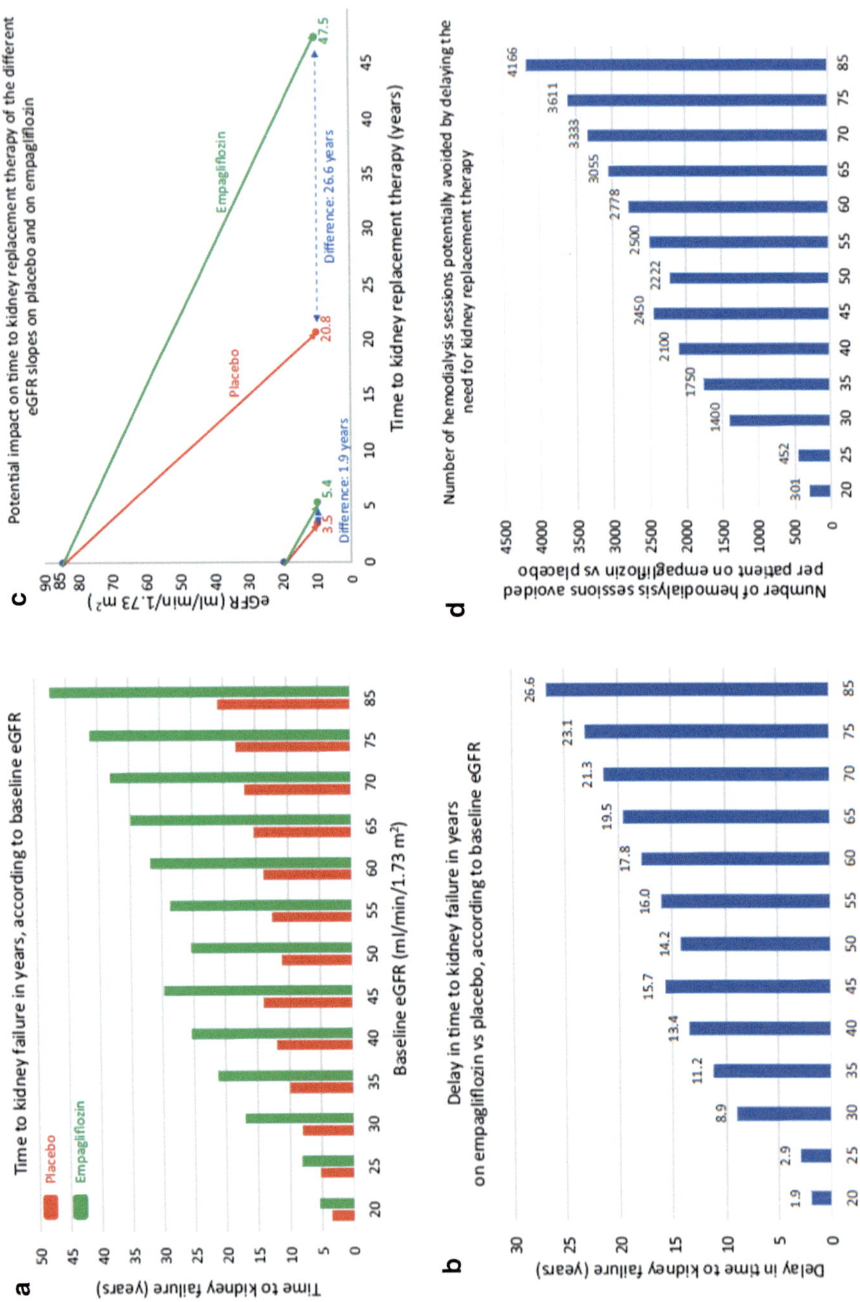

Fig. 2 (continued)

diverse CKD population, confirming the benefit of SGLT-2 inhibition on risk of a primary endpoint consisting of progression of kidney disease or death from cardiovascular causes in non-diabetic CKD. EMPA-KIDNEY enrolled patients with eGFR ≥20 mL/min/1.73 m^2 (a lower threshold than in the aforementioned trials) and with various baseline albuminuria levels (including also patients with UACR <30 mg/g while CREDENCE and DAPA-CKD only enrolled those with UACR >200 mg/g). A higher representation of non-diabetic participants was pre-specified in the trial, as patients with T2D, eGFR>60 mL/min/1.73 m^2 and previous atherosclerotic cardiovascular disease were excluded. Though initially included, the trial later excluded type 1 D (T1D). In addition, more liberal inclusion of participants not on RAS blockers was allowed in EMPA-KIDNEY, resulting in inclusion of about 1000 participants not on RAS blockers, either due to absence of proved kidney benefit in patients with normoalbuminuria or to previous intolerance. The primary outcome was first occurrence of a composite of kidney disease progression that included a sustained decline of ≥40% in eGFR from randomization, kidney replacement therapy, sustained decrease in eGFR to <10 mL/min/1.73 m^2 and cardiovascular death. The total study population consisted of 6609 participants (empagliflozin 10 mg vs placebo). This trial was also stopped early after 2.0 years because of efficacy. Empagliflozin had beneficial effect on the primary outcome (HR 0.72, 95% CI 0.64–0.82). In prespecified subgroups, the primary benefit of empagliflozin was consistent regardless of diabetes status, baseline eGFR, age, sex, CKD cause, cardiovascular disease, or RAS blocker. Effects appeared stronger with higher baseline UACR (P for trend = 0.02). No significant benefit was seen in the small subgroup with UACR <30 mg/g (HR 1.01, 95% CI 0.66–1.55), likely due to very low event rates (42 events vs 438 in the A3 group) and slower CKD progression in the placebo arm. Of note, in the analyses of chronic eGFR slopes, which account for long-term decline beyond the initial hemodynamic dip,showed that empagliflozin consistently slowed CKD progression across all eGFR and UACR strata, including normoalbuminuria. In those with UACR <30 mg/g, the mean chronic slope was −0.11 mL/min/1.73 m^2/year in empagliflozin groups versus −0.89 mL/min/1.73 m^2/year in the placebo, an eightfold slower decline versus placebo, resulting in the most stable on-treatment slope across albuminuria categories. These findings highlight that SGLT-2 inhibitors confer renal protection regardless of albuminuria status. A hypothetical transformation of chronic eGFR slopes into time to kidney failure (eGFR 10 mL/min/1.73 m^2) in the EMPA-KIDNEY trial is depicted in Fig. 2.

Interestingly, the post-trial follow-up (median of 2 additional years) of EMPA-KIDNEY confirmed sustained cardiorenal benefits of empagliflozin [39]. The study,

Fig. 2 Hypothetical transformation of chronic eGFR slopes into time to kidney failure (eGFR 10 mL/min/1.73 m^2) in the EMPA-KIDNEY trial. (**a**) Estimated time to kidney failure according to baseline eGFR, derived by applying chronic eGFR slopes from the 2 groups within prespecified eGFR subgroups (cut-offs: 30 and 45 mL/min/1.73 m^2) [9]. (**b**) Delay in time to kidney failure on empagliflozin vs placebo, calculated as the difference between groups for each baseline eGFR. (**c**) Graphical representation of representative chronic eGFR slopes, from baseline values of 20 and 85 mL/min/1.73 m^2 to kidney failure, for placebo and empagliflozin. The observed delay corresponds to the values shown in (**b**). (**d**) Estimated number of hemodialysis sessions potentially avoided by delaying the need for kidney replacement therapy with empagliflozin. (From Fernández-Fernandez et al. [38] with permission)

with a median additional follow-up of 2 years, found that empagliflozin continued to provide cardiorenal benefits for up to 12 months after discontinuation, with a carry-over effect of a 13% risk reduction in the primary composite outcome in the whole post-trial follow-up period. However, this benefit declined with time beyond the active-trial period (hazard ratio [HR] 0.72; 95% CI 0.64–0.82), indicating the need for long-term treatment to maximize benefits. The CV and kidney benefits (HR 0.79; 95% CI 0.72–0.87) were consistent across various eGFR and UACR categories and in different primary kidney disease etiologies (active-trial + post-trial follow-up periods).

Mechanistic Basis of the Renoprotective Effects of SGLT-2 Inhibitors

Multiple mechanisms have been proposed to explain the renoprotective effects of SGLT-2 inhibitors [15]. Key contributors may include reductions in body weight and visceral adiposity, lowering of serum uric acid, and improvements in blood pressure, endothelial function, and arterial stiffness [15]. Experimental data further suggest that SGLT-2 inhibition exerts anti-inflammatory and antifibrotic effects and may ameliorate renal hypoxia [37, 40–44]. The most clear mechanism, however, is their ability to reduce intraglomerular pressure (Fig. 3) [37, 40]. In diabetes, afferent arteriolar vasodilation leads to glomerular hyperfiltration, an increase in intraglomerular pressure, endothelial glomerular injury, and albuminuria [46, 47]. Upregulation of SGLT-2 expression and activity is a key contributor of afferent vasodilation. This process starts by increasing proximal sodium reabsorption, thereby reducing sodium chloride delivery to the macula densa; this triggers tubuloglomerular feedback, leading to dilation of the afferent arteriole [48, 49]. Evidence supporting this mechanism comes from a study in 27 patients with T1D and hyperfiltration, where empagliflozin for 8 weeks reduced inulin-measured GFR by 33 mL/min/1.73 m^2 and renal blood flow measured by para-aminohippurate clearance [50]. These findings suggest that SGLT-2 inhibition restores tubuloglomerular feedback, limiting afferent dilation, and thereby lowering intraglomerular pressure—a pathophysiological hallmark of proteinuric diabetic nephropathy. Such an effect of SGLT-2 inhibitors would explain the characteristic slight eGFR drop appearing within a few weeks of treatment initiation and being fully reversible after discontinuation of the drug [37]. In addition, this action would typically explain the reductions in intraglomerular pressure, albuminuria, and renal injury progression observed with these drugs. Reversal of afferent arteriole dilation would offer reductions in intraglomerular pressure that would be independent of the main nephroprotective mechanism of ACEIs and ARBs, that is efferent arteriole vasodilation through inhibition of the angiotensin-II action; thus a complementary renoprotective effect is expected to occur from the combination of an SGLT-2 inhibitor with an ACEI or an ARB, resulting in maximum renoprotection [15, 17].

Of note, a randomized trial of dapagliflozin in 44 patients with T2D provided further insights into renal hemodynamics. In this study, dapagliflozin reduced

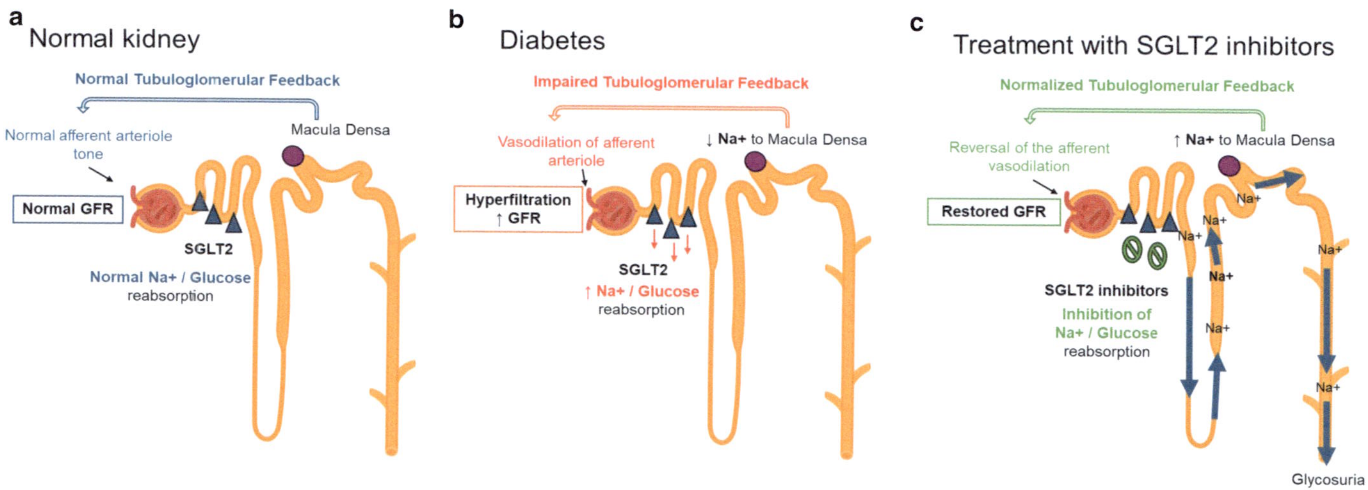

Fig. 3 Effects of SGLT-2 inhibitors on glomerular hemodynamics. Under physiological conditions, SGLT-2 co-transporters reabsorb ~90% of filtered glucose together with sodium, allowing the macula densa to regulate normal tubuloglomerular feedback and maintain stable GFR (**a**). In diabetes, upregulation of SGLT-2 expression and activity increases proximal tubular sodium reabsorption, reducing sodium chloride delivery to the macula densa. This suppresses tubuloglomerular feedback, promotes afferent arteriolar vasodilation, and drives glomerular hyperfiltration (**b**). By inhibiting SGLT-2, these drugs block proximal glucose and sodium reuptake, restoring sodium chloride delivery to the macula densa. This reactivation of tubuloglomerular feedback corrects afferent vasodilation, thereby lowering renal plasma flow, reducing intraglomerular pressure, and normalizing GFR (**c**). (From Sarafidis et al. [45] modified)

intraglomerular pressure and GFR without increasing renal vascular resistance, suggesting that the effect was mediated by efferent vasodilation rather than afferent vasoconstriction [51]. A number of limitations that may hamper the conclusions of the later study have been noted in the literature [52]. However, it cannot be excluded that in patients with T2D, particularly those of older age, the renal microcirculation has different regulatory mechanisms than those in young T1D patients and initially healthy kidneys and, thus, further research in this field is needed. Overall, even if the details on the actual underlying mechanism are still not fully understood, the fact that across large outcome trials, the consistent early and reversible "dip" in eGFR observed during the first weeks of SGLT-2 inhibitor therapy strongly supports a unifying mechanism of reduced intraglomerular hypertension and single-nephron hyperfiltration as the primary basis of renoprotection [15].

SGLT-2 Inhibitors for Cardioprotection in CKD

Cardioprotective Effects of SGLT-2 Inhibitors Observed in Cardiovascular Outcome Trials in Type 2 Diabetes

As mentioned before, the cardiovascular benefits of SGLT-2 inhibitors were first demonstrated in the major CVOT trials. The results were consistent also for the CKD subgroups; in the CKD subgroup of the EMPA-REG OUTCOME trial ($n = 2250$), a 29% lower risk for CV death, 24% for all-cause death, and 39% for hospitalization for heart failure (HHF) were observed, independent of eGFR or UACR strata [53, 54]. In the CANVAS program, canagliflozin reduced the primary CV outcome by 30% (HR 0.70), with consistent benefits across eGFR categories [32]. Similarly, in the DECLARE–TIMI 58 trial, subgroup data suggested consistent reductions in the combined endpoint of CV death or HHF across eGFR categories, with numerically greater benefit among patients with reduced kidney function [27]. In the Evaluation of Ertugliflozin Efficacy and Safety Cardiovascular Outcomes Trial (VERTIS-CV) trial, the composite of CV death or HHF was modestly reduced (HR 0.88, not statistically significant overall), yet subgroup analyses indicated significant benefit in CKD stage 3 patients, in those with albuminuria, and across higher Kidney Disease: Improving Global Outcomes (KDIGO) risk strata, especially for HHF reduction [55].

Cardioprotective Effects of SGLT-2 Inhibitors Observed in Trials in Heart Failure

Following the observation of substantial benefits in heart failure (HF) outcomes from the initial CVOTs, dedicated HF studies have since confirmed the efficacy of SGLT-2 inhibitors in patients with and without diabetes (Table 3). In the Study to Evaluate the Effect of Dapagliflozin on the Incidence of Worsening Heart Failure or Cardiovascular Death in Patients With Chronic Heart Failure (DAPA-HF), which

Table 3 Main clinical trials demonstrating reno- and cardioprotection in patients with heart failure receiving SGLT-2 inhibitors

Trial (year)	SGLT-2 inhibitor (dose)	Patient population	Number of patients	Mean eGFR (mL/min/1.73 m^2)	Median follow-up	Cardiovascular outcome (HR, 95% CI)	Kidney outcome (HR, 95% CI)
DAPA-HF (2019) [56]	Dapagliflozin (10 mg)	HFrEF	4744	66.0 ± 19.6 (65.5 ± 19.3 in the placebo group)	18.2 months	Worsening HF or CV death 0.74 (0.65–0.85) HHF or CV death 0.75 (0.65–0.85)	Sustained ≥50% eGFR decline, ESKD or renal death 0.71 (0.44 to 1.16)
DELIVER (2022) [57, 58]	Dapagliflozin (10 mg)	HF with EF >40%	6263	61 ± 19 (61 ± 19 in the placebo group)	2.3 years	HHF or urgent visit for HF or CV death 0.82 (0.73–0.92)	Post-hoc composite kidney outcome (first ≥50% decline in eGFR; first eGFR <15 mL/min/1.73 m^2; ESKD; renal death) 1.08 (0.79–1.49)
EMPEROR-Reduced (2020) [59]	Empagliflozin (10 mg)	HFrEF	3730	61.8 ± 21.7 (62.2 ± 21.5 in the placebo group)	16 months	CV death or HHF 0.75 (0.65–0.86); HHF 0.70 (0.58–0.85)	Dialysis or renal transplantation or sustained eGFR reduction 0.50 (0.32–0.77)
SOLOIST (2020) [60]	Sotagliflozin (200–400 mg)	T2D recently hospitalized for worsening HF	1222	Median 49.2 (39.5–61.2) [50.5 (40.5–64.6) in the placebo group]	9 months	Total CV deaths, HHF or urgent visits for HF 0.67 (0.52–0.85)	Least-squares mean change in eGFR −0.16 (−1.30 to 0.98)
EMPEROR-Preserved (2021) [61]	Empagliflozin (10 mg)	HFpEF	5988	60.6 ± 19.8	26.2 months	CV death or HHF 0.79 (0.69–0.90); HHF 0.73 (0.61–0.83)	Rate of eGFR decline (−1.25 vs −2.62 mL/min/1.73 m^2/year, $p < 0.001$ in SGLT-2i vs placebo)

CV cardiovascular, *CVD* cardiovascular disease, *CI* confidence interval, *CKD* chronic kidney disease, *eGFR* estimated glomerular filtration rate, *ESKD* end-stage kidney disease, *HF* heart failure, *HHF* hospitalization for heart failure, *HR* hazard ratio, *MACE* major adverse cardiovascular events, *KRT* kidney replacement therapy, *SGLT-2i* sodium-glucose co-transporter 2 inhibitors, *T2D* type 2 diabetes mellitus

enrolled 4744 patients with HF and reduced ejection fraction (HFrEF), dapagliflozin significantly lowered the risk of the primary composite endpoint of worsening HF or cardiovascular death compared with placebo [56]. The Empagliflozin Outcome Trial in Patients with Chronic Heart Failure with Reduced Ejection Fraction (EMPEROR-Reduced trial) (3730 patients with HFrEF) showed similar findings, with empagliflozin reducing the risk of cardiovascular death or HF hospitalization irrespective of diabetes status [59].

In Empagliflozin Outcome Trial in Patients with Chronic Heart Failure with Preserved Ejection Fraction (EMPEROR-Preserved), empagliflozin also reduced the composite of cardiovascular death or HF hospitalization in patients with HF and preserved ejection fraction (HFpEF), again independent of diabetes status. This trial established empagliflozin as the first therapy with proven benefit across the full spectrum of ejection fraction, leading to its U.S. approval for HF irrespective of EF. Importantly, the benefits of empagliflozin were consistent across the full range of kidney function in EMPEROR-Reduced [61].

The Dapagliflozin Evaluation to Improve the Lives of Patients with Preserved Ejection Fraction Heart Failure (DELIVER) trial further extended the evidence for SGLT-2 inhibitors in HF. In 6263 patients with HF and left ventricular ejection fraction >40%, dapagliflozin significantly reduced the risk of the primary composite endpoint of worsening HF or cardiovascular death compared with placebo (HR 0.82; 95% CI 0.73–0.92; $P < 0.001$) [57].

Given the high prevalence of HF—particularly HFpEF—among patients with CKD, these findings highlighted a new era for SGLT-2 inhibitors as agents providing integrated cardiorenal protection, with CKD patients likely to derive substantial benefit [55]. Based on event rates from CKD trials, treatment with an SGLT-2 inhibitor for 1000 patient-years is estimated to prevent 11 first hospitalizations for HF or cardiovascular deaths in patients with T2D, with even greater benefit expected in those with established HF [62].

Cardioprotective Effects of SGLT-2 Inhibitors Observed in Renal Outcome Trials in Diabetic and Non-Diabetic CKD

Beyond their established renoprotective properties, large renal outcome trials of SGLT-2 inhibitors have also provided compelling evidence of cardiovascular protection in patients with diabetic and non-diabetic CKD.

In CREDENCE, cardiovascular death was significantly reduced (HR 0.78; 95% CI 0.61–1.00). Importantly, despite early trial termination, canagliflozin consistently lowered the risk of both composite and individual cardiovascular endpoints compared with placebo (Table 2), including cardiovascular death or hospitalization for HF; the composite of CV death, MI, or stroke; the broader composite including HF or unstable angina; and HF hospitalization alone (HR 0.61; 95% CI 0.47–0.80). All-cause mortality displayed a decreasing trend (HR 0.83; 95% CI 0.68–1.02) [33]. A secondary analysis of this trial investigating the effects of canagliflozin versus placebo on eGFR subgroups (30 to <45, 45 to <60, and 60 to <90 mL/min/1.73 m^2)

showed that the canagliflozin cardiovascular effects were consistent across subgroups (*P* for interaction 0.25–0.74) [63].

With respect to cardiovascular outcomes in DAPA-CKD, dapagliflozin reduced the composite of cardiovascular death or HHF (HR 0.71; 95% CI 0.55–0.92) and showed a favorable trend for cardiovascular mortality alone (HR 0.81; 95% CI 0.58–1.12). All-cause mortality was also significantly lower with dapagliflozin (HR 0.69; 95% CI 0.53–0.88) [34]. In a secondary analysis stratified by history of cardiovascular disease, the benefits of dapagliflozin were consistent across subgroups for both cardiovascular outcomes and overall mortality. The largest effects were observed for first HHF, with risk reductions of 46% in patients with established cardiovascular disease (HR 0.54; 95% CI 0.35–0.82) and 69% in those without cardiovascular disease (HR 0.31; 95% CI 0.10–0.94) [64].

In EMPA-KIDNEY trial [36], the rate of first and subsequent hospitalizations from any cause was lower in the empagliflozin group than in the placebo group (HR 0.86; 95% CI, 0.78–0.95). No significant effect was observed with respect to hospitalization for heart failure or death from cardiovascular causes (composite outcome) (HR 0.84; 95% CI, 0.67–1.07). The hazard ratio for death from cardiovascular causes was 0.84 (95% CI, 0.60–1.19).

The Effect of Sotagliflozin on Cardiovascular and Renal Events in Patients With Type 2 Diabetes and Moderate Renal Impairment Who Are at Cardiovascular Risk (SCORED) trial randomized 10,584 T2D patients with CKD (eGFR 25–60 mL/min/1.73 m^2) and cardiovascular risk to sotagliflozin or placebo with a primary cardiovascular endpoint [35] (Table 2). The primary endpoint was modified during the trial to a composite of cardiovascular death, HHF and urgent visits for HF. The trial ended prematurely (median follow-up of 16 months) due to loss of funding. For the same reason, planned adjudication was not completed, and investigator-reported events were included in the analysis, which is a second limitation of the study. Nevertheless, the primary endpoint event rate was 5.6 events/100 patient-years in the sotagliflozin group and 7.5 events/100 patient-years in the placebo group (HR, 0.74; 95% CI, 0.63–0.88; $p < 0.001$). Sotagliflozin also reduced the original co-primary endpoints of cardiovascular death, nonfatal MI, or nonfatal stroke (HR, 0.84; 95% CI, 0.72–0.99) and cardiovascular death or HHF (HR, 0.77; 95% CI, 0.66–0.91) [35].

The cumulative cardiovascular benefits of SGLT-2 inhibitors in patients with CKD have also been confirmed in recent meta-analyses [65, 66]. A meta-analysis of 12 large trials including approximately 90,000 participants demonstrated a 32% lower risk of hospitalization for heart failure for SGLT-2 inhibitors compared to placebo (HR 0.68; 95% CI 0.63–0.73) (Fig. 4). Reduction in HF events with SGLT-2 inhibitors was more prominent in patients with eGFR <60 mL/min/1.73 m^2 (HR 0.68; 95% CI 0.62–0.74) than in those with eGFR ≥60 mL/min/1.73 m^2 (HR 0.76; 95% CI 0.69–0.83). Subgroup analysis according to type of SGLT-2 inhibitor showed a consistent treatment effect across all studied agents (*p* forsubgroup-analysis = 0.44) [65].

Study or Subgroup	log[Hazard Ratio]	SE	Weight	Hazard Ratio IV, Fixed, 95% CI
CANVAS Program	-0.5621	0.2069	3.6%	0.57 [0.38, 0.86]
CREDENCE	-0.4891	0.1357	8.3%	0.61 [0.47, 0.80]
DAPA-CKD	-0.6766	0.2052	3.6%	0.51 [0.34, 0.76]
DAPA-HF	-0.4231	0.1277	9.4%	0.66 [0.51, 0.84]
DECLARE-TIMI 58	-0.3086	0.1205	10.5%	0.73 [0.58, 0.93]
DELIVER	-0.2862	0.0979	16.0%	0.75 [0.62, 0.91]
EMPA-KIDNEY	-0.2263	0.1452	7.3%	0.80 [0.60, 1.06]
EMPA-REG OUTCOME	-0.5347	0.2076	3.6%	0.59 [0.39, 0.88]
EMPEROR-Preserved	-0.4095	0.1247	9.8%	0.66 [0.52, 0.85]
EMPEROR-Reduced	-0.312	0.1276	9.4%	0.73 [0.57, 0.94]
SCORED	-0.4005	0.1007	15.1%	0.67 [0.55, 0.82]
VERTIS CV	-0.6931	0.212	3.4%	0.50 [0.33, 0.76]
Total (95% CI)			**100.0%**	**0.68 [0.63, 0.73]**

Heterogeneity: Chi² = 9.03, df = 11 (P = 0.62); I² = 0%
Test for overall effect: Z = 10.03 (P < 0.00001)

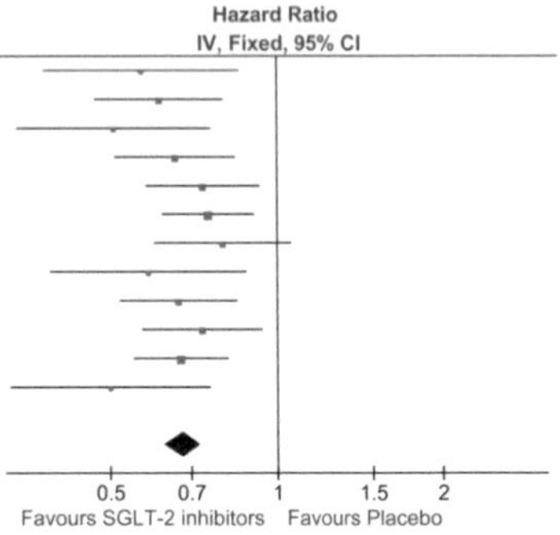

Fig. 4 Effect of SGLT-2 inhibitors compared to placebo on HF events (defined as HHF or urgent outpatient visit for worsening HF requiring ambulatory treatment with intravenous diuretics) in patients with CKD. (From Theodorakopoulou et al. [65] with permission). Abbreviations: HF heart failure, HHF hospitalization for heart failure

Safety Profile

The kidney safety profile of SGLT-2 inhibitors has been well characterized in meta-analyses [62]. Across 13 trials including over 90,000 participants, the only consistent excess risk was for mycotic genital infections (RR 3.57; 95% CI 3.14–4.06). No significant increase was observed for serious urinary tract infections, amputations, or fractures [62]. In patients with diabetes, the risk of ketoacidosis is approximately doubled, but the absolute risk remains low in T2D and is mainly relevant in the context of insulin deficiency or T1D.

Overall, the absolute harms of SGLT-2 inhibition are markedly outweighed by the substantial cardiorenal benefits, particularly in patients with CKD and especially in those without diabetes [62, 67]. Notably, meta-analyses of large placebo-controlled trials demonstrate that SGLT-2 inhibitors reduce the risk of acute kidney injury (HR 0.77; 95% CI 0.70–0.84) and lower the incidence of serious hyperkalemia events by 16% (HR 0.84; 95% CI 0.76–0.93) [67, 68]. No excess incidence of adverse events was observed with SGLT-2 inhibitors compared with placebo [62]. Reductions in serious hyperkalemia were consistent across trials and subgroups, irrespective of baseline kidney function, heart failure status, or concomitant therapy with RAS blockers, diuretics, or mineralocorticoid receptor antagonists (MRAs). Importantly, SGLT-2 inhibitors did not increase the risk of hypokalemia (HR 1.04; 95% CI 0.94–1.15) [69]. In HFrEF, the benefits of empagliflozin were unaffected by baseline MRA use in EMPEROR-Reduced, and empagliflozin treatment was associated with fewer MRA discontinuations, possibly reflecting reduced hyperkalemia risk [70]. In DAPA-HF, moderate/severe hyperkalemia (K^+ >6.0 mmol/L) was significantly less frequent with dapagliflozin versus placebo among patients on MRAs (HR 0.50; 95% CI 0.29–0.85) [71]. Multiple mechanisms have been proposed to explain how SGLT-2 inhibition mitigates hyperkalemia [68, 72].

Guidelines for Clinical Practice and Ongoing Research

In consideration of the remarkably consistent findings of cardiorenal benefit, SGLT-2 inhibitors are now recommended as first-line agents in treatment of patients with CKD by multiple societies including the American Diabetes Association (ADA), KDIGO, the European Society of Hypertension (ESH), the European Society of Cardiology (ESC)and other texts [12, 13, 73, 74]. Current guidance supports their use in patients with eGFR ≥20 mL/min/1.73 m^2, with discontinuation advised upon initiation of dialysis or after kidney transplantation. However, a potential therapeutic role of SGLT-2 inhibitors for these populations is under study. The Renal Lifecycle Trial (NCT05374291) is an ongoing study that evaluates the effects of dapagliflozin on kidney failure, HF, mortality and safety in patients with eGFR ≤25 mL/min/1.73 m^2, as well as in those under chronic dialysis or kidney transplant with an eGFR ≤45 mL/min/1.73 m^2.

Another emerging area is the role of SGLT-2 inhibitors in combination therapies for CKD [75, 76]. The complex pathophysiology of diabetic and non-diabetic CKD supports the rationale for using multiple evidence-based agents to reduce the lifetime risks of kidney failure, cardiovascular events, and mortality. In diabetic CKD, the strongest evidence exists, with four therapeutic classes already proven to improve renal, cardiovascular, and survival outcomes. A similar pillared approach is anticipated also for non-diabetic CKD, potentially incorporating disease-specific immunological therapies. Early data suggest additive efficacy and favorable safety with combination use, though further studies are needed to define the optimal sequencing and intensity of therapy. In the CONFIDENCE trial, 818 patients were randomized to empagliflozin+finerenone, finerenone monotherapy or empagliflozin monotherapy. At day 180, the reduction in the urinary albumin-to-creatinine ratio with combination therapy was 29% greater than that with finerenone alone (least-squares mean ratio of the difference in the change from baseline, 0.71; 95% CI 0.61–0.82) and 32% greater than that with empagliflozin alone (least-squares mean ratio of the difference in the change from baseline, 0.68; 95% CI, 0.59–0.79). Of note, neither agent, alone or in combination, led to unexpected adverse events. Symptomatic hypotension, acute kidney injury, and hyperkalemia leading to drug discontinuation were uncommon [77].

In this context, a growing number of large Phase III RCTs are now exploring the effects of combination therapy in CKD (Table 4). These include trials of aldosterone synthase inhibition plus SGLT-2 inhibitors versus SGLT-2 inhibitors alone, such as BAXDUO-ARCTIC (~2500 patients with albuminuric CKD, primary outcome change in eGFR at 2 years; NCT06268873) and BAXDUO-PACIFIC (~5000 patients with hypertension and CKD, composite primary outcome of sustained ≥50% eGFR decline, kidney failure, or CV death; NCT06742723). The EASi-KIDNEY trial is testing the safety and cardiorenal efficacy of vicadrostat in combination with empagliflozin versus empagliflozin alone in ~11,000 patients with CKD [78]. Finally, in the ZENITH-HP trial, the effect of zibotentan/dapagliflozin versus dapagliflozin alone is being studied in ~1500 patients with albuminuric CKD, with a primary outcome of change in eGFR over 24 months (NCT06087835).

Table 4 Future studies evaluating the effects of combination therapies in patients with CKD

Trial	Patient population	Number of patients	Intervention—comparison	Primary outcome
BAXDUO-ARCTIC (NCT06268873)	CKD and hypertension (eGFR≥30 and <90 mL/min/1.73 m^2 and UACR 200–5000 mg/g) Serum potassium ≤4.8 mmol/l (≤4.5 for eGFR<45 mL/min/1.73 m^2)	~2500 patients	Baxdrostat/dapagliflozin versus dapagliflozin/placebo	Change from baseline in eGFR to post treatment (at 2 years)
BAXDUO-PACIFIC (NCT06742723)	CKD and hypertension (eGFR ≥30 and <60 mL/min/1.73 m^2 and UACR 300-5000 mg/g or eGFR≥60 and < 75 mL/min/1.73 m^2 and UACR 500–5000 mg/g) Serum potassium ≤4.8 mmol/l (≤4.5 for eGFR<45 mL/min/1.73 m^2)	~5000 patients	Baxdrostat/dapagliflozin versus dapagliflozin/placebo	Time to the first occurrence of any of the components of the composite endpoint of ≥50% sustained decline in eGFR, kidney failure or CV death. (up to 41 months)
EASi-KIDNEY [78] (NCT06531824)	CKD (eGFR≥20 and <45 mL/min/1.73 m^2 or eGFR≥45 and <90 mL/min/1.73 m^2 and UACR ≥200 mg/g or UPCR ≥300 mg/g)	~11,000 patients	Vicadrostat/empagliflozin versus empagliflozin/placebo	Time to first occurrence of the primary composite outcome of kidney disease progression; or HHF; or CV death.
ZENITH-HP (NCT06087835)	CKD (eGFR≥20 and <90 mL/min/1.73 m^2 and UACR >700 mg/g or UPCR>1000 mg/g)	~1500 patients	Zibotentan/dapagliflozin versus dapagliflozin/placebo	Change in eGFR from baseline to month 24

CV cardiovascular, *CKD* chronic kidney disease, *eGFR* estimated glomerular filtration rate, *ESKD* end-stage kidney disease, *HHF* hospitalization for heart failure, *UACR* urine albumin-to-creatinine ratio, *UPCR* urine protein-to-creatinine ratio

Conclusions

SGLT-2 inhibitors have fundamentally changed the therapeutic landscape of CKD, demonstrating robust and consistent benefits across both diabetic and non-diabetic populations. Beyond their glucose-lowering effects, they provide complementary renoprotective and cardioprotective actions through hemodynamic, metabolic, and anti-inflammatory mechanisms. Large-scale outcome trials have shown that these agents slow CKD progression, reduce albuminuria, lower the risk of kidney failure, and substantially decrease cardiovascular morbidity and mortality, with a favorable safety profile and with benefits extending across a broad spectrum of kidney function and cardiovascular risk. Current guidelines endorse their use as first-line therapy in CKD with or without diabetes, while ongoing trials are investigating their role in patients with advanced CKD stages (i.e. dialysis, kidney transplantation) and in combination regimens.

References

1. Jager KJ, Kovesdy C, Langham R, Rosenberg M, Jha V, Zoccali C. A single number for advocacy and communication-worldwide more than 850 million individuals have kidney diseases. Kidney Int. 2019;96:1048–50.
2. US Renal Data System 2019 Annual Data Report: Epidemiology of Kidney Disease in the United States. Am J Kidney Dis. 2019:S0272-6386: 31008-X. Erratum in: Am J Kidney Dis. 2020;76:450.
3. Kramer A, Pippias M, Noordzij M, Stel VS, Andrusev AM, Aparicio-Madre MI, et al. The European renal association - European Dialysis and Transplant Association (ERA-EDTA) registry annual report 2016: a summary. Clin Kidney J. 2019;12:702–20.
4. Ortiz A, Wanner C, Gansevoort R, ERA Council. Chronic kidney disease as cardiovascular risk factor in routine clinical practice: a position statement by the Council of the European Renal Association. Clin Kidney J. 2023;16:403–7.
5. Go AS, Chertow GM, Fan D, McCulloch CE, Hsu C. Chronic kidney disease and the risks of death, cardiovascular events, and hospitalization. N Engl J Med. 2004;351:1296–305.
6. Kidney Disease: Improving Global Outcomes (KDIGO) CKD Work Group. KDIGO 2012 clinical practice guideline for the evaluation and management of chronic kidney disease. Kidney Int Suppl. 2013;3:1–150.
7. Foreman KJ, Marquez N, Dolgert A, Fukutaki K, Fullman N, McGaughey M, et al. Forecasting life expectancy, years of life lost, and all-cause and cause-specific mortality for 250 causes of death: reference and alternative scenarios for 2016–40 for 195 countries and territories. Lancet. 2018;392:2052–90.
8. Wanner C, Amann K, Shoji T. The heart and vascular system in dialysis. Lancet. 2016;388:276–84.
9. Afkarian M, Sachs MC, Kestenbaum B, Hirsch IB, Tuttle KR, Himmelfarb J, et al. Kidney disease and increased mortality risk in type 2 diabetes. J Am Soc Nephrol. 2013;24:302–8.
10. Levin A, Stevens PE, Bilous RW, Coresh J, Francisco ALMD, Jong PED, et al. Kidney disease: improving global outcomes (KDIGO) CKD work group. KDIGO 2012 clinical practice guideline for the evaluation and management of chronic kidney disease. Kidney Int Suppl. 2013;3:1–150.
11. Sarafidis PA, Ruilope LM. Aggressive blood pressure reduction and renin-angiotensin system blockade in chronic kidney disease: time for re-evaluation? Kidney Int. 2014;85:536–46.
12. Mancia G, Kreutz R, Brunström M, Burnier M, Grassi G, Januszewicz A, et al. 2023 ESH Guidelines for the management of arterial hypertension The Task Force For the management of arterial hypertension of the European Society of Hypertension: endorsed by theInternational Society of Hypertension (ISH) and the European renal association (ERA). J Hypertens. 2023;41:1874–2071.
13. Mark PB, Sarafidis P, Ekart R, Ferro CJ, Balafa O, Fernandez-Fernandez B, et al. SGLT2i for evidence based cardiorenal protection in diabetic and non-diabetic chronic kidney disease: a comprehensive review by EURECA-m and ERBP working groups of ERA. Nephrol Dial Transplant. 2023;38:gfad112.
14. Sarafidis PA, Stafylas PC, Kanaki AI, Lasaridis AN. Effects of renin-angiotensin system blockers on renal outcomes and all-cause mortality in patients with diabetic nephropathy: an updated meta-analysis. Am J Hypertens. 2008;21:922–9.

15. Sarafidis P, Ferro CJ, Morales E, Ortiz A, Malyszko J, Hojs R, et al. SGLT-2 inhibitors and GLP-1 receptor agonists for nephroprotection and cardioprotection in patients with diabetes mellitus and chronic kidney disease. A consensus statement by the EURECA-m and the DIABESITY working groups of the ERA-EDTA. Nephrol Dial Transplant. 2019;34:208–30.
16. Sarafidis P, Ortiz A, Ferro CJ, Halimi J-M, Kreutz R, Mallamaci F, et al. Sodium–glucose co-transporter-2 inhibitors for patients with diabetic and nondiabetic chronic kidney disease: a new era has already begun. J Hypertens. 2021;39:1090–7.
17. Loutradis C, Papadopoulou E, Angeloudi E, Karagiannis A, Sarafidis P. The Beneficial Hemodynamic Actions of SGLT-2 Inhibitors beyond the Management of Hyperglycemia. Curr Med Chem. 2020;27:6682–702
18. Piperidou A, Loutradis C, Sarafidis P. SGLT-2 inhibitors and nephroprotection: current evidence and future perspectives. J Hum Hypertens. 2021;35:12–25.
19. Imprialos KP, Sarafidis PA, Karagiannis AI. Sodium-glucose cotransporter-2 inhibitors and blood pressure decrease: a valuable effect of a novel antidiabetic class? J Hypertens. 2015;33:2185–97.
20. Mancia G, Cannon CP, Tikkanen I, Zeller C, Ley L, Woerle HJ, et al. Impact of Empagliflozin on blood pressure in patients with type 2 diabetes mellitus and hypertension by background antihypertensive medication. Hypertension. 2016;68:1355–64.
21. Papadopoulou E, Loutradis C, Tzatzagou G, Kotsa K, Zografou I, Minopoulou I, et al. Dapagliflozin decreases ambulatory central blood pressure and pulse wave velocity in patients with type 2 diabetes: a randomized, double-blind, placebo-controlled clinical trial. J Hypertens. 2021;39:749–58.
22. Jordan J, Tank J, Heusser K, Heise T, Wanner C, Heer M, et al. The effect of empagliflozin on muscle sympathetic nerve activity in patients with type II diabetes mellitus. J Am Soc Hypertens. 2017;11:604–12.
23. Chilton R, Tikkanen I, Cannon CP, Crowe S, Woerle HJ, Broedl UC, et al. Effects of empagliflozin on blood pressure and markers of arterial stiffness and vascular resistance in patients with type 2 diabetes. Diabetes Obes Metab. 2015;17:1180–93.
24. Piperidou A, Sarafidis P, Boutou A, Thomopoulos C, Loutradis C, Alexandrou ME, et al. The effect of SGLT-2 inhibitors on albuminuria and proteinuria in diabetes mellitus: a systematic review and meta-analysis of randomized controlled trials. J Hypertens. 2019;37:1334–43.
25. Zinman B, Wanner C, Lachin JM, Fitchett D, Bluhmki E, Hantel S, et al. Empagliflozin, cardiovascular outcomes, and mortality in type 2 diabetes. N Engl J Med. 2015;373:2117–28.
26. Neal B, Perkovic V, de Zeeuw D, Mahaffey KW, Fulcher G, Stein P, et al. Rationale, design, and baseline characteristics of the Canagliflozin Cardiovascular Assessment Study (CANVAS)–a randomized placebo-controlled trial. Am Heart J. 2013;166:217–223.e11.
27. Wiviott SD, Raz I, Bonaca MP, Mosenzon O, Kato ET, Cahn A, et al. Dapagliflozin and cardiovascular outcomes in type 2 diabetes. N Engl J Med. 2019;380:347–57.
28. Cannon CP, Pratley R, Dagogo-Jack S, Mancuso J, Huyck S, Masiukiewicz U, et al. Cardiovascular outcomes with Ertugliflozin in type 2 diabetes. N Engl J Med. 2020;383:1425–35.
29. Wanner C, Inzucchi SE, Lachin JM, Fitchett D, von Eynatten M, Mattheus M, et al. Empagliflozin and progression of kidney disease in type 2 diabetes. N Engl J Med. 2016;375:323–34.
30. Perkovic V, de Zeeuw D, Mahaffey KW, Fulcher G, Erondu N, Shaw W, et al. Canagliflozin and renal outcomes in type 2 diabetes: results from the CANVAS program randomised clinical trials. Lancet Diabetes Endocrinol. 2018;6:691–704.
31. Neal B, Perkovic V, Matthews DR, Mahaffey KW, Fulcher G, Meininger G, et al. Rationale, design and baseline characteristics of the CANagliflozin cardioVascular assessment study-renal (CANVAS-R): a randomized, placebo-controlled trial. Diabetes Obes Metab. 2017;19:387–93.
32. Neuen BL, Ohkuma T, Neal B, Matthews DR, de Zeeuw D, Mahaffey KW, et al. Cardiovascular and renal outcomes with Canagliflozin according to baseline kidney function. Circulation. 2018;138:1537–50.
33. Perkovic V, Jardine MJ, Neal B, Bompoint S, Heerspink HJL, Charytan DM, et al. Canagliflozin and renal outcomes in type 2 diabetes and nephropathy. N Engl J Med. 2019;380:2295–306.

34. Heerspink HJL, Stefánsson BV, Correa-Rotter R, Chertow GM, Greene T, Hou F-F, et al. Dapagliflozin in patients with chronic kidney disease. N Engl J Med. 2020;383:1436–46.
35. Bhatt DL, Szarek M, Pitt B, Cannon CP, Leiter LA, McGuire DK, et al. SCORED Investigators. Sotagliflozin in Patients with Diabetes and Chronic Kidney Disease. N Engl J Med. 2021;384:129–39.
36. The EMPA-KIDNEY Collaborative Group, Herrington WG, Staplin N, Wanner C, Green JB, Hauske SJ, et al. Empagliflozin in patients with chronic kidney disease. N Engl J Med. 2023;388:117–27.
37. Heerspink HJL, Kosiborod M, Inzucchi SE, Cherney DZI. Renoprotective effects of sodium-glucose cotransporter-2 inhibitors. Kidney Int. 2018;94:26–39.
38. Fernández-Fernandez B, Sarafidis P, Soler MJ, Ortiz A. EMPA-KIDNEY: expanding the range of kidney protection by SGLT2 inhibitors. Clin Kidney J. 2023;16:1187–98.
39. EMPA-KIDNEY Collaborative Group. Long-term effects of Empagliflozin in patients with chronic kidney disease. N Engl J Med. 2025;392:777–87.
40. Heerspink HJL, Perkins BA, Fitchett DH, Husain M, Cherney DZI. Sodium glucose cotransporter 2 inhibitors in the treatment of diabetes mellitus: cardiovascular and kidney effects, potential mechanisms, and clinical applications. Circulation. 2016;134:752–72.
41. Terami N, Ogawa D, Tachibana H, Hatanaka T, Wada J, Nakatsuka A, et al. Long-term treatment with the sodium glucose cotransporter 2 inhibitor, dapagliflozin, ameliorates glucose homeostasis and diabetic nephropathy in db/db mice. PLoS One. 2014;9:e100777.
42. O'Neill J, Fasching A, Pihl L, Patinha D, Franzén S, Palm F. Acute SGLT inhibition normalizes O2 tension in the renal cortex but causes hypoxia in the renal medulla in anaesthetized control and diabetic rats. Am J Physiol Renal Physiol. 2015;309:F227–34.
43. Chang Y-K, Choi H, Jeong JY, Na K-R, Lee KW, Lim BJ, et al. Dapagliflozin, SGLT2 inhibitor, attenuates renal ischemia-reperfusion injury. PLoS One. 2016;11:e0158810.
44. Górriz JL, Navarro-González JF, Ortiz A, Vergara A, Nuñez J, Jacobs-Cachá C, et al. Sodium-glucose cotransporter 2 inhibition: towards an indication to treat diabetic kidney disease. Nephrol Dial Transplant. 2020;35:i13–23.
45. Sarafidis P, Pella E, Kanbay M, Papagianni A. SGLT-2 inhibitors and nephroprotection in patients with diabetic and non-diabetic chronic kidney disease. Curr Med Chem. 2023;30:2039–60.
46. Sarafidis PA, Khosla N, Bakris GL. Antihypertensive therapy in the presence of proteinuria. Am J Kidney Dis. 2007;49:12–26.
47. Brenner BM, Lawler EV, Mackenzie HS. The hyperfiltration theory: a paradigm shift in nephrology. Kidney Int. 1996;49:1774–7.
48. Norton L, Shannon CE, Fourcaudot M, Hu C, Wang N, Ren W, et al. Sodium-glucose cotransporter (SGLT) and glucose transporter (GLUT) expression in the kidney of type 2 diabetic subjects. Diabetes Obes Metab. 2017;19:1322–6.
49. Solini A, Rossi C, Mazzanti CM, Proietti A, Koepsell H, Ferrannini E. Sodium-glucose cotransporter (SGLT)2 and SGLT1 renal expression in patients with type 2 diabetes. Diabetes Obes Metab. 2017;19:1289–94.
50. Cherney DZI, Perkins BA, Soleymanlou N, Maione M, Lai V, Lee A, et al. Renal hemodynamic effect of sodium-glucose cotransporter 2 inhibition in patients with type 1 diabetes mellitus. Circulation. 2014;129:587–97.
51. Van Bommel EJM, Muskiet MHA, van Baar MJB, Tonneijck L, Smits MM, Emanuel AL, et al. The renal hemodynamic effects of the SGLT2 inhibitor dapagliflozin are caused by post-glomerular vasodilatation rather than pre-glomerular vasoconstriction in metformin-treated patients with type 2 diabetes in the randomized, double-blind RED trial. Kidney Int. 2020;97:202–12.
52. Soler MJ, Porrini E, Fernandez-Fernandez B, Ortiz A. SGLT2i and postglomerular vasodilation. Kidney Int. 2020;97:805–6.
53. Wanner C, Lachin JM, Inzucchi SE, Fitchett D, Mattheus M, George J, et al. Empagliflozin and clinical outcomes in patients with type 2 diabetes mellitus, established cardiovascular disease, and chronic kidney disease. Circulation. 2018;137:119–29.

54. Levin A, Perkovic V, Wheeler DC, Hantel S, George JT, von Eynatten M, et al. Empagliflozin and cardiovascular and kidney outcomes across KDIGO risk categories: post hoc analysis of a randomized, double-blind, placebo-controlled, multinational trial. Clin J Am Soc Nephrol. 2020;15:1433–44.
55. Cherney DZI, McGuire DK, Charbonnel B, Cosentino F, Pratley R, Dagogo-Jack S, et al. VERTIS CV Investigators. Gradient of Risk and Associations With Cardiovascular Efficacy of Ertugliflozin by Measures of Kidney Function: Observations From VERTIS CV. Circulation. 2021;143:602–5.
56. McMurray JJV, Solomon SD, Inzucchi SE, Køber L, Kosiborod MN, Martinez FA, et al. Dapagliflozin in patients with heart failure and reduced ejection fraction. N Engl J Med. 2019;381:1995–2008.
57. Solomon SD, McMurray JJV, Claggett B, de Boer RA, DeMets D, Hernandez AF, et al. Dapagliflozin in heart failure with mildly reduced or preserved ejection fraction. N Engl J Med. 2022;387:1089–98.
58. Mc Causland FR, Claggett BL, Vaduganathan M, Desai AS, Jhund P, de Boer RA, et al. Dapagliflozin and kidney outcomes in patients with heart failure with mildly reduced or preserved ejection fraction: a prespecified analysis of the DELIVER randomized clinical trial. JAMA Cardiol. 2023;8:56–65.
59. Packer M, Anker SD, Butler J, Filippatos G, Pocock SJ, Carson P, et al. Cardiovascular and renal outcomes with Empagliflozin in heart failure. N Engl J Med. 2020;383:1413–24.
60. Bhatt DL, Szarek M, Steg PG, Cannon CP, Leiter LA, McGuire DK, et al. Sotagliflozin in patients with diabetes and recent worsening heart failure. N Engl J Med. 2021;384:117–28.
61. Anker SD, Butler J, Filippatos G, Ferreira JP, Bocchi E, Böhm M, et al. Empagliflozin in heart failure with a preserved ejection fraction. N Engl J Med. 2021;385:1451–61.
62. Nuffield Department of Population Health Renal Studies Group, SGLT2 inhibitor Meta-Analysis Cardio-Renal Trialists' Consortium. Impact of diabetes on the effects of sodium glucose co-transporter-2 inhibitors on kidney outcomes: collaborative meta-analysis of large placebo-controlled trials. Lancet. 2022;400:1788–801.
63. Jardine MJ, Zhou Z, Mahaffey KW, Oshima M, Agarwal R, Bakris G, et al. Renal, cardiovascular, and safety outcomes of Canagliflozin by baseline kidney function: a secondary analysis of the CREDENCE randomized trial. J Am Soc Nephrol. 2020;31:1128–39.
64. McMurray JJV, Wheeler DC, Stefánsson BV, Jongs N, Postmus D, Correa-Rotter R, et al. DAPA-CKD Trial Committees and Investigators. Effect of Dapagliflozin on Clinical Outcomes in Patients With Chronic Kidney Disease, With and Without Cardiovascular Disease. Circulation. 2021;143:438–48.
65. Theodorakopoulou MP, Alexandrou M-E, Tsitouridis A, Kamperidis V, Pella E, Xanthopoulos A, et al. Effects of sodium-glucose co-transporter 2 inhibitors on heart failure events in chronic kidney disease: a systematic review and meta-analysis. Eur Heart J Cardiovasc Pharmacother. 2024;10:329–41.
66. Karagiannidis AG, Theodorakopoulou MP, Alexandrou M-E, Iatridi F, Karkamani E, Anastasiou V, et al. Sodium-glucose co-transporter 2 inhibitors for all-cause and cardiovascular death in people with different stages of CKD: a systematic review and meta-analysis. Eur J Clin Investig. 2025;55:e14335.
67. Staplin N, Roddick AJ, Emberson J, Reith C, Riding A, Wonnacott A, et al. Net effects of sodium-glucose co-transporter-2 inhibition in different patient groups: a meta-analysis of large placebo-controlled randomized trials. EClinicalMedicine. 2021;41:101163.
68. Neuen BL, Oshima M, Agarwal R, Arnott C, Cherney DZ, Edwards R, et al. Sodium-glucose cotransporter 2 inhibitors and risk of hyperkalemia in people with type 2 diabetes: a meta-analysis of individual participant data from randomized, controlled trials. Circulation. 2022;145:1460–70.
69. Toyama T, Neuen BL, Jun M, Ohkuma T, Neal B, Jardine MJ, et al. Effect of SGLT2 inhibitors on cardiovascular, renal and safety outcomes in patients with type 2 diabetes mellitus and chronic kidney disease: a systematic review and meta-analysis. Diabetes Obes Metab. 2019;21:1237–50.

70. Ferreira JP, Zannad F, Pocock SJ, Anker SD, Butler J, Filippatos G, et al. Interplay of mineralocorticoid receptor antagonists and Empagliflozin in heart failure: EMPEROR-reduced. J Am Coll Cardiol. 2021;77:1397–407.
71. Shen L, Kristensen SL, Bengtsson O, Böhm M, de Boer RA, Docherty KF, et al. Dapagliflozin in HFrEF patients treated with mineralocorticoid receptor antagonists: an analysis of DAPA-HF. JACC Heart Fail. 2021;9:254–64.
72. Sampani E, Theodorakopoulou M, Iatridi F, Sarafidis P. Hyperkalemia in chronic kidney disease: a focus on potassium lowering pharmacotherapy. Expert Opin Pharmacother. 2023;24:1775–89.
73. de Boer IH, Khunti K, Sadusky T, Tuttle KR, Neumiller JJ, Rhee CM, et al. Diabetes management in chronic kidney disease: a consensus report by the American Diabetes Association (ADA) and Kidney Disease: Improving Global Outcomes (KDIGO). Kidney Int. 2022;102:974–89.
74. Kidney Disease: Improving Global Outcomes (KDIGO) CKD Work Group. KDIGO 2024 clinical practice guideline for the evaluation and management of chronic kidney disease. Kidney Int. 2024;105:S117–314.
75. Neuen BL, Yeung EK, Rangaswami J, Vaduganathan M. Combination therapy as a new standard of care in diabetic and non-diabetic chronic kidney disease. Nephrol Dial Transplant. 2025;40:i59–69.
76. Alicic RZ, Neumiller JJ, Tuttle KR. Combination therapy: an upcoming paradigm to improve kidney and cardiovascular outcomes in chronic kidney disease. Nephrol Dial Transplant. 2025;40:i3–i17.
77. Agarwal R, Green JB, Heerspink HJL, Mann JFE, McGill JB, Mottl AK, et al. Finerenone with Empagliflozin in chronic kidney disease and type 2 diabetes. N Engl J Med. 2025;393:533–43.
78. Judge PK, Tuttle KR, Staplin N, Hauske SJ, Zhu D, Sardell R, et al. The potential for improving cardio-renal outcomes in chronic kidney disease with the aldosterone synthase inhibitor vicadrostat (BI 690517): a rationale for the EASi-KIDNEY trial. Nephrol Dial Transplant. 2025;40:1175–86.

Mineralocorticoid Receptor Antagonists for Renoprotection and Cardioprotection in CKD

Fotini Iatridi and Marieta P. Theodorakopoulou

Introduction

Chronic kidney disease (CKD) is a growing public health concern, especially among individuals with type 2 diabetes (T2D) [1]. Approximately 30–40% of patients with T2D develop diabetic kidney disease (DKD), which represents the most common cause of kidney failure worldwide [2]. These patients are also at increased risk for cardiovascular events and have almost 3 times higher 10-year cumulative mortality than patients with T2D without CKD [3]. Despite the fact that inhibition of the renin–angiotensin system (RAS) using angiotensin-converting enzyme inhibitors (ACEis) or angiotensin receptor blockers (ARBs) has long been the foundation of therapy for albuminuric CKD, a significant residual risk for both kidney and cardiovascular progression remains [4, 5]. However, dual RAS blockade has not been proven effective and safe, posing increased risks of hyperkalemia and acute kidney injury (AKI) [6, 7].

Mineralocorticoid receptor antagonists (MRAs) have shown promise in bridging this therapeutic gap. Traditional steroidal MRAs such as spironolactone and eplerenone effectively reduce proteinuria [8, 9], but have not demonstrated consistent benefits in hard kidney or cardiovascular outcomes, while their use is often limited by side effects such as the risk of hyperkalemia and hormonal adverse events [10]. In recent years, non-steroidal MRAs have emerged as a therapeutic option with improved tissue selectivity and pharmacodynamic properties. Among these, finerenone has demonstrated significant benefits in large-scale randomized controlled trials (RCTs) in patients with CKD and T2D [11, 12]. This chapter provides a comprehensive review of the rationale for MRA use in CKD, the differences between steroidal and non-steroidal agents, the involved nephroprotective

F. Iatridi (✉) · M. P. Theodorakopoulou
1st Department of Nephrology, Aristotle University of Thessaloniki, Hippokration Hospital, Thessaloniki, Greece

P. Sarafidis, R. Pontremoli (eds.), *Hypertension and Chronic Kidney Disease*, Updates in Hypertension and Cardiovascular Protection,
https://doi.org/10.1007/978-3-032-29564-4_16

mechanisms, and the clinical evidence supporting their role in improving cardiorenal outcomes.

Pathophysiological Role of Mineralocorticoid Receptor Activation in Chronic Kidney Disease

Aldosterone is a steroidal hormone produced in the adrenal cortex that acts primarily through the mineralocorticoid receptor (MR), a nuclear receptor expressed in both epithelial and non-epithelial tissues [13]. In the distal nephron, aldosterone stimulates sodium reabsorption and potassium excretion by regulating the transcription of the epithelial sodium channel (ENaC), renal outer medullary potassium (ROMK) channel, and other transport proteins [14, 15]. In kidney epithelial cells such as podocytes [16] and proximal tubular cells [17], but also in non-epithelial tissues such as cardiomyocytes, vascular smooth muscle cells, macrophages in the heart [15, 16] and renal mesangial cells [18], MR activation drives inflammation, oxidative stress, and fibrosis [19, 20]. While aldosterone is the primary MR ligand, cortisol, which reaches much higher concentrations, also binds to the MR with equal affinity [19]. In distal tubular epithelial cells, the enzyme 11β-hydroxysteroid dehydrogenase type 2 (11β-HSD2) metabolizes cortisol to inactive cortisone [20]. However, in other cell types, such as cardiomyocytes, podocytes, and macrophages, where 11βHSD2 is absent or minimally expressed, cortisol acts as the main MR ligand [20].

Aldosterone exerts its biological effects through both genomic and non-genomic mechanisms. The classical genomic pathway involves ligand binding to cytosolic MR, followed by translocation of the receptor-ligand complex into the nucleus, where it can regulate gene expression (Fig. 1) [22, 23]. In the distal tubule, this leads to an increased synthesis of transport proteins such as ENaC and the Na^+-K^+-ATPase, typically observed 30–60 minutes after aldosterone release [24]. Recent advances have revealed the critical role of MR co-regulatory molecules in modulating the genomic response. Distinct ligand-dependent conformations of the MR will recruit specific coactivator or corepressor proteins, ultimately determining transcription of specific gene subsets [13, 22]. Thus, different agonist ligands induce unique transcriptional profiles. Various ligand-selective peptides with potent antagonistic activity on MR-mediated transcription that could represent future therapeutic options have already been developed [22]. In addition, aldosterone can also stimulate non-genomic effects, which occur more rapidly (within minutes) and are not inhibited by transcription blockers such as actinomycin D or classical MRAs [25]. These responses, which may or may not be MR-mediated, involve enhanced activity of membrane ion transporters, including Na^+-K^+-$2Cl^-$ co-transporter and Na^+-K^+-ATPase in cardiac tissue, and the Na^+-H^+ exchanger, ENaC, and Na^+-K^+-ATPase in renal tissue, and are linked to subcellular protein trafficking [25].

Several lines of evidence suggest that MR overactivation plays a key role in tissue injury and fibrosis. In the kidney, excessive MR signaling by aldosterone in podocytes, mesangial cells, and monocytes promotes macrophage infiltration [26],

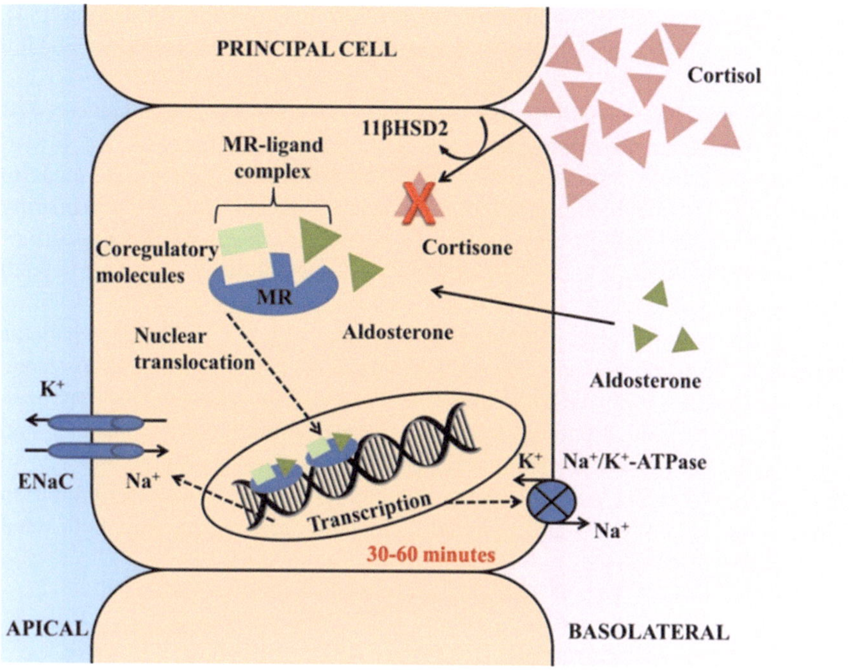

Fig. 1 Actions of aldosterone through activation of the mineralocorticoid receptor (MR) in principal cells of the distal nephron. The MR has comparable affinity for aldosterone and cortisol; however, ligand selectivity in the kidney is ensured by pre-receptor regulation. In tubular epithelial cells, the enzyme 11β-hydroxysteroid dehydrogenase type 2 (11β-HSD2) converts cortisol to inactive cortisone, allowing aldosterone to serve as the primary physiological MR ligand in the distal nephron, despite cortisol's much higher systemic concentrations. Aldosterone diffuses freely across the cell membrane and binds the MR ligand-binding domain, initiating a genomic cascade. Ligand binding prompts recruitment of co-regulatory proteins (coactivators or corepressors) and nuclear translocation of the MR-ligand complex. This ultimately upregulates synthesis of the epithelial sodium channel (ENaC) on the apical membrane and Na^+-K^+-ATPase on the basolateral membrane, promoting sodium reabsorption and potassium excretion. This classical genomic response typically occurs 30–60 minutes after aldosterone release or administration. (From Alexandrou et al. [21] under Creative Commons Attribution 4.0 International License)

collagen deposition, and the development of glomerulosclerosis and interstitial fibrosis [27]. These findings are supported by experimental data in streptozotocin-induced diabetic models, in which overexpression of MR, NADPH oxidase, and collagen I/IV lead to increased glomerular and tubulointerstitial collagen deposition [28]. Notably, stimuli such as angiotensin II, high glucose levels, and low-density lipoprotein (LDL) can induce local aldosterone synthesis in mesangial cells, suggesting a mechanism of autocrine/paracrine MR activation contributing to CKD pathogenesis, particularly in the diabetic setting [29]. Additionally, deficiency of Klotho, which can be present from early stages of CKD, can further enhance aldosterone synthesis [30–32]. MR inhibition with agents such as spironolactone, eplerenone, and finerenone in experimental models of DKD has shown to reduce collagen deposition [33], glomerulosclerosis and macrophage infiltration [34], podocyte injury [35], proteinuria and neutrophil gelatinase-associated lipocalin (NGAL) expression [36].

MR activation has deleterious effects beyond the kidney. In cardiomyocytes, MR signaling promotes hypertrophy, apoptosis, and interstitial fibrosis [24, 37]. In vascular smooth muscle cells and endothelial cells, overactivation of MR leads to impaired nitric oxide bioavailability, vasoconstriction, and vascular remodeling [38]. These systemic effects may explain the beneficial effects of MRAs in cardiovascular mortality in patients with heart failure (HF), which seems to extend beyond blood pressure (BP) reduction.

A key pathophysiological phenomenon associated with MR activation in patients treated with RAS inhibitors is "aldosterone breakthrough," in which aldosterone levels rise despite ACEi/ARB therapy [14, 39, 40]. This phenomenon has been observed in up to half of patients within one year of initiating RAS blockade and may underlie the persistent albuminuria and kidney disease progression seen in many patients receiving standard-of-care therapy [20]. Therefore, direct inhibition of MR signaling represents an important therapeutic target to mitigate both renal and cardiovascular injury.

Steroidal Mineralocorticoid Receptor Antagonists in Chronic Kidney Disease

Spironolactone and eplerenone have been used in clinical practice for several decades, particularly in the management of HF with reduced ejection fraction (HFrEF). Their nephroprotective effects have been extensively studied in patients with CKD and T2D, focusing primarily on their effects on urinary albumin excretion (UAE), a surrogate marker of long-term hard kidney outcomes [14, 41]. These agents act as competitive antagonists at the MR binding site, disrupting aldosterone-mediated transcriptional activity [42]. In the presence of aldosterone, they prevent recruitment of transcriptional coactivators, but in the absence of aldosterone, they exhibit partially agonistic coactivator recruitment properties [19]. Spironolactone is non-selective and binds also to androgen and progesterone receptors, leading to side effects such as gynecomastia, while eplerenone is more selective for MR but has a shorter half-life and lower potency (Table 1). Canrenone, the active metabolite of spironolactone, was expected to have fewer side effects than spironolactone by avoiding intermediate metabolites with antiandrogenic and progestational activity [43]. However, its use was limited by significant hyperkalemia due to low receptor selectivity, similar to first-generation MRAs [44].

Spironolactone

In a pivotal study including 45 T2D patients with urinary albumin to creatinine ratio (UACR) 30–300 mg/g and preserved kidney function (creatinine clearance >60 mL/

Table 1 Major pharmacodynamic properties of the main steroidal and non-steroidal MRAs

	Steroidal MR antagonists		Non-steroidal MR antagonist
	Spironolactone	Eplerenone	Finerenone
Structural properties	Flat (steroidal)	Flat (steroidal)	Bulky (non-steroidal)
Potency to MR	High	Moderate	High
Selectivity to MR	Low	Moderate	High
Tissue distribution	Kidney > heart (at least 6-fold)	Kidney > heart (~3-fold)	Balanced kidney: heart (1:1)
CNS penetration	Yes	Yes	No, based on preclinical data
Sexual side effects	Yes (gynecomastia)	Less than spironolactone	No signal, based on phase III data
Hyperkalemia	Yes	Yes	Moderately increased

min), 40% showed a rise in aldosterone and albuminuria levels, within 40 weeks of follow-up, despite ACEi therapy [45]. Among these, 13 received additional spironolactone 25 mg daily for 24 weeks, which led to notable reductions in albuminuria and left ventricular mass index (LVMI). Another randomized trial in 41 patients with overt proteinuria (>1.5 g/day) compared ramipril alone or in combination with irbesartan and/or spironolactone [46]. Addition of spironolactone to ramipril significantly improved proteinuria reduction (by 42%) compared to addition of irbesartan (by 15.7%), while addition of both agents did not result in further benefit over spironolactone/ramipril combination.

A parallel-group RCT randomized 81 patients on high-dose lisinopril (80 mg) to placebo, losartan 100 mg, or spironolactone 25 mg for 48 weeks [47]. A UACR decline of 34.0% was noted in the spironolactone group compared to a 16.8% in the losartan group, with no differences in creatinine clearance between groups and an increased risk of hyperkalemia for both active treatments. Several other trials confirmed the beneficial effects of spironolactone (25–50 mg) on top of ACEi/ARB therapy in DKD, showing decreases in albuminuria averaging 30–35%, reductions in BP (~6–7/3–4 mmHg), and a transient estimated glomerular filtration rate (eGFR) decline of approximately 3 mL/min/1.73 m^2 [48–57]. The PRIORITY (Proteomic Prediction and Renin Angiotensin Aldosterone System Inhibition Prevention Of Early Diabetic nephropathy In Type 2 Diabetic Patients With Normoalbuminuria) trial evaluated whether the urinary proteomic biomarker "CKD273" could identify T2D patients at high risk of kidney disease progression and whether spironolactone could mitigate this risk [58]. A total of 209 high-risk participants were assigned to spironolactone ($n = 102$) or placebo ($n = 107$), in addition to standard therapy, and were followed for a median of 2.5 years. A high-risk score from the proteomic classifier was indeed associated with increased risk of progression to moderately increased albuminuria (HR 2.48; 95% CI 1.80–3.42; $p < 0.0001$), while in the high-risk cohort, spironolactone did not significantly delay the onset of moderately increased albuminuria (HR 0.81; 95% CI 0.49–1.34). Finally, the recently published BARACK-D (Benefits of Aldosterone Receptor Antagonism in Chronic Kidney Disease) trial examined the effect of spironolactone 25 mg in addition of usual care compared to usual care alone, on cardiovascular outcomes in 1372 CKD patients with eGFR 30–49 mL/min/1.73 m^2 [59]. After 3 years of follow-up, there was no significant difference in the risk of the primary outcome (HR 1.05; 95% CI 0.81–1.37, for spironolactone vs usual care) or any of the individual components of the primary outcome. It should be noted that 62% of participants randomized to spironolactone stopped treatment within 6 months, mainly due to safety issues (eGFR decline, hyperkalemia, participants withdraw due to side effects), leading to the conclusion by the authors that spironolactone should not be used in stage 3b CKD without a specific treatment indication [59].

Eplerenone

In an RCT including 268 T2D patients with UACR ≥50 mg/g already on enalapril, eplerenone 50 and 100 mg reduced UACR by 41.0% and 48.4%, respectively, compared to 7.4% UACR reduction with placebo ($p < 0.001$ for both comparisons) [60]. Notably, there were no between-group BP differences, suggesting a BP-independent anti-proteinuric effect. A smaller trial in 75 T2D patients with UACR 30–300 mg/g compared ramipril or eplerenone monotherapies with their combination [61]. Dual drug therapy resulted in a 70% UACR reduction—significantly greater than monotherapy (37–38%)—though the risk of hyperkalemia was notably higher in patients with eGFR <60 mL/min/1.73 m^2. Similarly, in a secondary analysis of the MIRAD (Mineralocorticoid Receptor Antagonist in type 2 Diabetes) trial in 140 T2D patients with high cardiovascular risk, a 34% UACR decrease was observed with high-dose eplerenone (100 or 200 mg) versus placebo over 26 weeks [62]. Hyperkalemia (≥5.5 mmol/L) episodes did not differ between groups, although a small eGFR decline and a 0.26 mmol/L rise in serum potassium were evident in the eplerenone group.

Canrenone

In a study of 120 T2D patients with uncontrolled BP and UACR 60–300 mg/g, 24-week treatment with canrenone on top of background antihypertensive treatment reduced albuminuria by 45.3% versus 20.3% with hydrochlorothiazide ($p < 0.01$), with similar decreases in 24-h BP in both groups [43]. There was no significant effect on serum creatinine or potassium levels. Another study in 182 patients showed better eGFR preservation and neutral effect on potassium with canrenone compared to hydrochlorothiazide [63].

Non-steroidal Mineralocorticoid Receptor Antagonists in Chronic Kidney Disease

Finerenone is a third-generation, non-steroidal MRA with higher selectivity for the MR and more balanced tissue distribution between the heart and kidneys compared to steroidal MRAs (Table 1). It displays tissue- and ligand-specificity and is characterized by inhibiting the recruitment of co-regulatory molecules independently of aldosterone presence [14]. These properties contribute to more potent inhibition of pro-inflammatory and profibrotic signaling while minimizing the adverse effects typically seen with traditional MRAs, such as excessive potassium retention and BP lowering [19]. Differences in chemical structure between main steroidal and non-steroidal MRAs are shown in Fig. 2. Finerenone is licensed in Europe and United States for nephroprotection and cardioprotection in CKD and T2D. Esaxerenone, which is licensed in Japan for BP management, and apararenone are also selective non-steroidal MRAs with similar properties.

Finerenone

The safety and efficacy of finerenone in DKD were first evaluated in the ARTS-DN (Mineralocorticoid Receptor Antagonist Tolerability Study—Diabetic Nephropathy) study (Table 2). In this randomized, placebo-controlled trial of 821 patients with T2D and moderately or severely increased albuminuria on ACEi/ARB therapy, finerenone showed dose-dependent reductions in the placebo-corrected UACR at three months compared to baseline (0.79, 0.76, 0.67, and 0.62 for doses of 7.5, 10, 15, and 20 mg/day, respectively) [64]. Rates of hyperkalemia leading to discontinuation ranged from 0% to 3.2% across dose groups, indicating good tolerability. The ARTS-DN Japan study in 96 patients with DKD supported these findings, with similar UACR reductions from baseline for finerenone groups and no episodes of hyperkalemia >6.0 mmol/L [65].

Following these studies focusing on albuminuria reduction, two complementary large-scale phase 3 RCTs provided long-term data on hard cardiorenal outcomes, the Finerenone in reducing kidney failure and disease progression in Diabetic Kidney Disease (FIDELIO-DKD) [11] and the Finerenone in reducing cardiovascular mortality and morbidity in Diabetic Kidney Disease (FIGARO-DKD) [12]. FIDELIO-DKD included 5734 patients with T2D and either moderately increased albuminuria (30 to <300 mg/g) and eGFR 25 to <75 mL/min/1.73 m^2 or severely increased albuminuria (300 to ≤5000 mg/g) and eGFR 25 to <60 mL/min/1.73 m^2 and diabetic retinopathy, who received finerenone 10–20 mg or placebo on top of a maximum tolerated dose of RAS blocker [11]. During a median of 2.6 years, finerenone significantly reduced the primary composite kidney outcome (kidney failure, sustained ≥40% eGFR decline, or renal death) compared to placebo (HR 0.82; 95% CI 0.73–0.93), and also the main secondary kidney outcome of kidney failure, sustained ≥57% eGFR decrease or renal death (HR 0.76; 95% CI 0.65–0.90) and secondary cardiovascular outcome of nonfatal myocardial infarction (MI), nonfatal stroke, hospitalization for heart failure (HHF), or cardiovascular death (HR 0.86; 95% CI 0.75–0.99). The mean serum potassium increase in the finerenone group was 0.23 mmol/L and discontinuation due to hyperkalemia reported in 2.3% of patients.

FIGARO-DKD randomized 7437 patients with T2D and either UACR 30 to <300 mg/g and eGFR 25–90 mL/min/1.73 m^2 or UACR 300 to ≤5000 mg/g and

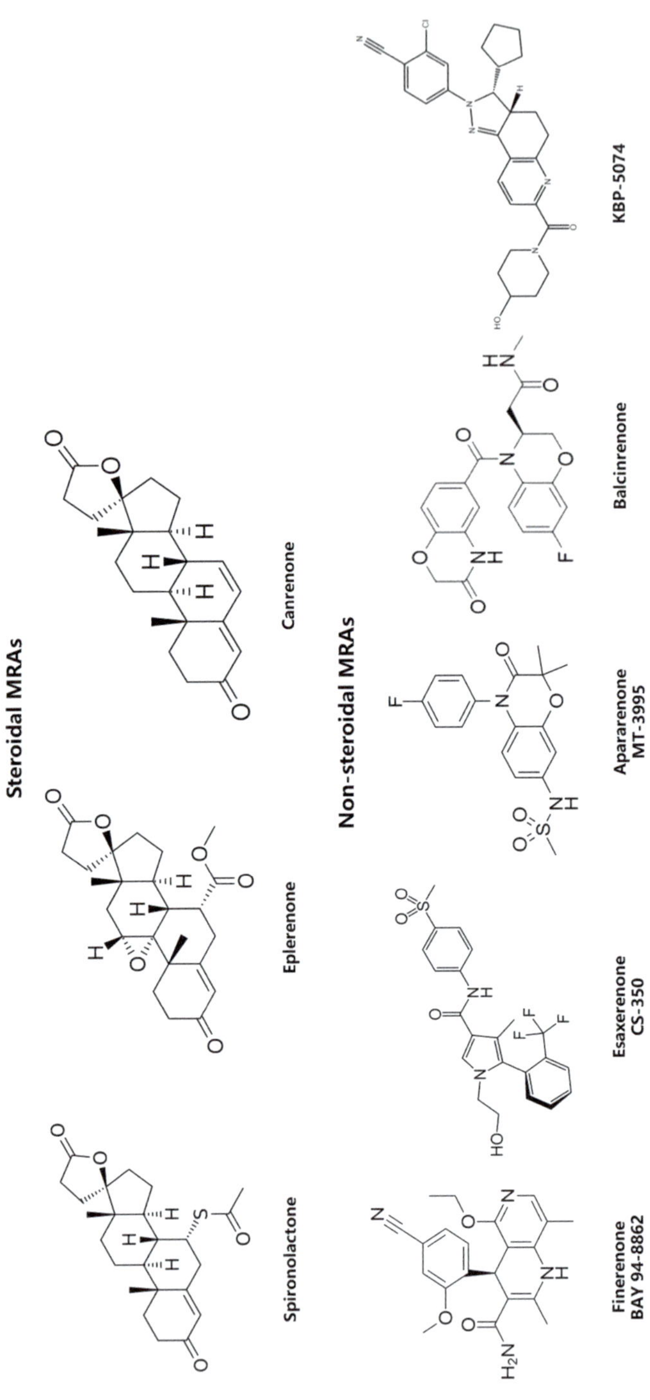

Fig. 2 Chemical structure of non-steroidal and steroidal mineralocorticoid receptor antagonists

Table 2 Main characteristics of RCTs examining the effects of finerenone, esaxerenone, and apararenone in albuminuria, renal, and cardiovascular outcomes in patients with DKD

Study	Study design	Population	No. of patients	Intervention	comparator	Follow up	Key findings
Bakris et al. 2015 (ARTS-DN) [64]	Double blind, parallel-group RCT	T2D and UACR 30 to <300 mg/g or >300 mg/g	821	Finerenone	Placebo	90 days	↓ placebo-corrected mean ratio of UACR at day 90 relative to baseline: Finerenone 7.5 mg 0.79 ($p = 0.004$); 10 mg 0.76 ($p = 0.001$); 15 mg 0.67 ($p < 0.001$); 20 mg 0.62 ($p < 0.001$) Significantly ↑ incidence of hyperK episodes leading to study discontinuation: Finerenone 7.5 mg 2.1%, 15 mg 3.2% and 20 mg 1.7% No difference in the risk of hyperK for placebo and finerenone 10 mg
Katayama et al. 2017 [65]	Double blind, parallel-group RCT	T2D and UACR 30 to <300 mg/g or >300 mg/g	96	Finerenone	Placebo	90 days	↓ LS mean ratio of finerenone to baseline (0.712); LS mean ratio of finerenone to placebo (0.670) for finerenone 20 mg ($p = 0.024$) ↑ K for finerenone (0.025-0.167 mmol/L) vs placebo (−0.075 mmol/L)

(continued)

Table 2 (continued)

Study	Study design	Population	No. of patients	Intervention	comparator	Follow up	Key findings
Bakris et al. 2020 (FIDELIO-DKD) [11]	Double blind, parallel-group RCT	T2D and: (a) UACR 300–5000 mg/g & eGFR 25–75 ml/min/1.73 m^2 or (b) UACR 30–300 mg/g, eGFR 25–60 ml/min/1.73 m^2, diabetic retinopathy	5734	Finerenone	Placebo	2.6 years	Primary composite of kidney failure (ESKD or eGFR <15 ml/min/1.73 m^2), ≥40% eGFR decrease, renal death: HR 0.82; 95% CI 0.73–0.93 Secondary composite of kidney failure (ESKD or eGFR <15 ml/min/1.73 m^2), ≥57% eGFR decrease, renal death: HR 0.76; 95% CI 0.65–0.90 Secondary composite of CV death, nonfatal MI/stroke, HHF: HR 0.86; 95% CI 0.75–0.99 Other secondary: kidney failure HR 0.87; 95% CI 0.72–1.05; ≥40% eGFR decrease HR 0.81; 95% CI 0.72–0.92; CV death HR 0.86; 95% CI 0.68–1.08; nonfatal MI HR 0.80; 95% CI 0.58–1.09; nonfatal stroke: HR 1.03; 95% CI 0.76–1.38; HHF HR 0.86; 95%CI 0.68–1.08 HyperK leading to drug discontinuation: 2.3% finerenone; 0.9% placebo

Pitt et al. 2021 (FIGARO-DKD) [12]	Double blind, parallel-group RCT	T2D and: (a) UACR 30–300 mg/g, eGFR ≥25–90 ml/min/1.73 m2 or (b) UACR 300–5000 mg/g, eGFR ≥60 ml/min/1.73 m2	7437	Finerenone	Placebo	3.4 years	Primary composite of CV death, nonfatal MI/stroke, HHF: HR 0.87; 95% CI 0.76–0.98 Secondary composite of kidney failure (ESKD or eGFR <15 ml/min/1.73 m^2), eGFR decrease of ≥40%, renal death: HR 0.87; 95% CI 0.76–1.01 Other secondary: HHF HR 0.71; 95% CI 0.56–0.90; ESKD HR 0.64, 95% CI 0.41–0.995 HyperK leading to drug discontinuation: 1.2% finerenone; 0.4% placebo
Agarwal et al. 2025 [66]	Double-blind, parallel-group RCT	T2D, UACR 100 to ≤5000 mg/g, eGFR 30–90 ml/min/1.73 m^2	807	Finerenone	Empagliflozin or placebo	6 months	↓ log-transformed UACR: 29% greater for combination than finerenone alone (LS mean ratio of the difference in the change from baseline, 0.71; 95% CI 0.61-0.82; $p < 0.001$); 32% greater for combination than empagliflozin alone (LS mean ratio of the difference in the change from baseline, 0.68; 95% CI 0.59-0.79; $p < 0.001$)
Ito et al. 2019 [67]	Double-blind, parallel-group RCT	T2D, UACR 45–300 mg/g, eGFR≥30 ml/min/1.73 m^2	365	Esaxerenone	Placebo	12 weeks	↓ UACR: −38% for esaxerenone 1.25 mg, −50% for 2.5 mg, −56% for 5 mg, −7% for placebo ($p < 0.001$) Remission of albuminuria: 21% for esaxerenone groups 2.5 and 5 mg; 3% for placebo ($p < 0.05$ for both comparisons) HyperK leading to drug discontinuation: 3% for esaxerenone 1.25 and 2.5 mg, 10% for 10 mg; 1% for placebo

(continued)

Table 2 (continued)

Study	Study design	Population	No. of patients	Intervention	comparator	Follow up	Key findings
Ito et al. 2020 (ESAX-DN) [68]	Double-blind, parallel-group RCT	T2D, UACR 45–300 mg/g, eGFR≥30 ml/min/1.73 m^2	455	Esaxerenone	Placebo	52 weeks	↓ UACR: −58% for esaxerenone; +8% for placebo ($p < 0.001$); eGFR: −11% for esaxerenone; −1% for placebo Remission of albuminuria: 22% for esaxerenone; 4% for placebo ($p < 0.001$) Time to first transition to overt proteinuria: HR 0.23; 95% CI 0.11–0.48 for esaxerenone HyperK episodes (>6.0 mmol/L or ≥5.5 mmol/L at two consecutive occasions): 9% for esaxerenone; 2% for placebo ($p = 0.002$) HyperK leading to drug discontinuation: 4% for esaxerenone; 1% for placebo
Ito et al. 2021 [69]	Open label, single-arm study	T2D,UACR ≥300 mg/g, eGFR≥30 ml/min/1.73 m^2	807	Esaxerenone	–	28 weeks	↓ UACR: −54.6% ($p < 0.001$); eGFR −8.3 mL/min /1.73 m2 for esaxerenone HyperK episodes (>6.0 mmol/L or ≥5.5 mmol/L at two consecutive occasions): 5.4% for esaxerenone

Wada et al. 2021 [70]	Double-blind, parallel-group RCT with open-label extension	T2D, UACR 50–300 mg/g	293	Apararenone	Placebo	24 weeks & 28 weeks	↓ UACR at 23 weeks: −62.9% for apararenone 2.5 mg; −50.8% for apararenone 5 mg; −46.5% for apararenone 10 mg; +113.7% for placebo ($p < 0.001$ versus placebo for all comparisons) Change in eGFR at 52 weeks: −5.3% (−22.0, +10.5) for apararenone 2.5 mg; −10.2% (−34.5, +14.6) for apararenone 5 mg; −10.80% (− 36.8, +19.1) for apararenone 10 mg ↑ K at 52 weeks: +0.14 mmol/L (0.006–0.22) for apararenone 2.5 mg; +0.18 mmol/L (0.1–0.26) for apararenone 5 mg; +0.25 mmol/L (0.16–0.33) for apararenone 10 mg

ACEi angiotensin converting enzyme inhibitor, *ARB* angiotensin receptor blocker, *CI* confidence interval, *CV* cardiovascular, *DKD* diabetic kidney disease, *eGFR* estimated glomerular filtration rate, *ESKD* end-stage kidney disease, *HHF* hospitalization for heart failure, *hyperK* hyperkalemia, *HR* hazard ratio, *K* potassium, *LS* least-squares, *MI* myocardial infarction, *RCT* randomized controlled trial, *T2D* type 2 diabetes, *UACR* urinary albumin creatinine ratio

eGFR ≥60 mL/min/1.73 m^2 to finerenone 10–20 mg or placebo [12]. After a follow-up of 3.4 years, finerenone significantly reduced the risk for the primary cardiovascular outcome (HR 0.87; 95% CI 0.76–0.98), including a notable 29% lower risk for HHF events (HR 0.71; 95% CI 0.56–0.90). A non-significantly lower risk for the key secondary kidney outcome was observed in the finerenone group compared to placebo (HR 0.87; 95% CI 0.76–1.01), with significantly lower rates of kidney failure (HR 0.64; 95% CI 0.41–0.995). Discontinuation due to hyperkalemia was 1.2% vs 0.4 in finerenone and placebo groups, respectively.

The pre-specified pooled analysis of both finerenone trials, FIDELITY, combining 13,171 participants, confirmed a significant 14% reduction in the risk for the composite cardiovascular outcome (HR 0.86; 95% CI 0.78–0.95) and a significantly 23% lower risk for the composite kidney outcome of kidney failure, sustained ≥57% eGFR decrease or renal death (HR 0.77; 95% CI 0.67–0.88) [71]. Among the individual components of the composite kidney outcome, there was evidence of a 30% risk reduction of sustained ≥57% eGFR decline from baseline (HR 0.70; 95% CI 0.60–0.83) and 20% of kidney failure (HR 0.80; 95% CI 0.64–0.99). Hyperkalemia-related drug discontinuation occurred in 1.7% vs 0.6% in the finerenone and placebo groups. Additionally, a FIDELITY on-treatment analysis reported reduced risk for all-cause (HR 0.82; 95% CI 0.70–0.96) and cardiovascular mortality (HR 0.82; 95% CI 0.67–0.99) with finerenone compared to placebo [72]. A recent pre-specified FIDELITY analysis examining the efficacy and safety of finerenone in 870 participants with stage 4 CKD showed a non-significantly lower risk for the composite cardiovascular outcome with finerenone compared to placebo (HR 0.78; 95% CI 0.57–1.07) and a significantly lower risk for the kidney composite outcome only for the first 2 years (after this time-point the direction of the association was inconsistent) [73].

Further secondary analyses from FIDELIO-DKD showed that apart from the benefit derived from HHF risk reduction, finerenone significantly reduced the risk of new-onset atrial fibrillation (AF) (HR 0.71; 95% CI 0.53–0.94), which is particularly important due to the high stroke risk associated with AF in CKD populations [74]. Finally, the potential influence of sodium-glucose co-transporter 2 inhibitors (SGLT2i), agents with proven cardiorenal benefits in this population, was explored in another FIDELITY subgroup analysis including patients on SGLT2i at baseline or during the trial. A similar risk for the primary kidney composite and secondary kidney and cardiovascular outcomes was observed between patients with or without SGLT2i use (p-interaction = 0.21, 0.54 and 0.46, respectively), while fewer hyperkalemia-related adverse events were reported with concomitant SGLT2i use [75]. In the recently published CONFIDENCE trial (Combination effect of finerenone and empagliflozin in participants with CKD and type 2 diabetes using a UACR Endpoint), examining the concomitant use of finerenone with empagliflozin, participants with eGFR 30–90 mL/min/1.73 m^2, UACR of 100 to ≤5000 mg/g and T2D were randomly assigned to a 1:1:1 ratio to receive finerenone, empagliflozin or both. Combination therapy led to a 29% greater UACR reduction after 6 months compared to finerenone alone and 32% compared to empaglifozin alone (Fig. 3), supporting the notion that these drug

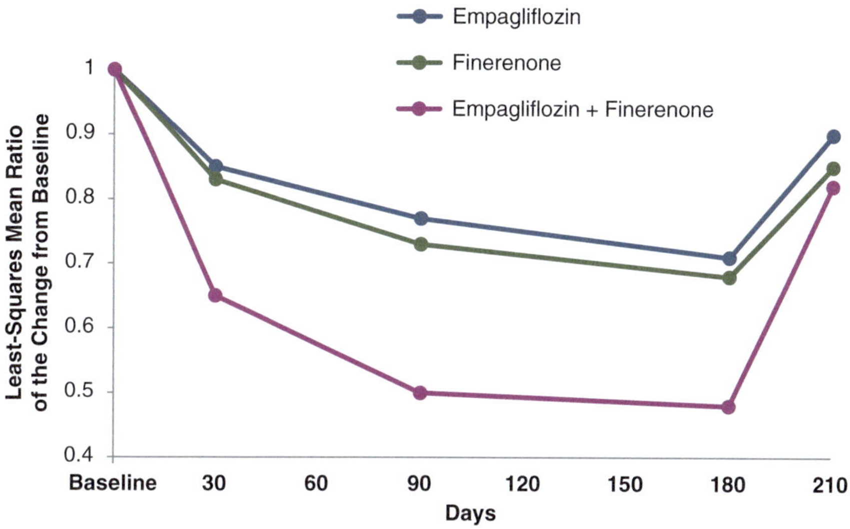

Fig. 3 Change in Urinary Albumin-to-Creatinine Ratio (UACR) in the three treatment groups examined in the CONFIDENCE trial. Note: trial medication was discontinued at 180 days after randomization and UACR was measured again 30 days later

classes have complementary actions and can offer additive benefits in patients with T2D and CKD [66]. Importantly, the combination was well tolerated; discontinuations due to symptomatic hypotension, AKI, or hyperkalemia were rare.

In the recently published Finerenone in Non-Diabetic CKD (FIND-CKD) trial, 1584 participants with CKD without diabetes, eGFR 25 to <90 mL/min/1.73 m² and UACR 200–3500 mg/g receiving RAS blockade were randomized to finerenone (10–20 mg daily) or placebo. Over 32 months, finerenone led to a significantly slower eGFR decline, with a total eGFR slope of −3.3 versus −4.0 mL/min/1.73 m²/year in the placebo group, corresponding to a between-group difference of 0.7 mL/min/1.73 m²/year (95% CI 0.3–1.1, $p < 0.001$). Finerenone also significantly reduced the risk of the composite kidney or cardiovascular outcome (sustained ≥57% eGFR decline, kidney failure, hospitalization for heart failure, or cardiovascular death) compared with placebo (HR 0.77; 95% CI 0.60–0.99). Hyperkalemia was more frequent with finerenone (17.0% vs 13.3%), although treatment discontinuation due to hyperkalemia remained uncommon (1.5% vs 0.1%), and hyperkalemia-related hospitalization was rare (0.9% vs 0.6%) [76]. A prespecified exploratory analysis of the 903 participants with glomerular diseases, demonstrated consistent effects; finerenone reduced the annualized eGFR decline by 0.73 mL/min/1.73 m² per year (95% CI 0.22–1.24), albuminuria by 42% at 12 months, and risk of kidney failure or sustained ≥40% eGFR decline by 26% (HR 0.74; 95% CI 0.57–0.97) compared with placebo [77]. Finally, in the prespecified INFINITY individual participant data pooled analysis, combining data from 14,574 participants, finerenone showed a 24% reduction in the composite kidney outcome of kidney failure or sustained ≥57% eGFR decline (HR 0.76; 95% CI 0.68–0.86), a 20% reduction in the composite cardiovascular outcome (HR 0.80; 95% CI 0.70–0.91), and a significant reduction in all-cause mortality (HR 0.88; 95% CI 0.79–0.99) versus placebo, with consistent treatment effects across CKD etiologies, baseline eGFR, albuminuria, glycemic status, and SGLT2 inhibitor use [78]. The above analyses confirm that the cardiorenal benefits of finerenone extend across a wide range of CKD aetiologies irrespective of diabetes status.

Other Non-steroidal MRAs

Esaxerenone has been previously tested in a phase 2b trial of 365 patients with T2D, UACR ≥45 to <300 mg/g and eGFR ≥30 mL/min/1.73 m^2 against placebo. A significant dose-dependent UACR decrease (21% to 56%) was found across esaxerenone groups (0.625 to 5 mg/day) compared to placebo [67]. In the ESAX-DN (Esaxerenone (CS-3150) in Patients with Type 2 Diabetes and Microalbuminuria) phase 3 trial, 455 patients received esaxerenone (1.25–2.5 mg/day) or placebo for 52 weeks. UACR decreased by 58% in the esaxerenone group versus an 8% increase in placebo ($p < 0.001$), while 22% of patients achieved remission of albuminuria. Hyperkalemia ≥6.0 mmol/L occurred in 9% of esaxerenone patients, leading to treatment discontinuation in 4% [68].

Apararenone was studied in a phase 2 RCT including 293 Japanese patients with T2D and UACR 50–300 mg/g [70]. Participants received apararenone 2.5, 5, or 10 mg/day or placebo and, after 24 weeks, significant UACR reductions were observed with apararenone, ranging from 46.5% to 62.9% across doses ($p < 0.001$ compared to placebo). Remission to UACR <30 mg/g and ≥30% reduction was observed in up to 29% of participants. The extension study confirmed sustained efficacy over 52 weeks. Serum potassium increased by 0.14–0.25 mmol/L with no severe adverse events [70].

Potential Mechanisms for the Nephroprotective Actions of Mineralocorticoid Receptor Antagonists

In contrast to conventional dual RAS blockade that failed to show additional cardiorenal benefit and was abandoned due to increased adverse events [6, 7], non-steroidal MRAs, and particularly finerenone, administered on top of single RAS blockade, demonstrated both safety and added efficacy. Two principal contributing mechanisms have been proposed. First, MRAs exert a modest hemodynamic effect that reduces intraglomerular pressure. In the FIDELIO-DKD trial, an early 40% decline in UACR in the finerenone group was accompanied by an early drop in eGFR, followed by a slower rate of eGFR decline. These findings are consistent with reduced intraglomerular hypertension [11], suggesting a similar mechanism of action with SGLT2i and ACEi/ARBs [79, 80]. The hemodynamic contribution of finerenone appears more substantial than that seen in dual RAS blockade trials, which typically lacked a consistent early eGFR dip and resulted in smaller UACR reductions

(11–20% difference between intervention and placebo groups) [6, 7]. In contrast, finerenone-induced UACR reductions ranged from 25–39%, suggesting a stronger impact on intraglomerular dynamics. Albuminuria reduction itself prevents activation of pro-inflammatory and profibrotic pathways in tubular cells, mitigates Klotho loss, and decreases proximal tubular metabolic burden [30, 81, 82].

The second mechanism involves the pro-inflammatory and profibrotic actions mediated by MR transcriptional activity. MR overactivation contributes to kidney inflammation and fibrosis via upregulation of pro-inflammatory gene transcription. In preclinical diabetic models, MRAs reduced collagen accumulation [33], prevented macrophage infiltration [34], and attenuated podocyte injury and glomerulosclerosis [35]. MR antagonism may also preserve Klotho expression, which is critical in limiting aldosterone-induced, RAS-independent cardiorenal damage [32, 83]. Finerenone can prevent aldosterone-induced nuclear MR accumulation and inhibit recruitment of steroid receptor coactivator-1 and RNA polymerase II to MR target genes, thereby modulating downstream gene expression differently than spironolactone or eplerenone [84]. Additionally, in contrast to steroidal MRAs, which paradoxically activate the S810L mutant MR associated with early-onset hypertension, finerenone acts as a pure antagonist, emphasizing its superior receptor profile. Comparative studies further support finerenone's superior anti-inflammatory and antifibrotic potency relative to natriuretic-equivalent doses of eplerenone [85].

Finally, preclinical data suggest a favorable role for non-steroidal MRAs in AKI settings. In ischemia/reperfusion models, MR antagonism decreased oxidative stress and restored endothelin-B receptor and endothelial nitric oxide synthase (eNOS) signaling [86]. MRAs also appeared to mitigate the AKI-to-CKD transition by reducing M1 macrophage infiltration and promoting IL-4-dependent polarization to M2 repair phenotypes, suggesting a protective immunomodulatory effect [87].

Clinical Applications and Future Perspectives

Several scientific societies have incorporated the use of finerenone in recent guidelines for patients with CKD and T2D. The 2023 European Renal Best Practice (ERBP) board of the European Renal Association (ERA) clinical practice document suggests use of finerenone in patients with CKD and T2D with eGFR >25 ml/min/1.73 m2, moderately or severely increased albuminuria and serum potassium ≤4.8 mmol/L, on top of an ACEi/ARB in maximum tolerated doses and independently of the use of an SGLT2i [88]. The 2023 ESH guidelines recommend finerenone, with class and level of evidence 1A, in patients with CKD and albuminuria associated with T2D if eGFR is at least 25 ml/min/1.73 m^2 and serum potassium <5.0 mmo/L [89]. The Kidney Disease: Improving Global Outcomes (KDIGO) 2022 guidelines for diabetes management in CKD [90], KDIGO 2024 guidelines for the evaluation and management of CKD [91], as well as American Diabetes Association (ADA) recommendations for cardiovascular disease and risk management [92], suggest the use of finerenone in patients with T2D, eGFR >25 ml/min per 1.73 m^2, normal serum potassium concentration, and albuminuria despite maximum tolerated dose of RAS blockade. The 2023 ESC Guidelines for the management of cardiovascular disease in patients with diabetes also recommend use of finerenone in patients with T2D and CKD to reduce CV events and kidney failure [93].

Future directions in MRA therapy may include broader indications beyond CKD patients with T2D and establishment of combination strategies with SGLT2i. The phase 3 Trial to Learn How Well Finerenone Works and How Safe it is in Adult Participants With Non diabetic Chronic Kidney Disease (FIND-CKD; NCT05047263) examined the effect of finerenone versus placebo on top of a RAS blocker in patients with non-diabetic albuminuric CKD [94]. The phase 3 Study to Learn How Well the Study Treatment Finerenone Works and How Safe it is in People With Long term Decrease in the Kidneys' Ability to Work Properly (Chronic Kidney Disease) Together With Type 1 Diabetes (FINE-ONE, NCT05901831) evaluated the efficacy of finerenone in patients with type 1 diabetes, UACR $\geq$200 to < 5000 mg/g and eGFR of $\geq$25 to < 90 ml/min/1.73 m^2, and the Study to Learn More About How Well the Study Treatment Finerenone Works, How Safe it is, How it Moves Into, Through, and Out of the Body, and the Effects it Has on the Body When Taken With an ACE Inhibitor or Angiotensin Receptor Blocker in Children With Chronic Kidney Disease and Proteinuria (FIONA, NCT05196035) will examine the use of finerenone in children with CKD and proteinuria. Additionally, following the recently published trial of finerenone in patients with HF and EF $\geq$40% [95], which demonstrated a significantly lower risk of a composite of worsening HF events and cardiovascular death than placebo and ongoing trials including patients with HF with preserved EF (A Study to Evaluate Finerenone on Clinical Efficacy and Safety in Patients with Heart Failure Who Are Intolerant or Not Eligible for Treatment with Steroidal Mineralocorticoid Receptor Antagonists, (FINALITY HF, NCT06033950); A Study to Determine the Efficacy and Safety of Finerenone and SGLT2i in Combination in Hospitalized Patients with Heart Failure, (CONFIDENCE-HF, NCT06024746)), non-steroidal MRAs may further expand their use in several clinical settings. Finally, long-term safety monitoring and real-world data will be essential to fully characterize the benefit-risk profile of MRAs in diverse populations.

Conclusions

Despite the widespread use of RAS blockers in patients with CKD as a standard-of-care for many decades, and the more recent recognition of SGLT2i as new agents with additional benefit, an important residual risk of adverse cardiovascular and kidney events remains in this population. MR antagonism represents a compelling strategy for reducing cardiorenal risk in patients with CKD, particularly those with T2D. While traditional steroidal MRAs provide important anti-albuminuric benefits limited by adverse effects, non-steroidal agents, and especially finerenone, have redefined the therapeutic landscape. Based on distinct pharmacodynamic properties, such as greater selectivity and better affinity for the MR, as well as more balanced distribution between heart and kidneys, and supported by robust clinical evidence, finerenone represents a safe and effective measure to slow CKD progression and reduce cardiovascular morbidity. Incorporation of finerenone into guideline-directed care marks a new era in the management of DKD, with ongoing research promising to extend these benefits to broader populations.

References

1. Jager KJ, Kovesdy C, Langham R, Rosenberg M, Jha V, Zoccali C. A single number for advocacy and communication-worldwide more than 850 million individuals have kidney diseases. Nephrol Dial Transplant. 2019;34:1803–5.
2. Saeedi P, Petersohn I, Salpea P, Malanda B, Karuranga S, Unwin N, et al. Global and regional diabetes prevalence estimates for 2019 and projections for 2030 and 2045: Results from the International Diabetes Federation Diabetes Atlas, 9th edition. Diabetes Res Clin Pract. 2019;157:107843.
3. Afkarian M, Sachs MC, Kestenbaum B, Hirsch IB, Tuttle KR, Himmelfarb J, et al. Kidney disease and increased mortality risk in type 2 diabetes. J Am Soc Nephrol. 2013;24:302–8.
4. Alicic RZ, Rooney MT, Tuttle KR. Diabetic kidney disease: challenges, Progress, and possibilities. Clin J Am Soc Nephrol. 2017;12:2032–45.
5. Sarafidis P, Papadopoulos CE, Kamperidis V, Giannakoulas G, Doumas M. Cardiovascular protection with sodium-glucose Cotransporter-2 inhibitors and mineralocorticoid receptor antagonists in chronic kidney disease: a milestone achieved. Hypertension. 2021;77:1442–55.
6. Parving HH, Brenner BM, McMurray JJ, de Zeeuw D, Haffner SM, Solomon SD, et al. Cardiorenal end points in a trial of aliskiren for type 2 diabetes. N Engl J Med. 2012;367:2204–13.
7. Fried LF, Emanuele N, Zhang JH, Brophy M, Conner TA, Duckworth W, et al. Combined angiotensin inhibition for the treatment of diabetic nephropathy. N Engl J Med. 2013;369:1892–903.
8. Mullens W, Damman K, Testani JM, Martens P, Mueller C, Lassus J, et al. Evaluation of kidney function throughout the heart failure trajectory – a position statement from the Heart Failure Association of the European Society of cardiology. Eur J Heart Fail. 2020;22:584–603.
9. Alexandrou M-E, Papagianni A, Tsapas A, Loutradis C, Boutou A, Piperidou A, et al. Effects of mineralocorticoid receptor antagonists in proteinuric kidney disease: a systematic review and meta-analysis of randomized controlled trials. J Hypertens. 2019;37:2307–24.
10. Trevisan M, de Deco P, Xu H, Evans M, Lindholm B, Bellocco R, et al. Incidence, predictors and clinical management of hyperkalaemia in new users of mineralocorticoid receptor antagonists. Eur J Heart Fail. 2018;20:1217–26.
11. Bakris GL, Agarwal R, Anker SD, Pitt B, Ruilope LM, Rossing P, et al. Effect of Finerenone on chronic kidney disease outcomes in type 2 diabetes. N Engl J Med. 2020;383:2219–29.
12. Pitt B, Filippatos G, Agarwal R, Anker SD, Bakris GL, Rossing P, et al. Cardiovascular events with Finerenone in kidney disease and type 2 diabetes. N Engl J Med. 2021;385:2252–63.
13. Gomez-Sanchez E, Gomez-Sanchez CE. The multifaceted mineralocorticoid receptor. Compr Physiol. 2014;4:965–94.
14. Sarafidis PA, Memmos E, Alexandrou M-E, Papagianni A. Mineralocorticoid receptor antagonists for Nephroprotection: current evidence and future perspectives. Curr Pharm Des. 2018;24:5528–36.
15. Shibata S, Rinehart J, Zhang J, Moeckel G, Castañeda-Bueno M, Stiegler AL, et al. Mineralocorticoid receptor phosphorylation regulates ligand binding and renal response to volume depletion and hyperkalemia. Cell Metab. 2013;18:660–71.
16. Shibata S, Nagase M, Yoshida S, Kawachi H, Fujita T. Podocyte as the target for aldosterone: roles of oxidative stress and Sgk1. Hypertension. 2007;49:355–64.

17. Patni H, Mathew JT, Luan L, Franki N, Chander PN, Singhal PC. Aldosterone promotes proximal tubular cell apoptosis: role of oxidative stress. Am J Physiol Renal Physiol. 2007;293:F1065–71.
18. Terada Y, Kobayashi T, Kuwana H, Tanaka H, Inoshita S, Kuwahara M, et al. Aldosterone stimulates proliferation of mesangial cells by activating mitogen-activated protein kinase 1/2, cyclin D1, and cyclin a. J Am Soc Nephrol. 2005;16:2296–305.
19. Agarwal R, Kolkhof P, Bakris G, Bauersachs J, Haller H, Wada T, et al. Steroidal and non-steroidal mineralocorticoid receptor antagonists in cardiorenal medicine. Eur Heart J. 2021;42:152–61.
20. Barrera-Chimal J, Girerd S, Jaisser F. Mineralocorticoid receptor antagonists and kidney diseases: pathophysiological basis. Kidney Int. 2019;96:302–19.
21. Alexandrou M-E, Theodorakopoulou MP, Sarafidis PA. Role of mineralocorticoid receptor antagonists in diabetic kidney disease. Kidney Dial. 2022;2:163–82.
22. Yang J, Chang C, Safi R, Morgan J, McDonnell DP, Fuller PJ, et al. Identification of ligand-selective peptide antagonists of the mineralocorticoid receptor using phage display. Mol Endocrinol. 2011;25:32–43.
23. Viengchareun S, Le Menuet D, Martinerie L, Munier M, Pascual-Le Tallec L, Lombès M. The mineralocorticoid receptor: insights into its molecular and (patho)physiological biology. Nucl Recept Signal. 2007;5:e012.
24. Hermidorff MM, de Assis LVM, Isoldi MC. Genomic and rapid effects of aldosterone: what we know and do not know thus far. Heart Fail Rev. 2017;22:65–89.
25. Ruhs S, Nolze A, Hübschmann R, Grossmann C. 30 years of the mineralocorticoid receptor: nongenomic effects via the mineralocorticoid receptor. J Endocrinol. 2017;234:T107–24.
26. Rocha R, Rudolph AE, Frierdich GE, Nachowiak DA, Kekec BK, Blomme EAG, et al. Aldosterone induces a vascular inflammatory phenotype in the rat heart. Am J Physiol Heart Circ Physiol. 2002;283:H1802–10.
27. Greene EL, Kren S, Hostetter TH. Role of aldosterone in the remnant kidney model in the rat. J Clin Invest. 1996;98:1063–8.
28. Taira M, Toba H, Murakami M, Iga I, Serizawa R, Murata S, et al. Spironolactone exhibits direct renoprotective effects and inhibits renal renin-angiotensin-aldosterone system in diabetic rats. Eur J Pharmacol. 2008;589:264–71.
29. Nishikawa T, Matsuzawa Y, Suematsu S, Saito J, Omura M, Kino T. Effect of atorvastatin on aldosterone production induced by glucose, LDL or angiotensin II in human renal mesangial cells. Arzneimittelforschung. 2010;60:445–51.
30. Fernandez-Fernandez B, Izquierdo MC, Valiño-Rivas L, Nastou D, Sanz AB, Ortiz A, et al. Albumin downregulates Klotho in tubular cells. Nephrol Dial Transplant. 2018;33:1712–22.
31. Voelkl J, Alesutan I, Leibrock CB, Quintanilla-Martinez L, Kuhn V, Feger M, et al. Spironolactone ameliorates PIT1-dependent vascular osteoinduction in klotho-hypomorphic mice. J Clin Invest. 2013;123:812–22.
32. Zhou X, Chen K, Wang Y, Schuman M, Lei H, Sun Z. Antiaging gene klotho regulates adrenal CYP11B2 expression and aldosterone synthesis. J Am Soc Nephrol. 2016;27:1765–76.
33. Fujisawa G, Okada K, Muto S, Fujita N, Itabashi N, Kusano E, et al. Spironolactone prevents early renal injury in streptozotocin-induced diabetic rats. Kidney Int. 2004;66:1493–502.
34. Han S-Y, Kim C-H, Kim H-S, Jee Y-H, Song H-K, Lee M-H, et al. Spironolactone prevents diabetic nephropathy through an anti-inflammatory mechanism in type 2 diabetic rats. J Am Soc Nephrol. 2006;17:1362–72.
35. Kang YS, Ko GJ, Lee MH, Song HK, Han SY, Han KH, et al. Effect of eplerenone, enalapril and their combination treatment on diabetic nephropathy in type II diabetic rats. Nephrol Dial Transplant. 2009;24:73–84.
36. Lachaux M, Barrera-Chimal J, Nicol L, Rémy-Jouet I, Renet S, Dumesnil A, et al. Short- and long-term administration of the non-steroidal mineralocorticoid receptor antagonist finerenone opposes metabolic syndrome-related cardio-renal dysfunction. Diabetes Obes Metab. 2018;20:2399–407.

37. Nagase M, Ayuzawa N, Kawarazaki W, Ishizawa K, Ueda K, Yoshida S, et al. Oxidative stress causes mineralocorticoid receptor activation in rat cardiomyocytes: role of small GTPase Rac1. Hypertension. 2012;59:500–6.
38. Chai W, Garrelds IM, de Vries R, Batenburg WW, van Kats JP, Danser AHJ. Nongenomic effects of aldosterone in the human heart: interaction with angiotensin II. Hypertension. 2005;46:701–6.
39. Bomback AS, Klemmer PJ. The incidence and implications of aldosterone breakthrough. Nat Clin Pract Nephrol. 2007;3:486–92.
40. Sarafidis PA, Ruilope LM. Cardiorenal disease development under chronic renin-angiotensin-aldosterone system suppression. J Renin-Angiotensin-Aldosterone Syst. 2012;13:217–9.
41. Sarafidis PA, Ruilope LM. Aggressive blood pressure reduction and renin-angiotensin system blockade in chronic kidney disease: time for re-evaluation? Kidney Int. 2014;85:536–46.
42. Rogerson FM, Yao Y, Smith BJ, Fuller PJ. Differences in the determinants of eplerenone, spironolactone and aldosterone binding to the mineralocorticoid receptor. Clin Exp Pharmacol Physiol. 2004;31:704–9.
43. Fogari R, Derosa G, Zoppi A, Lazzari P, D'Angelo A, Mugellini A. Comparative effect of canrenone or hydrochlorothiazide addition to valsartan/amlodipine combination on urinary albumin excretion in well-controlled type 2 diabetic hypertensive patients with microalbuminuria. Expert Opin Pharmacother. 2014;15:453–9.
44. Gomez-Sanchez EP. Third-generation mineralocorticoid receptor antagonists: why do we need a fourth? J Cardiovasc Pharmacol. 2016;67:26–38.
45. Sato A, Hayashi K, Naruse M, Saruta T. Effectiveness of aldosterone blockade in patients with diabetic nephropathy. Hypertension. 2003;41:64–8.
46. Chrysostomou A, Pedagogos E, MacGregor L, Becker GJ. Double-blind, placebo-controlled study on the effect of the aldosterone receptor antagonist spironolactone in patients who have persistent proteinuria and are on long-term angiotensin-converting enzyme inhibitor therapy, with or without an angiotensin II receptor blocker. Clin J Am Soc Nephrol. 2006;1:256–62.
47. Mehdi UF, Adams-Huet B, Raskin P, Vega GL, Toto RD. Addition of angiotensin receptor blockade or mineralocorticoid antagonism to maximal angiotensin-converting enzyme inhibition in diabetic nephropathy. J Am Soc Nephrol. 2009;20:2641–50.
48. Schjoedt KJ, Rossing K, Juhl TR, Boomsma F, Tarnow L, Rossing P, et al. Beneficial impact of spironolactone on nephrotic range albuminuria in diabetic nephropathy. Kidney Int. 2006;70:536–42.
49. Rossing K, Schjoedt KJ, Smidt UM, Boomsma F, Parving HH. Beneficial effects of adding spironolactone to recommended antihypertensive treatment in diabetic nephropathy: a randomized, double-masked, cross-over study. Diabetes Care. 2005;28:2106–12.
50. Schjoedt KJ, Rossing K, Juhl TR, Boomsma F, Rossing P, Tarnow L, et al. Beneficial impact of spironolactone in diabetic nephropathy. Kidney Int. 2005;68:2829–36.
51. van den Meiracker AH, Baggen RG, Pauli S, Lindemans A, Vulto AG, Poldermans D, et al. Spironolactone in type 2 diabetic nephropathy: effects on proteinuria, blood pressure and renal function. J Hypertens. 2006;24:2285–92.
52. Ziaee A, Abbas Vaezi A, Oveisi S, Javadi A, Hashemipour S, Kazemifar AM. Effects of additive therapy with spironolactone on albuminuria in diabetes mellitus: a pilot randomized clinical trial. Caspian J Intern Med. 2013;4:648–53.
53. Hase M, Babazono T, Ujihara N, Uchigata Y. Comparison of spironolactone and trichlormethiazide as add-on therapy to renin-angiotensin blockade for reduction of albuminuria in diabetic patients. J Diabetes Investig. 2013;4:316–9.
54. Esteghamati A, Noshad S, Jarrah S, Mousavizadeh M, Khoee SH, Nakhjavani M. Long-term effects of addition of mineralocorticoid receptor antagonist to angiotensin II receptor blocker in patients with diabetic nephropathy: a randomized clinical trial. Nephrol Dial Transplant. 2013;28:2823–33.
55. Oxlund CS, Henriksen JE, Tarnow L, Schousboe K, Gram J, Jacobsen IA. Low dose spironolactone reduces blood pressure in patients with resistant hypertension and type 2 diabetes mellitus: a double blind randomized clinical trial. J Hypertens. 2013;31:2094–102.

56. Kato S, Maruyama S, Makino H, Wada J, Ogawa D, Uzu T, et al. Anti-albuminuric effects of spironolactone in patients with type 2 diabetic nephropathy: a multicenter, randomized clinical trial. Clin Exp Nephrol. 2015;19:1098–106.
57. Chen Y, Liu P, Chen X, Li Y, Zhang F, Wang Y. Effects of different doses of Irbesartan combined with spironolactone on urinary albumin excretion rate in elderly patients with early type 2 diabetic nephropathy. Am J Med Sci. 2018;355:418–24.
58. Tofte N, Lindhardt M, Adamova K, Bakker SJL, Beige J, Beulens JWJ, et al. Early detection of diabetic kidney disease by urinary proteomics and subsequent intervention with spironolactone to delay progression (PRIORITY): a prospective observational study and embedded randomised placebo-controlled trial. Lancet Diabetes Endocrinol. 2020;8:301–12.
59. Hobbs FDR, McManus RJ, Taylor CJ, Jones NR, Rahman JK, Wolstenholme J, et al. Low-dose spironolactone and cardiovascular outcomes in moderate stage chronic kidney disease: a randomized controlled trial. Nat Med. 2024;30:3634–45.
60. Epstein M, Williams GH, Weinberger M, Lewin A, Krause S, Mukherjee R, et al. Selective aldosterone blockade with eplerenone reduces albuminuria in patients with type 2 diabetes. Clin J Am Soc Nephrol. 2006;1:940–51.
61. El Mokadem M, Abd El Hady Y, Aziz A. A prospective single-blind randomized trial of Ramipril, Eplerenone and their combination in type 2 diabetic nephropathy. Cardiorenal Med. 2020;10:392–401.
62. Brandt-Jacobsen NH, Johansen ML, Rasmussen J, Forman JL, Holm MR, Faber J, et al. Effect of high-dose mineralocorticoid receptor antagonist eplerenone on urinary albumin excretion in patients with type 2 diabetes and high cardiovascular risk: data from the MIRAD trial. Diabetes Metab. 2021;47:101190.
63. Derosa G, Gaudio G, Pasini G, D'Angelo A, Maffioli P. A randomized, double-blind clinical trial of canrenone vs hydrochlorothiazide in addition to angiotensin II receptor blockers in hypertensive type 2 diabetic patients. Drug Des Devel Ther. 2018;12:2611–6.
64. Bakris GL, Agarwal R, Chan JC, Cooper ME, Gansevoort RT, Haller H, et al. Effect of Finerenone on albuminuria in patients with diabetic nephropathy: a randomized clinical trial. JAMA. 2015;314:884–94.
65. Katayama S, Yamada D, Nakayama M, Yamada T, Myoishi M, Kato M, et al. A randomized controlled study of finerenone versus placebo in Japanese patients with type 2 diabetes mellitus and diabetic nephropathy. J Diabetes Complicat. 2017;31:758–65.
66. Agarwal R, Green JB, Heerspink HJL, Mann JFE, McGill JB, Mottl AK, et al. Finerenone with Empagliflozin in chronic kidney disease and type 2 diabetes. N Engl J Med. 2025; https://doi.org/10.1056/NEJMoa2410659. Published Online First: 5 June 2025
67. Ito S, Shikata K, Nangaku M, Okuda Y, Sawanobori T. Efficacy and safety of Esaxerenone (CS-3150) for the treatment of type 2 diabetes with microalbuminuria: a randomized, double-blind, placebo-controlled, phase II trial. Clin J Am Soc Nephrol. 2019;14:1161–72.
68. Ito S, Kashihara N, Shikata K, Nangaku M, Wada T, Okuda Y, et al. Esaxerenone (CS-3150) in patients with type 2 diabetes and microalbuminuria (ESAX-DN): phase 3 randomized controlled clinical trial. Clin J Am Soc Nephrol. 2020;15:1715–27.
69. Ito S, Kashihara N, Shikata K, Nangaku M, Wada T, Okuda Y, et al. Efficacy and safety of esaxerenone (CS-3150) in Japanese patients with type 2 diabetes and macroalbuminuria: a multicenter, single-arm, open-label phase III study. Clin Exp Nephrol. 2021;25:1070–8.
70. Wada T, Inagaki M, Yoshinari T, Terata R, Totsuka N, Gotou M, et al. Apararenone in patients with diabetic nephropathy: results of a randomized, double-blind, placebo-controlled phase 2 dose-response study and open-label extension study. Clin Exp Nephrol. 2021;25:120–30.
71. Agarwal R, Filippatos G, Pitt B, Anker SD, Rossing P, Joseph A, et al. Cardiovascular and kidney outcomes with finerenone in patients with type 2 diabetes and chronic kidney disease: the FIDELITY pooled analysis. Eur Heart J. 2022;43:474–84.
72. Filippatos G, Anker SD, August P, Coats AJS, Januzzi JL, Mankovsky B, et al. Finerenone and effects on mortality in chronic kidney disease and type 2 diabetes: a FIDELITY analysis. Eur Heart J Cardiovasc Pharmacother. 2023;9:183–91.

73. Sarafidis P, Agarwal R, Pitt B, Wanner C, Filippatos G, Boletis J, et al. Outcomes with Finerenone in participants with stage 4 CKD and type 2 diabetes: a FIDELITY subgroup analysis. Clin J Am Soc Nephrol. 2023; https://doi.org/10.2215/CJN.0000000000000149. Published Online First: 17 March 2023
74. Filippatos G, Bakris GL, Pitt B, Agarwal R, Rossing P, Ruilope LM, et al. Finerenone reduces new-onset atrial fibrillation in patients with chronic kidney disease and type 2 diabetes. J Am Coll Cardiol. 2021;78:142–52.
75. Rossing P, Anker SD, Filippatos G, Pitt B, Ruilope LM, Birkenfeld AL, et al. Finerenone in patients with chronic kidney disease and type 2 diabetes by sodium-glucose cotransporter 2 inhibitor treatment: the FIDELITY analysis. Diabetes Care. 2022;45:2991–8.
76. Heerspink HJL, Neuen BL, Agarwal R, et al. Finerenone in persons with chronic kidney disease without diabetes. N Engl J Med. 2026. https://doi.org/10.1056/NEJMoa2604625.
77. Neuen BL, Perkovic V, Agarwal R, et al. Finerenone in patients with chronic kidney disease due to glomerular diseases: a randomized clinical trial. JAMA. 2026:e269923. https://doi.org/10.1001/jama.2026.9923.
78. Neuen BL, Heerspink HJL, Perkovic V, et al. Efficacy and safety of finerenone in patients with chronic kidney disease: an individual participant data pooled analysis (INFINITY). Lancet. 407:2375–86.
79. Fernandez-Fernandez B, Fernandez-Prado R, Górriz JL, Martinez-Castelao A, Navarro-González JF, Porrini E, et al. Canagliflozin and renal events in diabetes with established nephropathy clinical evaluation and study of diabetic nephropathy with Atrasentan: what was learned about the treatment of diabetic kidney disease with canagliflozin and atrasentan? Clin Kidney J. 2019;12:313–21.
80. Fernandez-Fernandez B, Sarafidis P, Kanbay M, Navarro-González JF, Soler MJ, Górriz JL, et al. SGLT2 inhibitors for non-diabetic kidney disease: drugs to treat CKD that also improve glycaemia. Clin Kidney J. 2020;13:728–33.
81. Zoja C, Benigni A, Remuzzi G. Cellular responses to protein overload: key event in renal disease progression. Curr Opin Nephrol Hypertens. 2004;13:31–7.
82. Fernández-Fernández B, Valiño-Rivas L, Sánchez-Niño MD, Ortiz A. Albuminuria downregulation of the anti-aging factor klotho: the missing link potentially explaining the Association of Pathological Albuminuria with premature death. Adv Ther. 2020;37:62–72.
83. Kanbay M, Demiray A, Afsar B, Covic A, Tapoi L, Ureche C, et al. Role of klotho in the development of essential hypertension. Hypertension. 2021;77:740–50.
84. Amazit L, Le Billan F, Kolkhof P, Lamribet K, Viengchareun S, Fay MR, et al. Finerenone impedes aldosterone-dependent nuclear import of the mineralocorticoid receptor and prevents genomic recruitment of steroid receptor Coactivator-1. J Biol Chem. 2015;290:21876–89.
85. Kolkhof P, Delbeck M, Kretschmer A, Steinke W, Hartmann E, Bärfacker L, et al. Finerenone, a novel selective nonsteroidal mineralocorticoid receptor antagonist protects from rat cardiorenal injury. J Cardiovasc Pharmacol. 2014;64:69–78.
86. Fiorentino M, Grandaliano G, Gesualdo L, Castellano G. Acute kidney injury to chronic kidney disease transition. Contrib Nephrol. 2018;193:45–54.
87. Barrera-Chimal J, Rocha L, Amador-Martínez I, Pérez-Villalva R, González R, Cortés-González C, et al. Delayed spironolactone administration prevents the transition from acute kidney injury to chronic kidney disease through improving renal inflammation. Nephrol Dial Transplant. 2019;34:794–801.
88. Sarafidis P, Iatridi F, Ferro C, Alexandrou M-E, Fernandez-Fernandez B, Kanbay M, et al. Mineralocorticoid receptor antagonist use in chronic kidney disease with type 2 diabetes: a clinical practice document by the European renal best practice (ERBP) board of the European renal association (ERA). Clin Kidney J. 2023;16:1885–907.
89. Mancia Chairperson G, Kreutz C-CR, Brunström M, Burnier M, Grassi G, Januszewicz A, et al. ESH guidelines for the management of arterial hypertension The Task Force for the management of arterial hypertension of the European Society of Hypertension Endorsed by the European Renal Association (ERA) and the International Society of Hypertension (ISH). J Hypertens. 2023, 2023; https://doi.org/10.1097/HJH.0000000000003480. Published Online First: 21 June 2023

90. Kidney Disease: Improving Global Outcomes (KDIGO) Diabetes Work Group. KDIGO 2022 Clinical practice guideline for diabetes Management in Chronic Kidney Disease. Kidney Int. 2022;102:S1–S127.
91. Kidney Disease: Improving Global Outcomes (KDIGO) CKD Work Group. KDIGO 2024 Clinical practice guideline for the evaluation and management of chronic kidney disease. Kidney Int. 2024;105:S117–314.
92. American Diabetes Association professional practice committee. 10. Cardiovascular disease and risk management: standards of care in diabetes-2024. Diabetes Care. 2024;47:S179–218.
93. Marx N, Federici M, Schütt K, Müller-Wieland D, Ajjan RA, Antunes MJ, et al. 2023 ESC guidelines for the management of cardiovascular disease in patients with diabetes. Eur Heart J. 2023;44:4043–140.
94. Heerspink HJL, Agarwal R, Bakris GL, Cherney DZI, Lam CSP, Neuen BL, et al. Design and baseline characteristics of the Finerenone, in addition to standard of care, on the progression of kidney disease in patients with non-diabetic chronic kidney disease (FIND-CKD) randomized trial. Nephrol Dial Transplant. 2025;40:308–19.
95. Solomon SD, McMurray JJV, Vaduganathan M, Claggett B, Jhund PS, Desai AS, et al. Finerenone in heart failure with mildly reduced or preserved ejection fraction. N Engl J Med. 2024;391:1475–85.

Hypertension After Kidney Transplantation

Francesca Viazzi, Elisabetta Bussalino, Lucia Macciò, Elisa Russo, Cecilia Barnini, Giovanna Leoncini, Maria Carla Ghinatti, and Roberto Pontremoli

Introduction

Definition of Hypertension in Kidney Transplant Recipients

The prevalence of hypertension (HT) in kidney transplant recipients (KTRs) has been described between 70 and 95% [1–3]. The source of variability in estimates of prevalence, control, and different phenotypes of hypertension among KTRs is

F. Viazzi (✉) · L. Macciò · E. Russo
Unit of Nephrology, Dialysis and Transplantation, IRCCS AOM Azienda Ospedaliera Metropolitana Plesso Ospedale San Martino, Genoa, Italy

Department of Internal Medicine and Medical Specialties (DiMI), University of Genoa, Genoa, Italy
e-mail: francesca.viazzi@unige.it; lucia.maccio@aomliguria.it; elisa.russo@unige.it

E. Bussalino
Unit of Nephrology, Dialysis and Transplantation, IRCCS AOM Azienda Ospedaliera Metropolitana Plesso Ospedale San Martino, Genoa, Italy
e-mail: elisabetta.bussalino@aomliguria.it

C. Barnini
Department of Internal Medicine IV, Nephrology and Hypertension, Medical University Innsbruck, Innsbruck, Tirol, Austria
e-mail: Cecilia.Barnini@i-med.ac.at

G. Leoncini · R. Pontremoli
Department of Internal Medicine and Medical Specialties (DiMI), University of Genoa, Genoa, Italy

Internal Medicine Unit, IRCCS AOM Azienda Ospedaliera Metropolitana Plesso Ospedale San Martino, Genoa, Italy
e-mail: giovanna.leoncini@unige.it; roberto.pontremoli@unige.it

M. C. Ghinatti
Internal Medicine Unit, IRCCS AOM Azienda Ospedaliera Metropolitana Plesso Ospedale San Martino, Genoa, Italy
e-mail: maria.carla.ghinatti@aomliguria.it

P. Sarafidis, R. Pontremoli (eds.), *Hypertension and Chronic Kidney Disease*, Updates in Hypertension and Cardiovascular Protection,
https://doi.org/10.1007/978-3-032-29564-4_17

attributed to differences in the definitions used for HT diagnosis and in the type of blood pressure (BP) measurement used (in-office vs out-of-office setting) across various studies.

The cutoff values for HT diagnosis proposed by the 2021 Kidney Disease Improving Global Outcomes BP guidelines [4] were an office BP ≥ 130/80 mmHg. While for most patients with chronic kidney disease (CKD), the recommended target is systolic BP <120 mm Hg, for KTRs, the target BP is <130/80 mm Hg. More recently, a synopsis of the sections of the European Society of Hypertension (ESH) Guidelines judged relevant for the daily clinical practice of nephrologist, prepared by experts from ESH and European Renal Association (ERA), recommends that in all patients with CKD, the primary goal is to lower office systolic BP to <140/90 mmHg and that in most CKD patients, included KTRs, office BP may be lowered to <130/80 mmHg if tolerated and not below 120/70 mm Hg because of the absence of relevant evidence and the potential to induce harm [5].

Accordingly, the recently updated European Society of Cardiology guidelines retaining the definition of HT as blood pressure ≥ 140/90 mmHg for office BP, recommended to target systolic BP to 120–129 mmHg in CKD patients with the caution to individualize BP target for those with renal transplantation [6].

Although it has been shown that a BP ≥ 140/90 mm Hg significantly reduces kidney graft and patients' survival [3], the extent to which BP levels should be lowered is not known. As a matter of fact, Randomized Controlled Trials (RCTs) investigating the effect of BP on long-term graft and patient survival are not available, and BP targets for HT management in these individuals are extrapolated from data in CKD populations showing as patients in the intensive treatment arms had higher rates of mild acute kidney injury, incidence of CKD, and loss of estimated glomerular filtration rate (eGFR) [7, 8] Table 1.

Effects of Kidney Transplantation on Blood Pressure

Most KTRs have hypertension prior to transplant, or develop HT post-transplant.

Notably, some data suggest that donor with HT increases the risk of post-transplant HT among renal transplant recipients and is associated with higher rates of allograft failure. While only a few studies examining BP changes in KTRs receiving kidneys from hypertensive or normotensive donors are included in this meta-analysis, the incidence of HT among recipients from normotensive donors ranges from 8% to 18%, whereas from hypertensive donors it ranges from 3% to 25%, with a 31% higher risk of graft loss [9].

Risk factors for post-transplant HT include *recipient factors present before transplantation*, such as longstanding hypertension, age, male sex, increased body mass index, higher than recommended sodium intake, endocrine factors, African-American ethnicity and genetic profile. They also include *donor-related factors*, such as low nephron mass, poor allograft quality, donor age, donor's pre-transplantation hypertension, and genetic profile. Finally, have been described factors *related to the transplantation itself* such as delayed graft function, renal

Table 1 Summary of guidelines for the proposed cut off values for hypertension diagnosis in KTRs

Ref.	Definition of Hypertension	Target blood pressure in CKD	Recommendations for KTRs
KDIGO Blood Pressure Work Group [4], 2021	≥130/80 mmHg using standardized office BP measurement	For most CKD patients, the recommended target is SBP <120 mmHg using standardized office BP measurement	For KTRs the target BP is <130/80 mmHg
ERA synopsis of the 2023 ESH Guidelines for the Management of Arterial Hypertension [5], 2024	≥140/90 mmHg using standardized office BP measurement	Office BP may be lowered to <130/80 mmHg if tolerated and not below 120/70 mmHg because of the absence of relevant evidence and the potential to induce harm	In KTRs with hypertension, office BP may be lowered to <130 mmHg systolic and <80 mmHg diastolic
ESC Guidelines for the management of elevated blood pressure and hypertension [6], 2024	≥140/90 mmHg using standardized office BP measurement	In CKD patients, SBP may be targeted to 120-129 mmHg, if toleratd	Caution to individualize BP target for those patients with renal transplantation

KTR kidney transplant recipient, *KDIGO* kidney disease improving global outcome, *BP* blood pressure, *CKD* chronic kidney disease, *ERA* European Renal Association, *ESH* European Society of Hypertension, *ESC* European Society of Cardiology

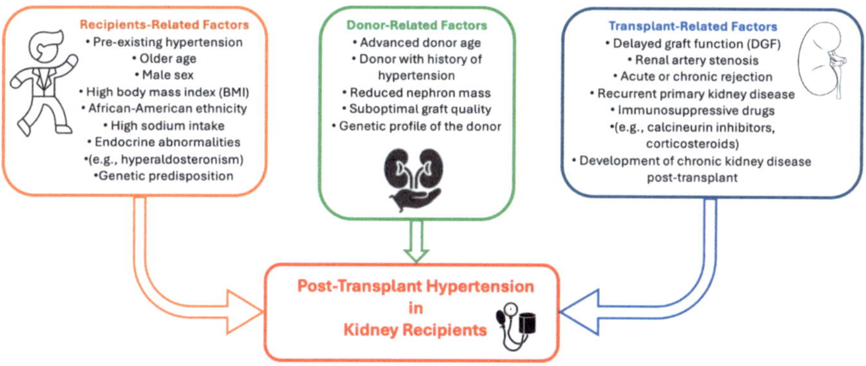

Fig. 1 Risk factors for post-transplant hypertension

transplant artery stenosis, immunosuppressive medications, particularly calcineurin inhibitors (CNI) and steroids, acute or chronic allograft rejection, recurrent disease and CKD [10–12] Fig. 1.

As for transplant recipients from living donors, kidney transplant (KT) per se has been described to be associated with significant improvement in office and ambulatory blood pressure monitoring (ABPM) values (8/5 mm Hg) in the short- and mid-term post-transplant periods along with reduction in antihypertensive agents [13]. The positive impact of KT on ABPM values was shown even in children [14]. The decrease in BP values is gradual and persistent at 3 and 12 months, leading to a better BP control despite a reduction in the average number of antihypertensive medication used [15]. Several pathogenetic mechanisms, including lowering of the activity of the renin-angiotensin-aldosterone-system (RAAS) and sympathetic system, improvement in endothelial function and arterial stiffness and decrease in sodium and volume overload, have been proposed for the favorable impact of KT on BP. KT from a living donor is the best treatment option for patients with end stage kidney disease and the safety of living donors is of paramount importance. While data available from the literature are concordant with the conclusion that kidney donation does not significantly affect BP levels up to 10 years of donation [15, 16], lifelong monitoring including management of BP values are mandatory.

Assessment of Hypertension in Kidney Transplant Recipients

The rate of BP control in kidney transplantation ranges around 50% [17]. As expected, using ABPM, the prevalence of uncontrolled hypertension increases to 64–66% of patients [18, 19]. Several lines of evidence support the use of out-of-office BP measurements in KT patients. For example, office and out-of-office BP measurements were compared in 260 KTRs followed for an average of 3.9 years. Overall, 25% of outpatient visits showed inadequate BP control when assessed by office BP, but not by 24-hour ABPM, indicating white-coat hypertension (WCH). Conversely, 12% of visits revealed masked hypertension (MHT). Ultimately, reliance on office BP measurements could lead to inappropriate therapeutic decisions in up to 37% of outpatient visits [20]. While Pisano et al. [17] in their systematic review reported an average prevalence of MHT in KTRs of 26%, compared to 10% for WCH, the prevalence of MHT appears to be significantly higher—up to 45%—in a cohort of KTRs with relatively preserved kidney function [19]. Interestingly, this increased proportion of MHT is justified by the fact that about 90% of this cohort of patients showed an abnormal nocturnal dipping pattern (non dipper or reverse dipper).

The main goal of post-transplant care is to improve graft and patient survival. Since a more effective strategy for identify HT and monitoring BP levels could promote this goal, the guidelines advocated increasing the use of ABPM in KTRs for diagnosis and management of HT [5]. In fact, although HBPM demonstrated the highest diagnostic accuracy compared to the gold standard 24-hour ABPM, 21% of patients were still misclassified as "controlled hypertensive" by HBPM [19]. This fact that altered circadian BP profile and nocturnal hypertension represent the norm, rather than the exception, in the transplant population underscores the evidence in favor of integration of ABPM in KTRs. Furthermore, it has been shown that nigh-time BP, as compared with office BP readings, correlates better with subclinical organ damage and CV events in this setting [21]. In particular, high ABPM metric and abnormal night-day profiles but non high office BP associate with left ventricular hypertrophy, increased intima media thikness, CV events and eGFR evolution overtime [21]. Certainly, the unique advantages of HBPM such as availability, tolerability, reproducibility and related improvement in patient adherence encourage the large adoption of HBPM in KTRs care.

Hypertension and Outcomes in KTRs

Effects of Blood Pressure Load on Cardiovascular Morbidity and Mortality

While transplantation is the treatment of choice for patients needing kidney replacement treatment, and is associated with reduced CV diseases and all-cause mortality, the population of KTRs is at higher CV risk as compared to the general population. Several retrospective studies showed that a 10-year KTR survival rates vary from 67% to 97% depending on the transplantation center, investigated time periods, race and ethnicity [22–24]. In Europe, average recipient age has increased from 44 years between 1986 and 1995, to 54 years in 2006–2015 and the proportion of KT candidates over 65 years old in United States represented a quarter of the wait list in 2018 and is constantly growing [6]. Such changes are likely to have affected the incidence and causes of death with graft functioning. Although there has been a downtrend in mortality of KTRs over the past 2 decades, CV disease remains the leading cause of death and inadequate control of post-transplant HT is associated with an increased risk of CV morbidity other that being an independent risk factor for mortality [25, 26].

The largest study investigating the relationship between BP goals and outcomes in KTRs is a retrospective analysis of data from 62,556 KTRs across 209 centers in 39 countries describing as patient mortality was significantly increased in those with BP $\geq$ 140/90 mm Hg [3].

An analysis in Acid for Vascular Outcome Reduction in Transplantation (FAVORIT) trial found that among 3474 KTRs, those with baseline systolic BP below 110 mm Hg had lower mortality than those with systolic BP 120–129 mmHg during a mean follow-up of 4.5 years [27] demonstrating that there is no notable J-shaped association between systolic BP level and cardiovascular or mortality outcomes. By contrast, lower levels of diastolic BP levels <70 mmHg were associated with a higher risk of CV diseases and all-cause mortality, reflecting an association between lower diastolic BP, or a wider pulse pressure as expression of increased vascular stiffness and more severe underlying comorbid conditions, including arteriosclerotic vascular disease [27].

Effects of Blood Pressure Load on Graft Function

Several retrospective studies show that a 10-year graft survival rate ranges between 50% and 77% and that the USA results are lower than those reported by other countries [24].

Graft survival depends on many factors, including inadequate control of post-transplant HT [26]. In experimental studies, HT accelerates the progression of kidney failure by elevating glomerular capillary hydrostatic pressure and glomerular hyper-filtration. Notably, grafted kidneys are likely to be susceptible to mechanical injury, which accelerates immune-mediated injury [28]. Because chronic allograft nephropathy may be, in part, mediated by renal ischemia, one could theorize that higher BP and thereby better kidney perfusion may be beneficial for graft survival. Nevertheless, several clinical studies have shown the negative effect of HT on graft outcomes. After a 6-years follow-up, 85 out of 808 subjects from Korean Cohort Study for Outcome in Patients with Kidney Transplantation (KNOW-KT) developed ≥50% decline in eGFR from baseline values or graft loss. This composite outcome was significantly more frequent in patients with systolic BP ≥ 140 mm Hg whether assessed at 1-year post-transplantation or as a time varying measure. Furthermore, the patients with stable systolic BP showed better outcomes than those with increasing systolic BP [29]. However, the effects of more intensive BP lowering on allograft function remain largely unknown. A cautious approach is advised given that the transplanted kidney is de-nervated, and KTRs are often managed with CNIs to prevent rejection. These factors may impair the myogenic response, reducing the transplanted kidney's ability to auto-regulate, thereby increasing the risk of acute kidney injury and accelerating the decline of renal function, particularly at lower blood pressure levels. Nevertheless, contrary to this a priori hypothesis, the secondary analysis of the multinational FAVORIT trial found no evidence for "J"- or "U"-shaped associations between either BP parameter and either outcome in stable KTRs. Therefore, reliable studies are needed to evaluate whether a threshold exists below which the risk of allograft dysfunction may increase.

Parameters of Blood Pressure Behavior and Cardiovascular and Overall Outcomes in Kidney Transplant Recipients

Recent guidelines recommend the use of out-of-office BP measurements as a complementary tool for improving the management of hypertension. In KTRs, the wider use of ABPM has led to the recognition of abnormal diurnal BP patterns and BP phenotypes. The rates of non-dipping status have been reported to range between 36%–95% and that of nocturnal hypertension between 69 and 77% [19].

The identification of a higher prevalence of uncontrolled MHT in KTRs as compared to CKD patients (26% vs 8%) is of extraordinary clinical relevance due to the fact that this condition predicts an increased risk for CV and kidney outcomes (50 and 70%, respectively) in CKD patients [30]. Furthermore, targeting nocturnal HT might be useful for the reduction of the burden of CV risk in KTRs, as confirmed by the observation that reverse dipper pattern was a risk factor for CV events in a prospective study on 126 KTRs [31]. Clinical trials are needed to determine whether treatment based on out of office BP levels will be able to reduce adverse outcome in patients with WCH and MHT, especially in KTRs.

Despite ongoing debate regarding the optimal BP target, the findings of some recent observational studies underscore the critical importance of not only achieving optimal BP levels but also implementing regular monitoring and management of BP in KTRs in response to fluctuations in blood pressure [29]. All the available types of BP variability (BPV) are used to describe the BP fluctuations overtime and have been associated with CV and kidney outcomes and total mortality in several settings including KT. In particular, KTRs showed lower short-term BPV compared to haemodialysis patients [15] and similar indices as compared to pre-dialysis CKD patients [32]. Disappointingly, despite a reduction in BP values, a corresponding decrease in BPV was not observed [33]. This might be explained with the occurrence of additional factors that are specific for these individuals such as activation of immune system response against graft and the effects of various immunosuppressive drugs. Recently, we provided the first evidence that long-term BPV constitutes an independent risk factor for CV events in KTRs [34]. An increase in systolic BPV assessed over a baseline period of 18 months was associated with a graded rise in the risk of both fatal and nonfatal CV events during a subsequent median follow-up of 67 months. In this cohort of 272 KTRs, patients in the highest systolic BPV tertile (>13 mm Hg) exhibited a fourfold increase in the incidence of fatal and nonfatal cardiovascular events (HR = 4.09 [95% CI, 1.34–12.43]; $P = 0.01$), independently of blood pressure load [34]. From a practical standpoint, our study underscores the importance of developing therapeutic strategies aimed at achieving long-term stabilization of BP levels, in order to reduce the significant CV burden in KT patients.

Therapeutic Options

Aiming to achieve the generally accepted target of <130/80 mm Hg, lifestyle modifications recommended for CKD should be adopted in KTRs, while most patients will likely require a combination of antihypertensive agents. Currently, no data are available regarding the effects of antihypertensive drugs on long-term kidney outcomes in KTRs, and therefore the guidelines avoid making specific recommendation about preferred agents [35].

A prior Cochrane systematic review suggested that ACEIs may pose a higher risk of hyperkalemia in transplant recipients and that CCBs could be associated with better renal protection [36]. Another comprehensive systematic review and meta-analysis, including 71 RCTs involving 6832 patients [37], concluded that CCBs appear significantly superior to placebo and to ACEIs or ARBs for several renal outcomes reducing graft loss by at least 40%. However, none of the antihypertensive agents assessed in this meta-analysis demonstrated a significant reduction in mortality or the occurrence of fatal or nonfatal CV events in this context.

RAAS inhibitors exhibited contrasting effects. While their use was associated with increased graft survival, lower BP and, in most cases, reduced proteinuria, they were also linked to a higher risk of hyperkalemia and decreased GFR. Although the available evidence is not yet conclusive, CCBs and/or RAAS inhibitors appear to be important components of an effective antihypertensive regimen. In addition, patients at increased risk of coronary artery disease may derive further benefit from beta-blocker therapy [37]. Moreover, thiazide/thiazide-like diuretics are effective in counteracting CNI mediated sodium-retention.

It should be taken in mind that the overall quality of available evidence remains limited. Furthermore, the substantial heterogeneity of the studies hampers definitive conclusions regarding long-term outcomes and limits the generalizability of findings to the whole KT population.

Therefore, well-designed RCTs are warranted to provide more robust evidence for the optimal selection and use of antihypertensive agents in KTRs.

Hypertension is a highly prevalent and clinically significant complication in KTRs, adversely affecting both patient survival and graft longevity. Despite evidence highlighting its impact on CV and renal outcomes, optimal BP targets specific to this population remain unclear. Routine use of ABPM is essential for accurate diagnosis and tailored management, given the unique BP profiles in transplant recipients. Future research is needed to develop personalized therapeutic strategies aimed at reducing blood pressure variability and improving long-term outcomes, ultimately enhancing patient quality of life and graft function.

References

1. Alexandrou ME, Ferro CJ, Boletis I, Papagianni A, Sarafidis P. Hypertension in kidney transplant recipients. World J Transplant. 2022;12:211–22. https://doi.org/10.5500/wjt.v12.i8.211.
2. Korogiannou M, Sarafidis P, Theodorakopoulou MP, Alexandrou ME, Xagas E, Boletis IN, Marinaki S. Diagnostic performance of office versus ambulatory blood pressure in kidney transplant recipients. Am J Nephrol. 2021;52:548–58. https://doi.org/10.1159/000517358.
3. Speer C, Benning L, Morath C, Zeier M, Frey N, Opelz G, Döhler B, Tran TH, Collaborative Transplant Study. Blood pressure goals and outcomes in kidney transplant recipients in an analysis of the collaborative transplant study. Kidney Int Rep. 2024;10:780–90. https://doi.org/10.1016/j.ekir.2024.12.004.
4. Kidney Disease: Improving Global Outcomes (KDIGO) Blood Pressure Work Group. KDIGO 2021 Clinical practice guideline for the Management of Blood Pressure in chronic kidney disease. Kidney Int. 2021;99:S1–S87.
5. Sarafidis P, Schmieder R, Burnier M, Persu A, Januszewicz A, Halimi JM, Arici M, Ortiz A, Wanner C, Mancia G, Kreutz R. A European Renal Association (ERA) synopsis for nephrology practice of the 2023 European Society of Hypertension (ESH) guidelines for the management of arterial hypertension. Nephrol Dial Transplant. 2024;39:929–43.
6. McEvoy JW, McCarthy CP, Bruno RM, Brouwers S, Canavan MD, Ceconi C, Christodorescu RM, Daskalopoulou SS, Ferro CJ, Gerdts E, Hanssen H, Harris J, Lauder L, McManus RJ, Molloy GJ, Rahimi K, Regitz-Zagrosek V, Rossi GP, Sandset EC, Scheenaerts B, Staessen JA, Uchmanowicz I, Volterrani M, Touyz RM, ESC Scientific Document Group. 2024 ESC guidelines for the management of elevated blood pressure and hypertension. Eur Heart J. 2024;45(38):3912–4018. https://doi.org/10.1093/eurheartj/ehae178. Erratum in: Eur Heart J. 2025;46:1300. doi:10.1093/eurheartj/ehaf031
7. Beddhu S, Rocco MV, Toto R, Craven TE, Greene T, Bhatt U, Cheung AK, Cohen D, Freedman BI, Hawfield AT, Killeen AA, Kimmel PL, Lash J, Papademetriou V, Rahman M, Rastogi A, Servilla K, Townsend RR, Wall B, Whelton PK, SPRINT Research Group. Effects of intensive systolic blood pressure control on kidney and cardiovascular outcomes in persons without

kidney disease: a secondary analysis of a randomized trial. Ann Intern Med. 2017;167:375–83. https://doi.org/10.7326/M16-2966.
8. Rocco MV, Sink KM, Lovato LC, Wolfgram DF, Wiegmann TB, Wall BM, Umanath K, Rahbari-Oskoui F, Porter AC, Pisoni R, Lewis CE, Lewis JB, Lash JP, Katz LA, Hawfield AT, Haley WE, Freedman BI, Dwyer JP, Drawz PE, Dobre M, Cheung AK, Campbell RC, Bhatt U, Beddhu S, Kimmel PL, Reboussin DM, Chertow GM, SPRINT Research Group. Effects of intensive blood pressure treatment on acute kidney injury events in the Systolic Blood Pressure Intervention Trial (SPRINT). Am J Kidney Dis. 2018;71:352–61. https://doi.org/10.1053/j.ajkd.2017.08.021.
9. Altheaby A, Al Dalbhi S, Alghamdi Y, Almigbal TH, Alotaibi KN, Batais MA, Alodhayani A, Alkhushail A, Alhantoushi M, Alsaad SM. Effect of donor hypertension on renal transplant recipients' blood pressure, allograft outcomes and survival: a systematic review and meta-analysis. Am J Cardiovasc Dis. 2019;9:49–58.
10. Mangray M, Vella JP. Hypertension after kidney transplant. Am J Kidney Dis. 2011;57:331–41. https://doi.org/10.1053/j.ajkd.2010.10.048.
11. Halimi JM, Ortiz A, Sarafidis PA, Mallamaci F, Wuerzner G, Pisano A, London G, Persu A, Rossignol P, Sautenet B, Ferro C, Boletis J, Kanaan N, Vogt L, Bolignano D, Burnier M, Zoccali C. Hypertension in kidney transplantation: a consensus statement of the 'hypertension and the kidney' working group of the European Society of Hypertension. J Hypertens. 2021;39:1513–21. https://doi.org/10.1097/HJH.0000000000002879.
12. Weir MR, Burgess ED, Cooper JE, Fenves AZ, Goldsmith D, McKay D, Mehrotra A, Mitsnefes MM, Sica DA, Taler SJ. Assessment and management of hypertension in transplant patients. J Am Soc Nephrol. 2015;26(6):1248–60. https://doi.org/10.1681/ASN.2014080834. Epub 2015 Feb 4. PMID: 25653099; PMCID: PMC4446882
13. Buus NH, Carlsen RK, Hughes AD, Skov K. Influence of renal transplantation and living kidney donation on large artery stiffness and peripheral vascular resistance. Am J Hypertens. 2020;33:234–42. https://doi.org/10.1093/ajh/hpz175.
14. Hamdani G, Nehus EJ, Hanevold CD, VanSickle JS, Hooper DK, Blowey D, Warady BA, Mitsnefes MM. Ambulatory blood pressure control in children and young adults after kidney transplantation. Am J Hypertens. 2017;30(10):1039–46. https://doi.org/10.1093/ajh/hpx092.
15. Xagas E, Sarafidis PA, Theodorakopoulou MP, Alexandrou ME, Korogiannou M, Argyris A, Protogerou A, Boletis IN, Marinaki S. A parallel evaluation of short- and mid-term changes of ambulatory blood pressure in kidney transplant recipients and kidney donors. Clin Kidney J. 2022;15:2097–106. https://doi.org/10.1093/ckj/sfac162.
16. Yalin SF, Trabulus S, Seyahi N, Cengiz M, Cicik ME, Altiparmak MR. Ambulatory blood pressure monitoring in living kidney donors: what changes in 10 years? Clin Transpl. 2018;32:e13224. https://doi.org/10.1111/ctr.13224.
17. Pisano A, Mallamaci F, D'Arrigo G, Bolignano D, Wuerzner G, Ortiz A, Burnier M, Kanaan N, Sarafidis P, Persu A, Ferro CJ, Loutradis C, Boletis IN, London G, Halimi JM, Sautenet B, Rossignol P, Vogt L, Zoccali C. Assessment of hypertension in kidney transplantation by ambulatory blood pressure monitoring: a systematic review and meta-analysis. Clin Kidney J. 2021;15(1):31–42. https://doi.org/10.1093/ckj/sfab135.
18. Fernandez Fresnedo G, Franco Esteve A, Gómez Huertas E, Cabello Chaves V, Díz Gómez JM, Osorio Moratalla JM, Gallego Samper R, Gallego Valcárcel E, Campistol Plana JM, Marín Iranzo R, Arias Rodríguez M, RETENAL Group. Ambulatory blood pressure monitoring in kidney transplant patients: RETENAL study. Transplant Proc. 2012;44(9):2601–2. https://doi.org/10.1016/j.transproceed.2012.09.037. PMID: 23146468
19. Eleftheriadis G, Naik MG, Osmanodja B, Halleck F, Schrezenmeier E, Liefeldt L, Choi M, Bachmann F, Avaniadi DP, von Hoerschelmann E, Lücht C, Zaks M, Duettmann W, Budde K. Office or home versus 24-h blood pressure measurement in stable kidney transplant recipients. Nephrol Dial Transplant. 2024;39:1890–9. https://doi.org/10.1093/ndt/gfae076.
20. Mallamaci F, Tripepi R, D'Arrigo G, Porto G, Versace MC, Marino C, Sanguedolce MC, Testa A, Tripepi G, Zoccali C. Long-term blood pressure monitoring by office and 24-h ambulatory

blood pressure in renal transplant patients: a longitudinal study. Nephrol Dial Transplant. 2019;34(9):1558–64. https://doi.org/10.1093/ndt/gfy355.
21. Pisano A, Mallamaci F, D'Arrigo G, Bolignano D, Wuerzner G, Ortiz A, Burnier M, Kanaan N, Sarafidis P, Persu A, Ferro CJ, Loutradis C, Boletis IN, London G, Halimi JM, Sautenet B, Rossignol P, Vogt L, Zoccali C. Blood pressure monitoring in kidney transplantation: a systematic review on hypertension and target organ damage. Nephrol Dial Transplant. 2021;25:gfab076. https://doi.org/10.1093/ndt/gfab076.
22. Ghelichi-Ghojogh M, Ghaem H, Mohammadizadeh F, Vali M, Ahmed F, Hassanipour S, Nikbakht HA, Rezaei F, Fararouei M. Graft and patient survival rates in kidney transplantation, and their associated factors: a systematic review and meta-analysis. Iran J Public Health. 2021;50:1555–63. https://doi.org/10.18502/ijph.v50i8.6801.
23. Poggio ED, Augustine JJ, Arrigain S, Brennan DC, Schold JD. Long-term kidney transplant graft survival-making progress when most needed. Am J Transplant. 2021;21:2824–32. https://doi.org/10.1111/ajt.16463.
24. Hariharan S, Israni AK, Danovitch G. Long-term survival after kidney transplantation. N Engl J Med. 2021;385:729–43.
25. Malhotra R, Katz R, Weiner DE, Levey AS, Cheung AK, Bostom AG, Ix JH. Blood pressure, chronic kidney disease progression, and kidney allograft failure in kidney transplant recipients: a secondary analysis of the FAVORIT trial. Am J Hypertens. 2019;32:816–23. https://doi.org/10.1093/ajh/hpz095.
26. Pilecki T, Czarkowska-Pączek B, Lisik W, Nazarewski S, Pączek L. Impact of blood pressure on risk of graft failure or death among patients after kidney transplantation in a 10-year observational period: a single-center retrospective analysis. Ann Transplant. 2023;28:e939472. https://doi.org/10.12659/AOT.939472.
27. Carpenter MA, John A, Weir MR, Smith SR, Hunsicker L, Kasiske BL, Kusek JW, Bostom A, Ivanova A, Levey AS, Solomon S, Pesavento T, Weiner DE. Blood pressure, cardiovascular disease, and death in the folic acid for vascular outcome reduction in transplantation trial. J Am Soc Nephrol. 2014;25:1554–62.
28. Raij L, Azar S, Keane WF. Role of hypertension in progressive glomerular immune injury. Hypertension. 1985;7:398–404.
29. Kim HJ, Kim KW, Joo YS, Ryu J, Jung HY, Jeong KH, Kim MG, Ju MK, Han S, Lee JS, Kang KP, Ro H, Lee KW, Huh KH, Kim MS, Kim BS, Yang J. Impact of blood pressure on allograft function and survival in kidney transplant recipients. Transpl Int. 2024;37:12574. https://doi.org/10.3389/ti.2024.12574.
30. Rahman M, Wang X, Bundy JD, Charleston J, Cohen D, Cohen J, Drawz PE, Ghazi L, Horowitz E, Lash JP, Schrauben S, Weir MR, Xie D, Townsend RR, CRIC Study Investigators. Prognostic significance of ambulatory BP monitoring in CKD: a report from the Chronic Renal Insufficiency Cohort (CRIC) study. J Am Soc Nephrol. 2020;31:2609–21. https://doi.org/10.1681/ASN.2020030236.
31. Ibernon M, Moreso F, Sarrias X, Sarrias M, Grinyó JM, Fernandez-Real JM, Ricart W, Serón D. Reverse dipper pattern of blood pressure at 3 months is associated with inflammation and outcome after renal transplantation. Nephrol Dial Transplant. 2012;27:2089–95. https://doi.org/10.1093/ndt/gfr587.
32. Korogiannou M, Theodorakopoulou M, Sarafidis P, Alexandrou ME, Pella E, Xagas E, Argyris A, Protogerou A, Papagianni A, Boletis IN, Marinaki S. Ambulatory blood pressure trajectories and blood pressure variability in kidney transplant recipients: a comparative study against chronic kidney disease patients. Kidney Res Clin Pract. 2022;41:482–91. https://doi.org/10.23876/j.krcp.21.250.
33. Xagas E, Sarafidis P, Iatridi F, Theodorakopoulou MP, Pella E, Korogiannou M, Argyris A, Protogerou A, Boletis IN, Marinaki S. Kidney transplantation and kidney donation do not affect short-term blood pressure variability. Blood Press. 2023;32:2181640. https://doi.org/10.1080/08037051.2023.2181640.
34. Bussalino E, Picciotto D, Macciò L, Parodi A, Gandolfo MT, Viazzi F. Visit-to-visit systolic blood pressure variability independently predicts cardiovascular events in a kidney

transplant Recipients' cohort. J Am Heart Assoc. 2024;13:e034108. https://doi.org/10.1161/JAHA.124.034108.

35. Mancia G, Kreutz R, Brunström M, Burnier M, Grassi G, Januszewicz A, Muiesan ML, Tsioufis K, Agabiti-Rosei E, Algharably EAE, Azizi M, Benetos A, Borghi C, Hitij JB, Cifkova R, Coca A, Cornelissen V, Cruickshank JK, Cunha PG, Danser AHJ, Pinho RM, Delles C, Dominiczak AF, Dorobantu M, Doumas M, Fernández-Alfonso MS, Halimi JM, Járai Z, Jelaković B, Jordan J, Kuznetsova T, Laurent S, Lovic D, Lurbe E, Mahfoud F, Manolis A, Miglinas M, Narkiewicz K, Niiranen T, Palatini P, Parati G, Pathak A, Persu A, Polonia J, Redon J, Sarafidis P, Schmieder R, Spronck B, Stabouli S, Stergiou G, Taddei S, Thomopoulos C, Tomaszewski M, Van de Borne P, Wanner C, Weber T, Williams B, Zhang ZY, Kjeldsen SE. 2023 ESH guidelines for the management of arterial hypertension the task force for the management of arterial hypertension of the European Society of Hypertension: endorsed by the International Society of Hypertension (ISH) and the European renal association (ERA). J Hypertens. 2023;41:1874–2071. https://doi.org/10.1097/HJH.0000000000003480.
36. Cross NB, Webster AC, Masson P, O'Connell PJ, Craig JC. Antihypertensive treatment for kidney transplant recipients. Cochrane Database Syst Rev. 2009;2009(3):CD003598. https://doi.org/10.1002/14651858.CD003598.pub2. Update in: Cochrane Database Syst Rev. 2024 Jul 31;7:CD003598. doi:10.1002/14651858.CD003598
37. Pisano A, Bolignano D, Mallamaci F, D'Arrigo G, Halimi JM, Persu A, Wuerzner G, Sarafidis P, Watschinger B, Burnier M, Zoccali C. Comparative effectiveness of different antihypertensive agents in kidney transplantation: a systematic review and meta-analysis. Nephrol Dial Transplant. 2020;35:878–87. https://doi.org/10.1093/ndt/gfz092.

Renovascular Hypertension

Tom Robberechts, Patricia Van der Niepen, Belen Ponte, and Alexandre Persu

Introduction

Renal artery stenosis (RAS) is quite common. However, the prevalence of true renovascular hypertension (RVH) is rather low (<1%) in patients with mild hypertension, while it can be as high as 40% in patients with severe, refractory, or acute hypertension [1]. There are two major causes of RAS: atherosclerotic disease and fibromuscular dysplasia (FMD). Atherosclerotic RAS (ARAS) accounts for approximately 90% of cases of RAS and is more common in patients ≥45 years, with other atherosclerotic lesions or cardiovascular (CV) risk factors (hypercholesterolemia, smoking, diabetes, arterial hypertension) [2–4]. Atherosclerosis mainly affects the proximal main renal artery or the aortic orifice, in continuation with aortic lesions,

T. Robberechts
Department of Nephrology and Hypertension, Universitair Ziekenhuis Brussel, Vrije Universiteit Brussel (VUB), Brussels, Belgium

Department of Cardiology, Cliniques Universitaires Saint-Luc, Université Catholique de Louvain, Brussels, Belgium

P. Van der Niepen
Department of Nephrology and Hypertension, Universitair Ziekenhuis Brussel, Vrije Universiteit Brussel (VUB), Brussels, Belgium

B. Ponte
Nephrology and Hypertension Division, Department of Medicine, University Hospitals of Geneva, Genève, Switzerland

A. Persu (✉)
Department of Cardiology, Cliniques Universitaires Saint-Luc, Université Catholique de Louvain, Brussels, Belgium

Pole of Cardiovascular Research, Institut de Recherche Expérimentale et Clinique, Université Catholique de Louvain, Brussels, Belgium
e-mail: alexandre.persu@uclouvain.be

P. Sarafidis, R. Pontremoli (eds.), *Hypertension and Chronic Kidney Disease*, Updates in Hypertension and Cardiovascular Protection,
https://doi.org/10.1007/978-3-032-29564-4_18

with segmental and intrarenal branch involvement in more advanced stages. FMD-RAS usually affects women younger than 50 years, although >10% of lesions are nowadays diagnosed at an age ≥65 years. It more frequently affects the mid/distal main renal artery or its intrarenal branches [5]. Both atherosclerosis and FMD can affect one or both renal arteries.

If left untreated, atherosclerotic lesions will continue to progress [6–9]. However, reliable data on risk of progression and progression rates are lacking. Moreover, ARAS is associated with high rates of CV disease (CVD), chronic kidney disease (CKD) and mortality [10–12].

Following an expert consensus statement of the Society for Cardiovascular Angiography and Interventions, severe RAS is defined as a > 70% diameter stenosis by visual estimation, or 50% to 70% visually estimated stenosis with a mean resting or hyperemic translesional pressure gradient of ≥10 mmHg or a systolic resting or hyperemic translesional gradient of ≥20 mmHg, or a renal fractional flow reserve (Pd/Pa) of ≤0.8. Moderate RAS is defined as a visually estimated stenosis of 50% to 70% without measurement of a translesional pressure gradient, or with a resting or hyperemic translesional mean gradient <10 mmHg or a translesional systolic resting or hyperemic gradient of <20 mmHg [13].

Medical treatment of CV risk factors should follow general guidelines to prevent and reduce CV risk. However, the optimal management of RAS remains a subject of debate due to the conflicting results obtained from case series, observational studies and randomized controlled trials [14–16].

Atherosclerotic Renal Artery Disease (ARAD)

Pathophysiology

Renal artery stenosis causes a reduction in blood flow and perfusion pressure toward the nephrons, initiating successive pathophysiological changes and compensatory mechanisms. Hypoperfusion of the juxtaglomerular apparatus activates the release of renin, thereby increasing the production and secretion of angiotensin II and aldosterone in order to restore renal perfusion. Simultaneously, this compensatory hormonal cascade increases sympathetic nerve activity, induces arterial remodeling and vasoconstriction, activates inflammatory and oxidative stress pathways, and promotes sodium/water retention. Rarefaction of microvessels, cortical hypoxia, stimulation of inflammatory cytokines, and recruitment of progenitor and inflammatory cells may eventually lead to the development of glomerulosclerosis and tubulointerstitial fibrosis [14, 16–18].

These hemodynamic effects and hormonal system activation are not restricted to severe RAS [14, 16, 17]. Even a small number of ischemic nephrons can cause RVH, as supported by numerous cases of segmental RAS with excessive unilateral renin release, hyperplasia of the juxtaglomerular apparatus, and cure of hypertension by partial nephrectomy or use of angiotensin-converting enzyme (ACE) inhibitors [19]. In addition, renal autoregulation may be compromised with secondary impact on renal flow [20, 21]. Chronic subclinical ischemia may further impair kidney function by activating systemic inflammation [21]. Therefore, restoring renal arterial blood flow may not reverse ischemic nephropathy and improve kidney function, especially in the presence of longstanding RAS. However, the optimal timeframe for revascularization remains unclear.

In unilateral RAS, the healthy kidney initially compensates for the adverse effects of renin-dependent hypertension through pressure-natriuresis. Hence, hypertension is mainly mediated by Angiotensin II elevation. However, in bilateral RAS, compensatory mechanisms no longer apply, precipitating sodium/volume retention and leading to a volume-dependent hypertension and increased risk of "flash" pulmonary edema [22]. In this situation, Angiotensin II may be normal or even low due to volume inhibition.

Prevalence

The number of patients diagnosed with ARAS has increased over the past decades due to an aging population, increased awareness, and improvements and increased use of imaging tools [23]. Incidental ARAS is a common finding [24, 25]. Atherosclerotic RAS is prevalent in patients with hypertension with or without diabetes (20% and 14% respectively). It is more common in patients aged 45 years and older and in patients with CKD, other atherosclerotic lesions, or CV risk factors [2, 23–29]. Many patients with ARAS are current or ex- smokers [30] or have dyslipidemia [31, 32]. Atherosclerotic RAS diagnosis is increasingly common in patients aged ≥65 years at the start of dialysis. Its prevalence in middle-aged patients with advanced CKD ranges from 5 to 24% and is doubled in dialysis patients [12]. Atherosclerotic RAS is found in approximately 10% of patients with acute kidney injury [23]. Therefore, screening for ARAS in patients with hypertension with a more severe phenotype is recommended by several international guidelines [17, 18, 33].

Atherosclerotic Renal Artery Stenosis (ARAS) as a Marker of Cardiovascular Risk

Atherosclerotic RAS is considered a marker of significant atheromatous burden. Indeed, several population-based data show an association between atherosclerotic renal artery disease and coronary artery disease (5–67%) [17, 29], heart failure (up to 68%) [22, 26, 27], aorta-iliac and distal peripheral arterial disease (12–56%) [23, 25, 34], abdominal aortic aneurysms (33%) [26, 35], and carotid artery stenosis and cerebrovascular disease (5.2–22%) [28]. Moreover, the presence of ARAS increases the mortality risk by 1.5-fold in pre-dialysis patients and by 3.3-fold in those on dialysis compared to non-atherosclerotic causes of CKD [36].

Atherosclerotic Renal Artery Stenosis and the Heart

The increased activation of the renin-angiotensin-aldosterone system (RAAS) with elevated levels of angiotensin II and aldosterone in patients with RAS plays an important role in the pathogenesis of CV remodeling and left ventricular hypertrophy (LVH) by generating reactive oxygen species and vascular inflammation, followed by fibroblasts and myofibroblasts proliferation, collagen production, perivascular and interstitial fibrosis [37–45]. In 95% of ARAS patients, abnormal cardiac structure and/or function are present with LVH and diastolic dysfunction being the predominant abnormalities [37, 38].

In particular, patients with CKD and ARAS are characterized by a significantly higher prevalence of LVH, increased left ventricular mass index (LVMI), and decreased LV diastolic function compared to CKD patients without ARAS even after matching for age, glomerular filtration rate (GFR), and 24-hour ambulatory blood pressure (BP) levels [37]. Compared to patients with primary hypertension, marked cardiac structural and both systolic and diastolic functional abnormalities are observed in patients with RVH with and without significant renal dysfunction (serum creatinine levels >2 or <2 mg/dL). While patients with primary hypertension and patients with RVH and serum creatinine <2 mg/dL have concentric LVH, patients with more severe CKD have predominantly eccentric LVH [46]. The latter is probably due to a more pronounced volume overload in patients with severe renal impairment, which is known to be associated with systolic dysfunction [38]. These differences in myocardial changes might contribute to the higher morbidity and mortality rates observed in patients with atherosclerotic renovascular CKD compared to non-atherosclerotic causes of CKD [17]. Moreover, in patients with ARAS undergoing revascularization, diastolic dysfunction was common and associated with increased mortality during follow-up [47]. These changes seem to be specific to ARAS and not encountered in all causes of RAS. In contrast to studies in ARAS, Dobrowolski et al. observed no difference in LV morphology and function between patients with FMD-RAS and matched controls with primary hypertension [48]. However, BP was well controlled, and the majority of patients did not have actually significant RAS.

Atherosclerotic Renal Artery Stenosis and the Kidney

Renal artery stenosis can lead to progressive loss of GFR and development of ischemic nephropathy. Although many patients with ARAS have CKD, the causal relationship between stenosis and the development of CKD is not always clear. A stenosis can be found incidentally in patients with CKD caused by other disorders. Additionally, other causes of a decreased renal blood flow (vasculitis, thrombotic microangiopathy, ischemic acute tubular necrosis) may also induce ischemia of the kidneys. Finally, true histological diagnosis of CKD is often unknown. Therefore, the true incidence and prevalence of ARAS-related CKD is unclear.

In contrast to mild stenosis, lumen stenosis of 70% and more leads to cortical hypoxia, as has been shown by BOLD-MRI [49, 50]. Tissue hypoxia induces microvascular rarefaction, activation of oxidative pathways, stimulation of inflammatory cytokines and recruitment of progenitor and inflammatory cells, leading to fibrosis of glomeruli, tubuli, and interstitium [16–18]. Lesser degrees of stenosis may compromise renal autoregulation, reduce renal blood flow and GFR, but without the development of severe hypoxia [16, 20, 50]. In such cases, kidney damage may be due to activation of the inflammatory pathway triggered by chronic subclinical ischemia, rather than to the reduced blood flow itself [21, 51]. Patients with ischemic nephropathy may present with a persistent and progressive decrease in GFR. Fluctuations in renal function can be seen after BP reduction or administration of antihypertensive agents, particularly RAAS blockers, or changes in volume status. Progressive decline in GFR can result from underlying significant degree of stenosis (typically a high-grade stenosis of both renal arteries or a unilateral stenosis in a solitary functional kidney), or from hypertensive nephrosclerosis, or atheroembolic events.

Diagnosis of ARAS

When to Screen for ARAS?

Screening for ARAS is warranted if clinical findings suggest a secondary cause of hypertension, and other causes of secondary hypertension are excluded. Development of acute kidney injury after introduction of RAAS blockers, renal asymmetry, and flash pulmonary edema are some of the possible signs of underlying RAS (Table 1). Before screening, the potential risks of contrast studies and invasive procedures (i.e., contrast-induced acute kidney injury, cholesterol embolism, etc.) should be considered. Theoretically, invasive testing is only recommended when renal revascularization is being considered and patients are likely to benefit from revascularization (Table 2). To date, however, no absolute clinical, laboratory, or radiological features can predict outcome after renal artery revascularization [53].

Which Diagnostic Tests Should Be Used?

The gold standard for diagnosing RAS remains conventional catheter-based angiography. However, several non-invasive tests can be used for initial testing, especially when it is uncertain that renal revascularization will be necessary (Table 3a and 3b). The choice of the initial test should be based upon patient characteristics and institutional expertise.

Duplex Doppler Ultrasonography

Duplex Doppler ultrasonography (DDUS) is often used as screening test for RAS, due to its low cost and easy availability. However, it is operator-dependent and consequently subject to inter- and intra-observer variability.

Renal artery peak systolic velocity (PSV) and renal-aortic ratio (RAR) are two key parameters to define hemodynamic significance of stenotic lesions. If PSV is increased

Table 1 Clinical findings suggestive of secondary hypertension

Disorder	Suggestive clinical features
General indicators of secondary hypertension	Severe or drug resistant hypertension Sudden BP rise in a patient with an otherwise stable controlled hypertension Elevated BP in young adults (<30 y) with no family history of hypertension Hypertension in children before puberty and without obesity
Renovascular disease	Acute kidney injury (>30% increase in serum creatinine) ≤1 week after initiating an ACE-inhibitor or ARB; or after BP lowering Hypertension (≥160/≥100 mmHg) in patients with diffuse atherosclerosis Hypertension in patients with renal asymmetry (size difference >1.5 cm) or a unilateral small kidney without a causative urological abnormality Hypertension in patients with recurrent acute 'flash' pulmonary oedema Chronic kidney disease Decompensated heart failure, particularly in patients with CKD grade 3–5 and hypertension
Primary kidney disease	Decreased GFR and/ or abnormal urinalysis Morphologic structural abnormalities
Endocrine disorders	
Primary aldosteronism	Unexplained hypokalemia
Pheochromocytoma	Paroxysmal elevations of BP accompanied with headache, palpitations and sweating
Cushing syndrome	Cushingoid appearance
Hypothyroidism	Symptoms of hypothyroidism and elevated TSH
Primary hyperparathyroidism	Elevated serum calcium and PTH
Sleep apnea syndrome	In overweight or obese patients, loud snoring or apneic episodes, daytime somnolence
Drug-induced hypertension	Oral contraceptives, NSAIDs, chemotherapeutic agents, cocaine and other stimulants, anabolic steroids, vasoconstrictive agents, calcineurin inhibitors, erythropoietin stimulating agents, antidepressants, …

ACE angiotensin converting enzyme, *ARB* angiotensin receptor blocker, *BP* blood pressure, *CKD* Chronic kidney disease, *GFR* glomerular filtration rate, *NSAIDs* nonsteroidal anti-inflammatory drugs, *PTH* parathyroid hormone, *TSH* thyroid stimulating hormone

Table 2 Clinical syndromes likely to benefit from revascularization in the presence of a renal artery stenosis >70% and a viable kidney parenchyma (renal diameter >8 cm, cortical thickness >0.5 cm, RRI <0.8)

Clinical syndromes likely to benefit from revascularization	
Definite indications	Possible indications
Resistant hypertension	Chronic heart failure
ACE-i or ARB-induced AKI AKI induced by BP lowering	Coexistence of progressive CKD and uncontrolled hypertension
Acute pulmonary edema or acute decompensation of heart failure	Asymptomatic high-grade RAS (either bilateral or solitary kidney) with viable renal parenchyma
Progressive CKD in high-grade RAS (bilateral stenosis or solitary kidney)	New (<3 months) dialysis patients with non-functioning but possibly viable kidney parenchyma
AKI due to acute renal artery occlusion or high-grade RAS with anuria	
Kidney transplant with RAS (symptomatic or asymptomatic)	Higher likelihood to benefit from revascularization A short duration (<5 y) of BP elevation [52] Fibromuscular dysplasia

ACE angiotensin converting enzyme, *AKI* acute kidney injury, *ARB* angiotensin receptor blocker, *CKD* Chronic kidney disease, *RAS* renal artery stenosis

≥180 to 200 cm/s and the RAR ≥ 3.5, a high probability of significant stenosis (≥60% reduction in diameter) is reported [54]. Those are called "direct" signs for RAS, as they are measured directly in the main arteries. Their sensitivity and specificity vary between 79–91% and 73–97%, respectively. The examination can also show turbulences as focal color aliasing on the Doppler, or a characteristic color bruit. Besides some anatomic features, DDUS provides functional assessment criteria of the renal arteries. From the Doppler waveforms of the intra-renal arteries a renal resistive index (RRI) can be calculated (RRI = peak systolic velocity–end-diastolic velocity). RRI has high sensitivity and specificity for detecting severe stenosis (95–97%, respectively). In case of a significant stenosis, the RRI is expected to be low initially, typically less than 0.5, indicating a potential for reversibility. On the contrary, when the stenosis is already long-standing and kidney tissue remodeling has already occurred, RRI is high. Therefore, RRI can be used as a surrogate marker of the parenchymal viability and is useful to predict the outcome after revascularization (RRI ≥0.8: low likelihood of benefit). Other parameters like End-Diastolic Velocity (EDV) ≥150 cm/s, Acceleration Time (AT) >0.07 s or Acceleration Index (AI) < 300 cm/s^2 can further increase the likelihood of diagnosing a significant stenosis. However, these parameters are less well described in clinical practice and actually reflect the Doppler "tardus parvus" waveform, as it is more commonly referred to nowadays [54].

Duplex Doppler ultrasonography can be used for serial measurements to detect progression of RAS or restenosis after a revascularization procedure. However, a negative DDUS does not exclude RAS. Consequently, in case of high suspicion, additional testing should be performed [17, 18].

Computed Tomography Angiography

Computed tomography angiography (CTA) with intravenous iodinated contrast is an accurate diagnostic test with a high sensitivity and specificity. However, both are

Table 3a Diagnostic tests in renal artery stenosis

Diagnostic test	Diagnostic criteria	Advantages	Disadvantages
Duplex ultrasound	Direct criteria: PSV >180–200 cm/s Renal/aorta PSV ratio $\geq$ 3.5	High sensitivity and specificity in experienced hands Non-invasive Widely available	Time consuming Operator dependent Technically challenging, esp. if obesity
CT-angiography	Stenosis >70% Stenosis ≥50% with post stenotic dilation	High sensitivity and specificity Non-invasive Widely available Fast Visualization of arterial calcification	Contrast-induced nephropathy Exposure to ionizing radiation
MR-angiography	Stenosis >70% Stenosis ≥50% with post stenotic dilatation	High sensitivity and specificity Non-invasive Renal artery ostium visibility better than in DSA	Contra-indicated if non-compatible metallic implants Artifacts from respiration Hard to achieve if claustrophobia Risk of nephrogenic systemic fibrosis with group 1 gadolinium agents if low GFR
Conventional angiography (DSA)	Stenosis >70% Stenosis ≥50% with post stenotic dilatation Translesional pressure gradient >10%	Accurate assessment of degree of RAS Possibility of concomitant treatment with PTRA+S	Invasive Costly Only 2D images Bleeding risk due to arterial puncture Risk of contrast nephropathy Risk of atheroembolism
Captopril renography		Non-invasive Provides relative function of each kidney	No information on renal artery anatomy or degree of stenosis Less reliable if CKD or bilateral RAS

CKD chronic kidney disease, *DSA* digital subtraction angiography, *PSV* peak systolic velocity, *PTRA+S* percutaneous transluminal renal angioplasty with stenting, *RA* renal artery, *RAS* renal artery stenosis, *RRI* renal resistive index

Table 3b Diagnostic criteria for renal artery stenosis in duplex ultrasound

Direct signs(main renal artery)	Indirect signs (intra-renal arteries waveform)
Focal color aliasing	AT >0.07 sec
Color bruit	AI <3 m/sec^2
Turbulence	ΔRRI R-L > 5% (>0.05)
PSV >180–200 cm/sec	Tardus parvus
Renal-aortic ratio > 3.5	Kidney asymmetry (>1.5 cm)

AI acceleration index, *AT* acceleration time, *PSV* peak systolic velocity, *RRI* renal resistive index

lower in patients with a smaller degree of stenosis or with stenosis of distal arterial segments, as in FMD.

Magnetic Resonance Angiography

Contrast-enhanced magnetic resonance angiography (MRA) is an accurate diagnostic test with a high sensitivity and specificity for detecting proximal RAS. However, due to its lower spatial resolution, MRA may miss stenosis (esp. in accessory renal arteries). Conversely, false positive results are also possible, due to motion or respiration artifacts. MRA can be a good alternative to CTA if exposure to iodinated contrast or radiation should be avoided.

Captopril Renography

A radionuclide renography is a functional test, which compares blood flow and filtration between the two kidneys. A potential difference between the kidneys can be enhanced by administration of captopril. Although a captopril renogram may suggest hemodynamic significance of a stenosis, it is no longer considered suitable for initial testing because of its poor sensitivity and specificity.

Renin Sampling

Plasma renin activity (PRA) and selective renal vein renin measurements are not useful as diagnostic tests. Dietary sodium intake, hydration status, bilateral RAS and various antihypertensive drugs can influence PRA values.

Conventional Angiography (DSA)

Catheter-based or digital subtraction angiography is the gold standard for diagnosing RAS. It should mainly be used when there is a strong suspicion of significant stenosis for which angioplasty (+/− stenting) is considered. Given its invasive nature, risk of complications and cost, it is not advised as first-line screening tool.

New imaging technologies, such as functional MRI [55] or contrast-enhanced ultrasonography [56, 57], hold promise as non-invasive tools to characterize RAS and its hemodynamic impact. They may therefore be valuable in pre-treatment counseling of RAS patients who may benefit from endovascular treatment (Fig. 1).

Management

Since ARAS is a marker of atheromatous burden and associated with increased risk of CV events, optimal CV risk management should be offered to all patients. Smoking cessation, optimal BP control and diabetic treatment, optimization of lipid profile, weight loss in case of overweight/obesity, regular physical exercise and reduced sodium consumption are essential [17, 18, 58]. In some patients, revascularization by percutaneous transluminal renal angioplasty with stenting (PTRAS) may be indicated. Selected patients may be eligible for surgery, depending on the severity of the stenosis, the hemodynamic impact, the clinical characteristics of the patient and the likelihood of BP control and kidney function recovery.

What Is the Optimal Medical Management?

Targets for control of BP and selection of antihypertensive drugs in ARAS follow the general BP management guidelines [18, 33]. However, since reduced renal perfusion triggers RAAS activation, the use of RAAS blockers is considered the first-line choice to treat hypertension in this setting [17, 18, 59]. They are well tolerated even in bilateral mild ARAS and have been shown to reduce mortality [60, 61]. However, there are some concerns about their use in severe, bilateral ARAS or in a single kidney with a significant ARAS, due to a potential decline in GFR [62, 63]. After initiation of a RAAS blocker, kidney function should be monitored, and in case of a significant decline in GFR (>25% drop), renal artery revascularization should be considered [62, 64]. Observational studies in patients with ARAS suggest that the use of low-dose aspirin is also associated with reduced risk of mortality [65]. As patients with ARAS are considered at high CV risk, lipid-lowering drugs should be part of their treatment with low LDL targets.

Despite optimal medical treatment, little is known about the progression risk of established ARAS. Stenosis may progress and eventually lead to complete occlusion of the renal artery, or chronic renal ischemia with GFR loss. In studies mainly dating from the period before 2000, progression of RAS has been observed in 11–44% of patients after respectively 2.6–4 years of follow-up, using repeated renal

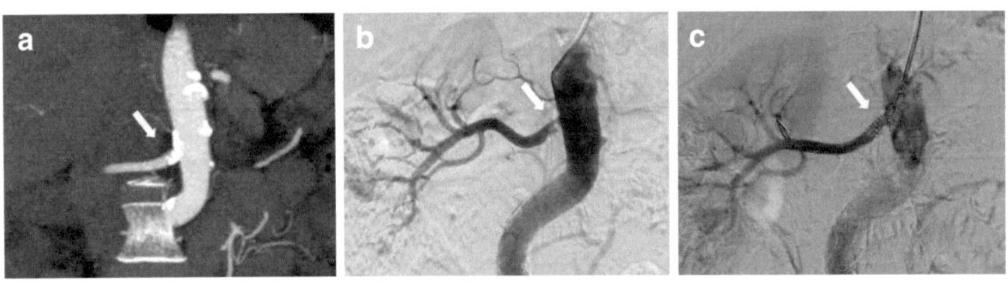

Fig. 1 (**a**) Computed tomography angiography showing an atheromatous aspect of the aorta and renal artery, with atherosclerotic renal artery stenosis. (**b**) Catheter-based angiography confirming the presence of a high-grade stenosis at the proximal right renal artery. (**c**) Catheter-based angiography after angioplasty with stenting of the right renal artery, showing improved patency post-stenting

angiograms and up to 52% at five years using serial DDUS [66–68]. Progression was more likely to occur in patients with more severe stenosis at baseline [67]. Progression to end-stage kidney disease was rare in patients with unilateral disease [69]. The highest risk of kidney mass loss, measured by repeat DUS and defined as a reduction in kidney length of more than 1 cm, was associated with greater degree of stenosis and higher BP [70]. However, in the cited studies—dating from an era with less stringent BP and lipid targets and lack of newer nephroprotective drugs such as SGLT2-inhibitors—medical management was probably not comparable to nowadays standards. Indeed, a more recent study showed lower progression risk (progression in 14% of kidneys on 8 years follow-up), possibly due to improved control of CV risk factors [9]. Therefore, the aforementioned cited progression rates cannot be simply extrapolated to current practice. New techniques have the potential to advance research into the complex pathophysiology of RAS and mechanistic-based treatments for RAS, targeting disease mechanisms, such as oxidative stress, inflammation, mitochondrial damage, and cellular senescence [51].

Renal Artery Revascularization

Whereas in the distant past only surgery was an option for revascularization, the development of percutaneous interventional techniques gave rise to much broader treatment indications in RAS. Based on observational data regarding efficacy and safety, an important increase in the number of percutaneous interventions for the treatment of ARAS was observed in the late 90s [71]. However, opinion on the efficacy of renal artery revascularization changed considerably since the 2000s as several randomized controlled trials (RCTs) failed to demonstrate a significant benefit of PTRA on BP, renal function, and survival in patients with ARAS compared to medical therapy alone (Table 4) [35, 52, 72–75]. Subsequently, initial enthusiasm regarding PTRA for ARAS was tempered by the failure of these trials, and its use decreased drastically (Table 5) [14, 15]. Despite substantial methodological shortcomings of these trials, which limit their generalizability, there is now a more nuanced consensus that revascularization may still be beneficial for selected patients [14, 15, 17, 18]. Indication for revascularization depends on the severity of the stenosis, hemodynamic impact, clinical characteristics of the patient, and the likelihood of BP response and recovery of kidney function [14, 15, 76]. Patients with a short-standing hypertension have a higher likelihood of benefiting from revascularization. However, the duration of BP elevation after which revascularization is no longer useful is unclear. Only one study suggested that surgical revascularization has no effect on BP if hypertension has been present for >5 years [77].

Kidney viability is an important positive predictor of revascularization outcome. A kidney length of ≥8 cm, a renal cortical thickness of ≥0.5 cm, and a renal resistive index of less than 0.8 are associated with a higher likelihood of renal recovery and BP improvement after revascularization [17, 18, 78, 79]. Reversible hypoxic kidney damage or the so-called hibernating kidney parenchyma can be detected using BOLD-MRI, and may probably respond better to revascularization [80, 81]. The availability of new diagnostic techniques, such as intravascular ultrasound, BOLD-MRI, radiomics analysis, and artificial intelligence, opens up opportunities

Table 4 Prospective, randomized, clinical trials of balloon angioplasty, with and without stenting, versus medical therapy in atherosclerotic renal artery stenosis

Author	Patients (*n*)	Follow-up (months)	Randomization	Difference in BP outcome between treatment arms	Difference in renal functional outcome	Other key clinical outcomes
Plouin et al. *(EMMA study) 1998* [72]	49	6	23 PTRA 26 medical treatment	Significant reduced anti-hypertensive drugs in PTRA group		26% complications in PTRA group
Webster et al. *(SNRASCG) 1998* [73]	55	3–54	25 PTRA 30 medical treatment	Significant BP reduction Only if BL-RAS; no significant difference in CV events or renal function	No	No significant difference in survival
Van Jaarsveld et al. *(DRASTIC study) 2000* [35]	106	12	56 PTRA 50 medical treatment	Significant reduced anti-hypertensive drugs in PTRA group	No	
Bax et al. (star) *2009* [52]	140	24	76 medical treatment 64 medical treatment + PTRAS	No	No	Significant number of PTRAS-related complications No significant difference in CV mortality and morbidity
Wheatley et al. (astral) *2009* [74]	806	33.6 (median)	403 medical treatment403 medical treatment + PTRAS (95%) or PTRA	No	No	No s significant difference in CV events and mortality. PTRAS associated with 6.7% serious adverse events

(continued)

Table 4 (continued)

Author	Patients (*n*)	Follow-up (months)	Randomization	Difference in BP outcome between treatment arms	Difference in renal functional outcome	Other key clinical outcomes
Cooper et al. (CORAL) *2014* [75]	947	43 (median)	480 medical treatment 467 medical treatment + PTRAS (95%) or PTRA	No	No	No significant difference in fatal and non-fatal CV and renal events or all-cause mortality

BP blood pressure, *CrCl* creatinine clearance, *CVE* cardiovascular events, *PTRA* percutaneous transluminal renal angioplasty, *PTRAS* percutaneous transluminal renal artery stenting

Table 5 Design weaknesses and limitations of the major randomized clinical trials

Author/study	Weakness and limitations
Plouin et al. *(EMMA study), 1998* [67]	No blinding of intervention, 27% crossover; 8.7% PTRA+S Mean baseline stenosis grade: not reported Mean baseline n° drugs: 1.333 (DDD) Exclusion criteria: Diastolic BP > 109 mmHg, Malignant HTN, Acute pulmonary edema.
Webster et al., *Scottish and Newcastle Renal Artery Stenosis Collaborative Group, 1998* [68]	No blinding of intervention, 20% participants assigned to PTRA had surgery Mean baseline stenosis grade: 50.9% Mean baseline n° drugs: 2.6 Different grades of kidney function
Van Jaarsveld et al., *(DRASTIC study), 2000* [32]	No blinding of intervention, 44% participants assigned to medical therapy had PTRA at 3 months; 3.6% PTRA+S Mean baseline n° drugs: 2.0
Bax et al., (STAR study), *2009* [69]	No blinding of intervention; 28% participants allocated to PTRA did not undergo revascularization, mainly due to minimal stenosis; 1.3% crossover Mean baseline stenosis grade: not reported Mean baseline n° drugs: 2.9 BP inclusion criterion: Stable BP (<140/90 mmHg) for 1 month prior to randomization Different grades of kidney function
Wheatley et al., (ASTRAL study), *2009* [71]	No blinding of intervention; 17% participants allocated to PTRA did not undergo revascularization; 6% crossover Mean baseline n° drugs: 2.8 Non standardized medical treatment BP inclusion criterion: no clear definition was given Patients were only enrolled if their physician was uncertain as to whether revascularization would be of clinical benefit, which led to exclusion of patients most likely to benefit from revascularization
Cooper et al., (CORAL study), *2014* [70]	No blinding of intervention; 5.4% participants allocated to PTRA did not undergo revascularization; 4% crossover Problems with recruiting changed the inclusion criteria: the threshold of 155 mmHg for defining systolic HTN was abandoned, and patients with controlled BP were enrolled Mean baseline stenosis grade: 67% Mean baseline n° drugs: 2.1 Small kidneys (>7 cm) allowed Drop outs: 17%

BP blood pressure, *CKD* chronic kidney disease, *DDD* defined daily dose, *HTN* hypertension, *PTRA* percutaneous transluminal renal angioplasty, *PTRA+S* percutaneous transluminal renal artery angioplasty with stenting

to identify ischemic lesions responsive to renal revascularization [82]. However, these techniques are not yet widely used in daily clinical practice. On the other hand, underlying CKD with an elevated urine albumin-to-creatinine ratio (UACR) >300 mg/g (30 mg/mmol) may be a negative predictor of successful revascularization [83].

Nevertheless, well-conducted, observational studies have shown substantial benefit from revascularization in selected clinical phenotypes, including BP improvement, preserved kidney function, reduced risk of acute and chronic CV events, improved cardiac remodeling and/or reduced mortality [14, 15, 17, 18, 84–90]. A meta-analysis by Cuspidi et al. suggests that renal artery revascularization, added to antihypertensive therapy, has a beneficial effect on LV structure, as evidenced by a significant reduction in LVMI and a 40% reduction in the risk of LVH. The lower the systolic BP after the intervention, the greater the regression of LVH [91]. In another study, the decrease in LVMI and the regression rate of LVH were greater in FMD-RAS than in ARAS after PTRA. FMD, severe RAS, and higher baseline LVMI were independent predictors of a LVMI reduction of at least 20%. In FMD-RAS, regression of LVM after PTRA tended to be associated with lower number of CV events, which was not observed in ARAS [92]. Observational data suggest that recurrent acute pulmonary edema can be prevented by successful revascularization with stenting of the affected renal arteries [93]. In patients with refractory hypertension, flash pulmonary edema, heart failure, or rapidly declining kidney function, revascularization is associated with a significant reduction in mortality and CV events compared to medical therapy [14]. Therefore, proper selection of patients who may benefit from revascularization is crucial in clinical decision-making.

Globally, three major criteria have to be checked prior to therapeutic decision:

1. Confirmation of a clinical syndrome likely to benefit from revascularization (Table 2), such as therapy-resistant hypertension; RAAS-inhibitor-induced AKI; progressive CKD; flash pulmonary edema or heart failure [17, 18].
2. Confirmation of a high-grade (>70%) stenosis—benefit is unlikely if stenotic degree <50%.
3. Confirmation of renal parenchymal viability (renal diameter >8 cm, cortical thickness >0.5 cm, RRI <0.8).

Main Criticisms and Limitations of Relevant RCT's

Although the importance of these RCTs within the field of ARAS should not be underestimated, they had important shortcomings. Many of the available RCTs included subjects who were unlikely to benefit from revascularization such as mild RAS, mild hypertension or advanced CKD with small kidneys. Conversely, those with a more critical presentation (in either clinical or radiological parameters) were excluded from study participation. Furthermore, the trials were hindered by a lack of pre-specified subgroups, enrollment delays, variability in study protocols regarding imaging techniques for RAS diagnosis and evaluation, poor assessment and overestimation of the degree of stenosis, multiple protocol revisions, high crossover rates, and low event rates (Table 5) [14, 15, 85].

These limitations should be taken into consideration for clinical decision-making.

What to Expect from Revascularization?

The technical success rate varies according to the lesion site and the degree of stenosis. Incomplete occlusions of the main renal artery respond better to PTRA than total occlusions and ostial lesions. To avoid elastic recoil and restenosis, ARAS are treated with PTRA and primary stenting.

The clinical success rate depends on the anatomy of the stenosis and clinical phenotype. In responders, BP usually gradually decreases over the following weeks, allowing to reduce antihypertensive treatment. Yet, a rapid drop in BP within the first 48 h after PTRA may be seen, especially in case high-grade stenosis and recent hypertension.

The overall results of PTRA alone were inferior to those of PTRAS. A higher primary success rate as well as a higher patency rate and lower restenosis rate at six months have been observed [94, 95]. PTRAS was also more effective in improving BP and kidney function [95, 96]. For these reasons, current guidelines recommend stenting on top of PTRA in ARAS, unless the anatomy precludes stenting [17, 18, 97].

What Are the Possible Complications of Revascularization?

Most procedural complications are relatively minor and include puncture site hematoma or bruising. However, serious complications may occur, including renal artery dissection, perforation or thrombosis (1–9%) [74, 98]. Acute kidney injury can occur from cholesterol embolization or from the use of the radiocontrast agent. Advanced CKD or CVD and widespread atheromatosis increase the risk of these complications. Manipulation of the renal artery by dilation and stenting damages the arterial endothelium, which may cause restenosis. The rate of restenosis ranges between 11 and 39% during the first two years after revascularization [95, 99–101]. A rise in BP and/or a fall in GFR may indicate restenosis and justify immediate medical imaging. Doppler Duplex ultrasonography is an accurate technique to identify significant restenosis in stented renal arteries. The PSV and RAR cutoff values for detecting renal artery in-stent restenosis (ISR) are higher than those in native, non-stented renal arteries. Del Conde et al. reported a PSV of 382 ± 128 cm/s and a RAR of 5.3 ± 2.4 in a cohort of stented renal arteries with 60–99% restenosis [102]. Therefore, applying the cut-offs for non-stented stenotic lesions on stented arteries might overestimate the degree of restenosis. Whether routine follow-up with DDUS is necessary is not sufficiently studied, in contrast to clinical follow-up with regular measurements of BP and kidney function [101, 103–105]. To avoid complications, optimal sizing and deployment of the renal stent is of utmost importance. Repeat PTRA(S) may be performed to treat in-stent stenosis; however, the restenosis rate will be increased [106]. Therefore, surgical intervention may be indicated. Distal filter protection devices may increase the safety and effectiveness of revascularization by preventing cholesterol atheroembolization [107].

Surgical Revascularization

Since the expanded arsenal of antihypertensive drugs and the widespread adoption of PTRA(S), surgical revascularization is only performed in patients who have complex anatomic lesions (small renal arteries, early branching of the main RA, simultaneous surgery of the abdominal aorta) or in case of a complication (recurrent restenosis/dissection/perforation) [108, 109]. Surgical treatment can include bypassing of the stenosis, re-implantation of a whole kidney or removal of an atrophic kidney due to arterial occlusion. Overall, surgery is as effective as PTRA(S), but the primary success rate is slightly higher and the incidence of restenosis is lower than with PTRA(S). On the other hand, the mortality rate is higher [110, 111].

Proposed Future Research in Atherosclerotic RAS

- Investigating the natural evolution of ARAS and the impact of current pharmacological standard of care.
- Optimizing patient selection: to identify high-risk patient profiles who will benefit most from revascularization on pre-specified outcomes (BP control, renal function preservation, CV outcome).
- Confirming optimal imaging techniques and cut-offs for hemodynamic significance of RAS.
- Improving techniques to assess renal parenchymal viability and microvascular disease, including functional imaging and/or biomarkers.
- Confirming benefits of revascularization compared to medical modern standard CV prevention strategies (including SGLT2 inhibition, mineralocorticoid antagonism, and more stringent lipid and BP targets).
- Assessing patient-reported outcomes as well as cost-effectiveness of medical vs interventional treatment strategies.

Renal Artery Stenosis Due to Fibromuscular Dysplasia (FMD)

Introduction

FMD is a non-atherosclerotic, non-inflammatory arterial disease of medium- and small-sized muscular arteries throughout the body. A variety of genetic, mechanical, hormonal and environmental factors may play a role in its pathogenesis. Arterial stenosis can be multifocal or focal, with multifocal subtype accounting for +/− 80% of cases (Fig. 2). Multivessel disease—with FMD lesions involving multiple vascular beds—is common. With prevalence rates of 66–91%, renal arteries are among the blood vessels most frequently affected. Multifocal FMD is characterized by the typical "string-of-beads" pattern (alternating dilatations and stenosis) and usually occurs in the mid and distal portions of the artery. Focal FMD may occur in any part of the artery. Dissection, aneurysm and tortuosity may also occur. However, to be considered as part of the FMD-spectrum, at least one multifocal or focal arterial

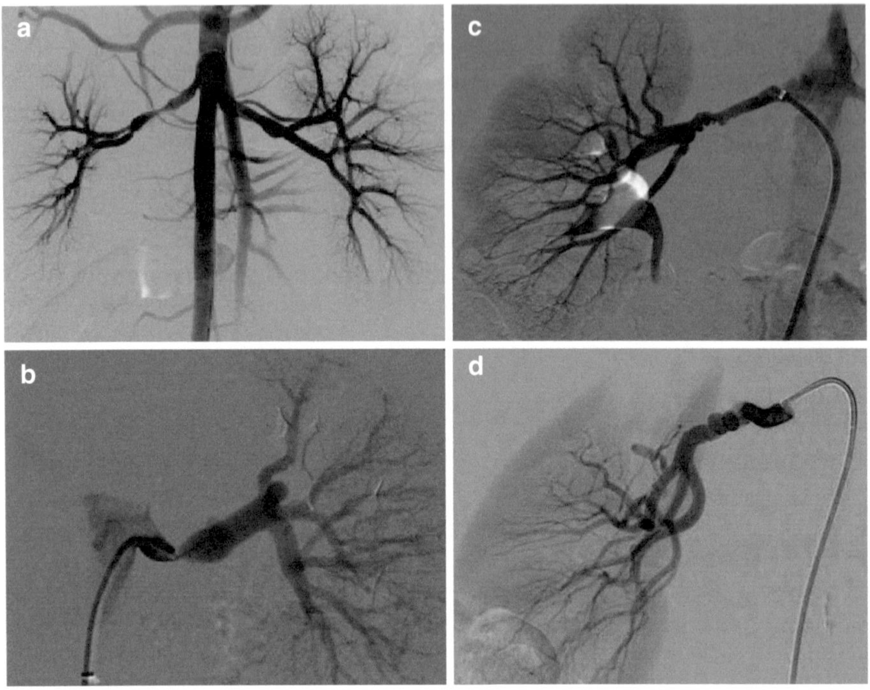

Fig. 2 Panel (**a**, **b**) showing conventional angiographic images of renal arteries with focal FMD. Panel (**c**, **d**) showing conventional angiographic images of renal arteries with a string-of-beads appearance, so-called multifocal FMD

stenotic lesion has to be present. FMD may occur at any age, but is generally seen in young and middle-aged adults with a mean age of diagnosis of 43–53 years. The overwhelming majority of patients with FMD are women (82–95%). Compared to women, men with FMD have higher rates of focal FMD and arterial dissection [5, 112–115].

Clinical Presentation of Renal FMD

Depending on the severity of arterial lesions, renal FMD may remain asymptomatic. If symptomatic, hypertension is the most frequent clinical manifestation of renal FMD. In particular, hypertension in younger patients, or severe or resistant hypertension should raise suspicion for underlying FMD.

Unlike ARAS, FMD lesions do not affect the integrity of the renal parenchyma, unless an acute ischemic event has occurred or long-standing hypertension has compromised parenchymal integrity (i.e., renal infarction post renal artery dissection) [116–118]. The heart is usually unaffected in FMD, except in the case of long-standing hypertension or spontaneous coronary artery dissection, which may be the first manifestation of FMD [48, 106, 119].

Diagnosis of Renal FMD

CT angiography is considered as the first-line diagnostic tool for renal FMD. MR angiography offers an alternative in case of contraindications for CTA. CT angiography has a better spatial resolution, especially for distal lesions, and may visualize small calcifications, which allows a more accurate discrimination between FMD-RAS and ARAS. Renal duplex may be preferred as initial investigation in expert centers and/or performed in parallel in order to obtain information on the hemodynamic significance of the arterial lesions. However, specific diagnostic cut-offs for FMD are lacking and the criteria applied for ARAS may not be as accurate to exclude FMD. During ultrasound examination, it is important to visualize the entire length of the artery and not just the ostium, as distal lesions are common. Therefore, FMD cannot be formally ruled out if the arteries have not been fully visualized and checked for tortuosity or turbulence. Conventional catheter-based angiography remains the gold standard, but is mainly used if the level of suspicion of significant stenosis is very high and revascularization is considered.

If a renal lesion is present, the First International FMD Consensus advises to perform a CTA or MRA from brain to pelvis in order to detect FMD-lesions in other vascular beds, including aneurysms or dissections. Systematic screening of all vascular beds may lead to supplementary interventions—mainly aneurysm repair and/or angioplasty—and thus improve long-term prognosis [5, 112, 113]. In the Polish ARCADIA-POL registry, systematic brain-to-pelvis screening led to discovery of new lesions with interventional treatment indication in 25% of cases [120].

Medical Management of Renal Artery FMD

In the absence of specific data, the general guidelines regarding target BP and preferred antihypertensive drug are applied in renal FMD [33, 112], with preference for RAAS blockers [121, 122]. These recommendations are based on extrapolation from ARAS and the tentative involvement of the RAAS system. Despite the lack of specific RCTs and in the absence of contraindication, antiplatelet therapy (i.e., aspirin 75–100 mg daily) may and is often prescribed, in view of assumed increased risk of thrombotic or thromboembolic events, due to blood flow disturbances resulting from string-of-beads or marked arterial tortuosity [112]. Lipid-lowering drugs are not routinely recommended in FMD and are only indicated in light of global CV risk management, where general lipid management guidelines apply [123, 124].

Smoking cessation should be strongly encouraged as smoking may be associated with a higher prevalence of aneurysms, progression rate and complications [125].

Because of the female predominance in FMD, it has been hypothesized that elevated estrogen levels play a role in its development. However, there are no data demonstrating whether high estrogen levels (i.e., pregnancy, oral contraceptive use, or exogenous female hormones) increase the prevalence of FMD-lesions or FMD-associated complications (aneurysm rupture, dissection). Nevertheless, it is important to screen hypertensive women of childbearing potential for FMD and, if indicated, perform renal angioplasty prior to pregnancy. Indeed, pregnant patients with FMD have a higher prevalence of gestational hypertension, preterm birth and, to a lesser extent, preeclampsia, which may be prevented by timely FMD diagnosis and adequate management [126, 127].

Revascularization of FMD-RAS

Is Revascularization of FMD-RAS Needed?

The natural course of FMD is unclear but it is generally considered a non-progressive disease, with a low recurrence rate, and low incidence of new arterial lesions [67, 128]. Studies from the 80's examining the evolution of lesions by follow-up angiography showed progression of lesions in majority of cases [129, 130]. Complete arterial occlusion and ischemic atrophy of the involved kidney was rare. However, since angiographic follow-up was presumably applied in the most severe cases with the highest risk of progression, these findings might have been subject to bias. More recent data do not confirm this risk of progression [128, 131]. A recent pilot study (however only published as abstract) showed no progression in known arterial lesions and development of new arterial lesions in less than 2% of patients after 2–3 years of follow-up with CTA [131]. However, in patients with cervical artery dissection, the presence of FMD was associated with a higher risk of dissection recurrence (hazard ratio: 3.4) [132]. Given the lack of clear data and uncertainty regarding risk factors for progression, the international consensus recommends at least annual follow-up by a health care provider experienced in FMD [112]. The timing of clinical and radiological follow-up should be individualized, depending on the clinical picture and severity of the disease. In patients with renal FMD, follow-up should include BP monitoring and assessment of renal function. Imaging follow-up can be done by renal DDUS in expert centers, without the need of repeating CTA [112].

When and How Should FMD-RAS Be Revascularized?

The international consensus recommends revascularization by angioplasty without stenting for hemodynamically significant stenosis. A translesional pressure gradient of at least 10% in mean aortic pressure (i.e., $Pd/Pa < 0.90$) is proposed as cutoff. However, the latter is extrapolated from data on ARAS since specific data in a FMD population are lacking [112, 133].

The international consensus recommends to perform translesional pressure gradient measurements during catheter-based angiography, particularly in case of multifocal FMD [112]. Due to a varying number of beads and degree of inter-bead stenosis, the hemodynamic significance of multifocal lesions is difficult to assess visually, potentially leading to over- or underestimation of true hemodynamic impact of stenosis. However, this implies an invasive, costly and time-consuming approach, which is not available or feasible in a majority of centers.

Duplex Doppler ultrasound may give some idea of the hemodynamic impact of FMD-related stenosis, and may be useful to assess recovery of hemodynamic changes after angioplasty and during follow-up. However, the diagnostic criteria for hemodynamic significance are extrapolated from ARAS and are not validated in FMD [112].

Renal artery stenting is reserved for management of associated aneurysms, or for the treatment of procedural complications, such as arterial dissection or rupture, as cases of stent kinking, fracture, in-stent restenosis a/o occlusion have been reported [134]. In restenosis, repeat angioplasty is possible. However, in recurrent restenosis, surgery is preferred to avoid jeopardizing future surgical options. Surgery is also the treatment of choice for complex FMD lesions [112, 135].

The reported outcomes after revascularization by PTRA or surgery are highly variable. A meta-analysis of 47 angioplasty studies reported a hypertension cure rate of 36%, with higher cure rates after surgery (54%) [136]. Hypertension cure has been associated with younger patient age at the time of treatment, shorter duration of hypertension, and focal stenosis (compared to multifocal FMD). A recent study showed that the use of pressure wire to guide renal artery procedures in multifocal FMD (reaching a residual systolic trans-stenotic gradient $\leq$10 mmHg) may result in better long-term outcomes [137].

A protocol for catheter-based angiography and angioplasty in patients with FMD-RAS is published in the International Consensus guidelines [112].

Proposed Future Research in FMD-RAS

Tools for non-invasive evaluation of renal artery hemodynamics to aid in selecting cases most likely to benefit from renal artery revascularization.
Effectiveness studies of hemodynamic-guided angioplasty to determine the clinical outcome.
Efficacy studies of antiplatelet therapy in renal FMD.
Identification of factors associated with disease progression, complications (dissection, aneurysm), and major cardiovascular events.

In addition, other topics for further research are proposed for FMD in general [112, 115].

Rare Causes of Renovascular Hypertension

Thanks to extensive use of non-invasive imaging techniques, less common causes of RVH are increasingly being identified. These include focal stenosis as in phakomatosis (neurofibromatosis type 1 and tuberous sclerosis), Williams-Beuren syndrome, Alagille syndrome, and Grange syndrome. Vascular malformations and aneurysms (arteriovenous fistula, atypical FMD, Loeys-Dietz syndrome) can also induce RVH, as can inflammatory connective tissue disorders (Takayasu and giant cell arteritis, polyarteritis nodosa, Behcet's syndrome) and collagen vascular disorders (vascular Ehlers-Danlos, Marfan syndrome). Additionally dissections—either isolated renal artery dissection or secondary forms (ex., segmental arterial mediolysis, pregnancy, malignant hypertension or post-mechanical trauma)—can cause RVH. Finally, post-radiation fibrosis, thrombotic or cholesterol embolization may also lead to impaired renal blood flow and RVH.

The clinical approach depends on the underlying condition and should thus be tailored individually [112, 138].

Conclusions

Renovascular hypertension is usually caused by ARAS. In non-atherosclerotic forms, FMD is the most likely etiology. Renal artery stenosis often contributes to hypertensive, renal, and CV disease burden. Effective treatment of RAS should be tailored to the individual patient by a multidisciplinary team consisting of nephrologists, cardiologists, and interventional radiologists among others. The decision to revascularize or to treat pharmacologically will depend on the severity of stenosis, patient's age, and overall CV risk, the duration of hypertension, the presence of ischemic kidney damage, and the response to medical therapy.

Atherosclerotic RAS should be considered as a manifestation of a usually diffuse atherosclerotic disease. Therefore, optimal medical treatment of all CV risk factors remains the cornerstone of management to improve the CV prognosis of patients. Although major clinical trials have failed to establish the role of revascularization as a universal first-line treatment for ARAS, revascularization remains a valid treatment option in selected patients with significant RAS, a specific clinical presentation (i.e., resistant hypertension, recent decline in kidney function, flash pulmonary edema/heart failure) and viable renal parenchyma.

In FMD-RAS, revascularization is recommended as first-line treatment in young/middle-aged patients with recent hypertension and hemodynamically significant stenosis. Use of low-dose aspirin is often advised to prevent complications, while pharmacological treatment of hypertension and hyperlipidemia follows general guidelines. FMD should be considered as a systemic disease, as the majority of patients present with lesions in two or more vascular beds. Therefore, at least once in a lifetime, a systematic screening of the arterial beds by CT- or MR angiography is recommended.

References

1. Safian RD, Textor SC. Renal-artery stenosis. N Engl J Med. 2001;344(6):431–42.
2. Hansen KJ, Edwards MS, Craven TE, Cherr GS, Jackson SA, Appel RG, et al. Prevalence of renovascular disease in the elderly: a population-based study. J Vasc Surg. 2002;36(3):443–51.
3. Edwards MS, Hansen KJ, Craven TE, Bleyer AJ, Burke GL, Levy PJ, et al. Associations between renovascular disease and prevalent cardiovascular disease in the elderly: a population-based study. Vasc Endovasc Surg. 2004;38(1):25–35.

4. Peng M, Jiang X-J, Dong H, Zou Y-B, Zhang H-M, Song L, et al. Etiology of renal artery stenosis in 2047 patients: a single-center retrospective analysis during a 15-year period in China. J Hum Hypertens. 2016;30(2):124–8.
5. Pappaccogli M, Di Monaco S, Warchoł-Celińska E, Lorthioir A, Amar L, Aparicio LS, et al. The European/International Fibromuscular Dysplasia Registry and Initiative (FEIRI)—clinical phenotypes and their predictors based on a cohort of 1000 patients. Cardiovasc Res. 2021;117(3):950–9.
6. Vassallo J, Green D, Alderson HV, Chiu D, Sinha S, Kalra PA. Risks for mortality and renal replacement therapy in atherosclerotic renovascular disease compared with other causes of chronic kidney disease. Nephrology. 2015;20(10):688–96.
7. Pearce JD, Craven BL, Craven TE, Piercy KT, Stafford JM, Edwards MS, et al. Progression of atherosclerotic renovascular disease: a prospective population-based study. J Vasc Surg. 2006;44(5):955–62.
8. Shafique S, Peixoto AJ. Renal artery stenosis and cardiovascular risk. J Clin Hypertens (Greenwich). 2007;9:201–8.
9. Peng M, Dong H, Jiang X, Che W, Zou Y, Zhang Y, et al. A randomized unblinded trial to compare effects of intensive versus conventional lipid-lowering therapy in patients undergoing renal artery stenting. J Cardiol. 2019;74:443–50.
10. Wright JR, Shurrab AE, Cheung C, Waldek S, O'Donoghue DJ, Foley RN, et al. A prospective study of the determinants of renal functional outcome and mortality in atherosclerotic renovascular disease. Am J Kidney Dis. 2002;39(6):1153–61.
11. Edwards MS. Renovascular disease and the risk of adverse coronary events in the elderly. Arch Intern Med. 2005;165(2):207–13.
12. Guo H, Kalra PA, Gilbertson DT, Liu J, Chen S-C, Collins AJ, et al. Atherosclerotic renovascular disease in older US patients starting dialysis, 1996 to 2001. Circulation. 2007;115(1):50–8.
13. Klein AJ, Jaff MR, Gray BH, Aronow HD, Bersin RM, Diaz-Sandoval LJ, et al. SCAI appropriate use criteria for peripheral arterial interventions: an update. Catheter Cardiovasc Interv. 2017;90(4):E90–E110.
14. Van der Niepen P, Rossignol P, Lengelé JP, Berra E, Sarafidis P, Persu A. Renal artery stenosis in patients with resistant hypertension: stent it or not? Curr Hypertens Rep. 2017;19(1):5.
15. Pappaccogli M, Robberechts T, Lengelé JP, Van der Niepen P, Sarafidis P, Rabbia F, et al. Endovascular versus medical Management of Atherosclerotic Renovascular Disease: update and emerging concepts. Hypertension. 2023;80(6):1150–61.
16. Textor SC, Lerman LO. Paradigm shifts in atherosclerotic renovascular disease: where are we now? J Am Soc Nephrol. 2015;26(9):2074–80.
17. Hicks CW, Clark TWI, Cooper CJ, et al. Atherosclerotic renovascular disease: a KDIGO (kidney disease: improving global outcomes) controversies conference. Am J Kidney Dis. 2022;79(2):289–301.
18. Sarafidis PA, Theodorakopoulou M, Ortiz A, Fernandez-Fernandez B, Nistor I, Schmieder R, et al. Atherosclerotic renovascular disease: a clinical practice document by the European Renal Best Practice (ERBP) board of the European Renal Association (ERA) and the Working Group Hypertension and the Kidney of the European Society of Hypertension (ESH). Nephrol Dial Transplant. 2023;38:2835–50.
19. Sarafidis PA, Georgianos PI, Germanidis G, Giavroglou C, Nikolaidis P, Lasaridis AN, et al. Hypertension and symptomatic hypokalemia in a patient with simultaneous unilateral stenosis of intrarenal arteries and mesangioproliferative glomerulonephritis. Am J Kidney Dis. 2012;59(3):434–8.
20. Hill GS, Heudes D, Bariéty J. Morphometric study of arterioles and glomeruli in the aging kidney suggests focal loss of autoregulation. Kidney Int. 2003;63(3):1027–36.
21. Wright JR, Duggal A, Thomas R, Reeve R, Roberts ISD, Kalra PA. Clinicopathological correlation in biopsy-proven atherosclerotic nephropathy: implications for renal functional outcome in atherosclerotic renovascular disease. Nephrol Dial Transplant. 2001;16(4):765–70.

22. Messerli FH, Bangalore S, Makani H, et al. Flash pulmonary oedema and bilateral renal artery stenosis: the Pickering syndrome. Eur Heart J. 2011;32(18):2231–5.
23. Kalra PA, Guo H, Kausz AT, Gilbertson DT, Liu J, Chen SC, et al. Atherosclerotic renovascular disease in United States patients aged 67 years or older: risk factors, revascularization, and prognosis. Kidney Int. 2005;68(1):293–301.
24. Leertouwer TC, Pattynama PM, van den Berg-Huysmans A. Incidental renal artery stenosis in peripheral vascular disease: a case for treatment? Kidney Int. 2001;59(4):1480–3.
25. Ozkan U, Oguzkurt L, Tercan F, Nursal TZ. The prevalence and clinical predictors of incidental atherosclerotic renal artery stenosis. Eur J Radiol. 2009;69(3):550–4.
26. de Mast Q, Beutler JJ. The prevalence of atherosclerotic renal artery stenosis in risk groups: a systematic literature review. J Hypertens. 2009;27(7):1333–40.
27. de Silva R, Loh H, Rigby AS, Nikitin NP, Witte KKA, Goode K, et al. Epidemiology, associated factors, and prognostic outcomes of renal artery stenosis in chronic heart failure assessed by magnetic resonance angiography. Am J Cardiol. 2007;100(2):273–9.
28. Kawarada O, Yokoi Y, Morioka N, Takemoto K. Renal artery stenosis in cardio-and cerebrovascular disease renal duplex ultrasonography as an initial screening examination. Circ J. 2007;71(12):1942–7.
29. Januszewicz A, Januszewicz M, Prejbisz A, Dobrowolski P, Persu A, Kreutz R. Atherosclerotic renovascular disease and cardiovascular risk: new concepts. Pol Arch Intern Med. 2022;132(12):16384. https://doi.org/10.20452/pamw.16384.
30. Plouin PF, Chatellier G, Darné B, Raynaud A. Blood pressure outcome of angioplasty in atherosclerotic renal artery stenosis. Hypertension. 1998;31(3):823–9.
31. Endo M, Kumakura H, Kanai H, Araki Y, Kasama S, Sumino H, et al. Prevalence and risk factors for renal artery stenosis and chronic kidney disease in Japanese patients with peripheral arterial disease. Hypertens Res. 2010;33(9):911–5.
32. van Jaarsveld BC, Krijnen P, Pieterman H, Derkx FH, Deinum J, Postma CT, et al. The effect of balloon angioplasty on hypertension in atherosclerotic renal-artery stenosis. Dutch Renal Artery Stenosis Intervention Cooperative Study Group. N Engl J Med. 2000;342(14):1007–14.
33. Mancia G, Kreutz R, Brunström M, Burnier M, Grassi G, Januszewicz A, et al. 2023 ESH guidelines for the management of arterial hypertension the task force for the management of arterial hypertension of the European Society of Hypertension. J Hypertens. 2023;41(12):1874–2071.
34. Missouris CG, Buckenham T, Cappuccio FP, MacGregor GA. Renal artery stenosis: a common and important problem in patients with peripheral vascular disease. Am J Med. 1994;96(1):10–4.
35. Lim J, Truong HD, Song TY, Giam WJH, Koh EL, Tan JKS. The interdependent hemodynamic influence between abdominal aortic aneurysm and renal artery stenosis. Sci Rep. 2024;14(1):31986.
36. Ritchie J, Green D, Alderson HV, Chiu D, Sinha S, Kalra PA. Risks for mortality and renal replacement therapy in atherosclerotic renovascular disease compared with other causes of chronic kidney disease. Nephrology. 2015;20(10):688–96.
37. Wright JR, Shurrab AE, Cooper A, Kalra PR, Foley RN, Kalra PA. Left ventricular morphology and function in patients with atherosclerotic Renovascular disease. J Am Soc Nephrol. 2005;16(9):2746–53.
38. Januszewicz A, Mulatero P, Dobrowolski P, Monticone S, Van der Niepen P, Sarafidis P, et al. Cardiac phenotypes in secondary hypertension: JACC state-of-the-art review. J Am Coll Cardiol. 2022;80:1480–97.
39. Rizzoni D, Muiesan ML, Porteri E, Salvetti M, Castellano M, Bettoni G, et al. Relations between cardiac and vascular structure in patients with primary and secondary hypertension. J Am Coll Cardiol. 1998;32(4):985–92.
40. Muiesan ML, Rizzoni D, Salvetti M, Porteri E, Monteduro C, Guelfi D, et al. Structural changes in small resistance arteries and left ventricular geometry in patients with primary and secondary hypertension. J Hypertens. 2002;20(7):1439–44.

41. Li Y, Chen Z, Lan R, Ran T, He J, Li J, et al. Atherosclerotic renal artery stenosis, mediating biomarkers, and risk of cardiac among individuals with hypertension: a real-world study. Int J Cardiol Heart Vasc. 2024;55:101556.
42. Matsumura K, Fujii K, Oniki H, Oka M, Iida M. Role of aldosterone in left ventricular hypertrophy in hypertension. Am J Hypertens. 2006;19(1):13–8.
43. Cuspidi C, Dell'Oro R, Sala C, et al. Renal artery stenosis and left ventricular hypertrophy. J Hypertens. 2017;35(12):2339–45.
44. Pickering TG, Herman L, Devereux RB, Sotelo JE, James GD, Sos TA, et al. Recurrent pulmonary oedema in hypertension due to bilateral renal artery stenosis: treatment by angioplasty or surgical revascularisation. Lancet. 1988;2(8610):551–2. https://doi.org/10.1016/s0140-6736(88)92668-2.
45. Sanga V, Bertoli E, Crimì F, Barbiero G, Battistel M, Seccia TM, Rossi GP. Pickering syndrome: an overlooked Renovascular cause of recurrent heart failure. J Am Heart Assoc. 2023;12(19):e030474. https://doi.org/10.1161/JAHA.123.030474.
46. Khangura KK, Eirin A, Kane GC, Misra S, Textor SC, Lerman A, et al. Cardiac function in renovascular hypertensive patients with and without renal dysfunction. Am J Hypertens. 2014;27(3):445–53.
47. Ghanami RJ, Rana H, Craven TE, Hoyle J, Edwards MS, Hansen KJ. Diastolic function predicts survival after renal revascularization. J Vasc Surg. 2011;54:1720–6.
48. Dobrowolski P, Januszewicz M, Klisiewicz A, Prejbisz A, Warchoł-Celińska E, Michałowska I, et al. Echocardiographic assessment of left ventricular morphology and function in patients with fibromuscular dysplasia. J Hypertens. 2018;36(6):1318–25.
49. Gloviczki ML, Glockner JF, Lerman LO, McKusick MA, Misra S, Grande JP, et al. Preserved oxygenation despite reduced blood flow in poststenotic kidneys in human atherosclerotic renal artery stenosis. Hypertension. 2010;55:961–6.
50. Abumoawad A, Saad A, Ferguson CM, Eirin A, Woollard JR, Herrmann SM, et al. Tissue hypoxia, inflammation, and loss of glomerular filtration rate in human atherosclerotic renovascular disease. Kidney Int. 2019;95(4):948–57.
51. Eirin A, Chade AR, Lerman LO. Kidney intrinsic mechanisms as novel targets in Renovascular hypertension. Hypertension. 2024;81(2):206–17.
52. Bax L, Woittiez AJ, Kouwenberg HJ, Mali WP, Buskens E, Beek FJ, et al. Stent placement in patients with atherosclerotic renal artery stenosis and impaired renal function: a randomized trial. Ann Intern Med. 2009;150:840–8.
53. Ronden RA, Houben AJ, Kessels AG, Stehouwer CD, de Leeuw PW, Kroon AA. Predictors of clinical outcome after stent placement in atherosclerotic renal artery stenosis: a systematic review and meta-analysis of prospective studies. J Hypertens. 2010;28(12):2370–7.
54. Harvin HJ, Verma N, Nikolaidis P, Hanley M, Dogra VS, Goldfarb S, et al. ACR Appropriateness Criteria® Renovascular Hypertension. J Am Coll Radiol. 2017;14(11):S540–9.
55. Fu J, Lin Z, Zhang B, Song L, Qin N, Qiu J, et al. Magnetic resonance imaging in atherosclerotic renal artery stenosis: the update and future directions from interventional perspective. Kidney Dis (Basel). 2023;10(1):23–31.
56. Shivgulam ME, Liu H, Kivell MJ, MacLeod JR, O'Brien MW. Effectiveness of contrast-enhanced duplex ultrasound for detecting renal artery stenosis: a systematic review. J Clin Ultrasound. 2024;52(6):763–72.
57. Li Y, Wang Y, Liu ZS, Ma N, Zhang WD, Ren JH. Clinical practice report of contrast-enhanced ultrasound in renal artery disease. J Ultrasound Med. 2024;43(1):117–25.
58. Sun D, Chen Z, Eirin A, Zhu XY, Lerman A, Textor SC, et al. Hypercholesterolemia impairs nonstenotic kidney outcomes after reversal of experimental Renovascular hypertension. Am J Hypertens. 2016;29(7):853–9.
59. Vassallo D, Kalra PA. Progress in the treatment of atherosclerotic renovascular disease: the conceptual journey and the unanswered questions. Nephrol Dial Transplant. 2016;31(10):1595–605.

60. Losito A, Errico R, Santirosi P, Lupattelli T, Scalera GB, Lupattelli L. Long-term follow-up of atherosclerotic renovascular disease. Beneficial effect of ACE inhibition. Nephrol Dial Transplant. 2005;20:1604–9.
61. Chrysochou C, Foley RN, Young JF, Khavandi K, Cheung CM, Kalra PA. Dispelling the myth: the use of renin-angiotensin blockade in atheromatous renovascular disease. Nephrol Dial Transplant. 2012;27(4):1403–9.
62. van de Ven PJ, Beutler JJ, Kaatee R, Beek FJ, Mali WP, Koomans HA. Angiotensin converting enzyme inhibitor-induced renal dysfunction in atherosclerotic renovascular disease. Kidney Int. 1998;53:986–93.
63. Hricik DE, Dunn MJ. Angiotensin-converting enzyme inhibitor-induced renal failure: causes, consequences, and diagnostic uses. J Am Soc Nephrol. 1990;1(6):845–58.
64. Bakris GL, Weir MR. Angiotensin-converting enzyme inhibitor-associated elevations in serum creatinine: is this a cause for concern? Arch Intern Med. 2000;160:685–93.
65. Ritchie J, Green D, Alderson HV, Chrysochou C, Vassallo D, Sinha S, et al. Associations of antiplatelet therapy and beta blockade with patient outcomes in atherosclerotic renovascular disease. J Am Soc Hypertens. 2016;10(2):149–58.
66. Crowley JJ, Santos RM, Peter RH, Puma JA, Schwab SJ, Phillips HR, et al. Progression of renal artery stenosis in patients undergoing cardiac catheterization. Am Heart J. 1998;136(5):913–8.
67. Pohl MA, Novick AC. Natural history of atherosclerotic and fibrous renal artery disease: clinical implications. Am J Kidney Dis. 1985;5(4):A120–30.
68. Caps MT, Perissinotto C, Zierler RE, Polissar NL, Bergelin RO, Tullis MJ, et al. Prospective study of atherosclerotic disease progression in the renal artery. Circulation. 1998;98(25):2866–72. https://doi.org/10.1161/01.cir.98.25.2866.
69. Chábová V, Schirger A, Stanson AW, McKusick MA, Textor SC. Outcomes of atherosclerotic renal artery stenosis managed without revascularization. Mayo Clin Proc. 2000;75(5):437–44.
70. Caps MT, Zierler RE, Polissar NL, Bergelin RO, Beach KW, Cantwell-Gab K, et al. Risk of atrophy in kidneys with atherosclerotic renal artery stenosis. Kidney Int. 1998;53(3):735–42.
71. Murphy TP, Soares G, Kim M. Increase in utilization of percutaneous renal artery interventions by medicare beneficiaries, 1996–2000. AJR Am J Roentgenol. 2004;183(3):561–8.
72. Plouin PF, Chatellier G, Darné B, Raynaud A. Blood pressure outcome of angioplasty in atherosclerotic renal artery stenosis: a randomized trial. Essai Multicentrique Medicaments vs Angioplastie (EMMA) study group. Hypertension. 1998;31:823–9.
73. Webster J, Marshall F, Andalla M, Dominiczak A, Edwards R, Isles CG, et al. Randomised comparison of percutaneous angioplasty vs continued medical therapy for hypertensive patients with atheromatous renal artery stenosis. Scottish and Newcastle Renal Artery Stenosis Collaborative Group. J Hum Hypertens. 1998;12:329–35.
74. Wheatley K, Ives N, Gray R, Kalra PA, Moss JG, Baigent C, ASTRAL Investigators, et al. Revascularization versus medical therapy for renal-artery stenosis. N Engl J Med. 2009;361:1953–62.
75. Cooper CJ, Murphy TP, Cutlip DE, Jamerson K, Henrich W, Reid DM, CORAL Investigators, et al. Stenting and medical therapy for atherosclerotic renal-artery stenosis. N Engl J Med. 2014;370:13–22.
76. Sarafidis PA, Stavridis KC, Loutradis CN, Saratzis AN, Pateinakis P, Papagianni A, et al. To intervene or not? A man with multidrugresistant hypertension, endovascular abdominal aneurysm repair, bilateral renal artery stenosis and end-stage renal disease salvaged with renal artery stenting. Blood Press. 2016;25(2):123–8.
77. Hughes JS, Dove HG, Gifford RW Jr, Feinstein AR. Duration of blood pressure elevation in accurately predicting surgical cure of renovascular hypertension. Am Heart J. 1981;101(4):408–13.
78. Radermacher J, Chavan A, Bleck J, Vitzthum A, Stoess B, Gebel MJ, et al. Use of Doppler ultrasonography to predict the outcome of therapy for renal-artery stenosis. N Engl J Med. 2001;344:410–7.

79. Viazzi F, Leoncini G, Derchi LE, Pontremoli R. Ultrasound Doppler renal resistive index: a useful tool for the management of the hypertensive patient. J Hypertens. 2014;32(1):149–53.
80. Chrysochou C, Green D, Ritchie J, Buckley DL, Kalra PA. Kidney volume to GFR ratio predicts functional improvement after revascularization in atheromatous renal artery stenosis. PLoS One. 2017;12(6):e0177178.
81. Ebrahimi B, Gandhi D, Alsaeedi MH, Lerman LO. Patterns of cortical oxygenation may predict the response to stenting in subjects with renal artery stenosis: a radiomics-based model. Cardiovasc Magn Reson. 2024;26(1):100993.
82. Simeoni M, Borrelli S, Garofalo C, Fuiano G, Esposito C, Comi A, et al. Atherosclerotic-nephropathy: an updated narrative review. J Nephrol. 2021;34(1):125–36.
83. Thadhani R, Pascual M, Tolkoff-Rubin N, Nickeleit V, Colvin R. Preliminary description of focal segmental glomerulosclerosis in patients with renovascular disease. Lancet. 1996;347(8996):231–3.
84. Green D, Ritchie JP, Chrysochou C, Kalra PA. Revascularisation of renal artery stenosis as a therapy for heart failure: an observational cohort study. Lancet. 2015;385(Suppl 1):S11.
85. Bhalla V, Textor SC, Beckman JA, Casanegra AI, Cooper CJ, Kim ESH, et al. Revascularization for Renovascular disease: a scientific statement from the American Heart Association. Hypertension. 2022;79(8):e128–43.
86. Vassallo D, Ritchie J, Green D, Chrysochou C, Kalra PA. The effect of revascularization in patients with anatomically significant atherosclerotic renovascular disease presenting with high-risk clinical features. Nephrol Dial Transplant. 2018;33(3):497–506.
87. Ritchie J, Green D, Chrysochou C, Chalmers N, Foley RN, Kalra PA. High-risk clinical presentations in atherosclerotic Renovascular disease: prognosis and response to renal artery revascularization. Am J Kidney Dis. 2014;63(2):186–97.
88. Kawarada O, Yokoi Y, Morioka N, Shiotani S, Higashimori A. Cardiac benefits of renal artery stenting. EuroIntervention. 2010;6(4):485–91.
89. Chrysochou C, Sharma R, Kalra PA, Kalra PR. Improved left ventricular filling following bilateral renal artery stenting. Int J Cardiol. 2011;150(1):e40.
90. Reinhard M, Schousboe K, Andersen UB, Buus NH, Rantanen JM, Bech JN, et al. Renal artery stenting in consecutive high-risk patients with atherosclerotic Renovascular disease: a prospective 2-center cohort study. J Am Heart Assoc. 2022;11(7):e024421.
91. Cuspidi C, Tadic M, Sala C, Quarti-Trevano F, Gherbesi E, Mancia G, Grassi G. Left ventricular mass reduction and hypertrophy regression following renal artery revascularization: a meta-analysis. J Hypertens. 2021;39:4–11.
92. Iwashima Y, Fukuda T, Horio T, Kusunoki H, Hayashi SI, Kamide K, et al. Impact of percutaneous revascularization on left ventricular mass and its relationship to outcome in hypertensive patients with renal artery stenosis. Am J Hypertens. 2020;33(6):570–80.
93. Bloch MJ, Trost DW, Pickering TG, Sos TA, August P. Prevention of recurrent pulmonary edema in patients with bilateral renovascular disease through renal artery stent placement. Am J Hypertens. 1999;12:1–7.
94. van de Ven PJ, Kaatee R, Beutler JJ, Beek FJ, Woittiez AJ, Buskens E, et al. Arterial stenting and balloon angioplasty in ostial atherosclerotic renovascular disease: a randomised trial. Lancet. 1999;353(9149):282–6.
95. Rocha-Singh K, Jaff MR, Rosenfield K, ASPIRE-2 Trial Investigators. Evaluation of the safety and effectiveness of renal artery stenting after unsuccessful balloon angioplasty: the ASPIRE-2 study. J Am Coll Cardiol. 2005;46(5):776–83.
96. Zeller T, Frank U, Müller C, Bürgelin K, Sinn L, Bestchorn HP, et al. Predictors of improved renal function after percutaneous stent-supported angioplasty of severe atherosclerotic ostial renal artery stenosis. Circulation. 2003;108(18):2244–9.
97. Hirsch AT, Haskal ZJ, Hertzer NR, Bakal CW, Creager MA, Halperin JL, et al. ACC/AHA 2005 practice guidelines for the management of patients with peripheral arterial disease (lower extremity, renal, mesenteric, and abdominal aortic): a collaborative report from the American Association for Vascular Surgery/Society for Vascular Surgery, Society for Cardiovascular Angiography and Interventions, Society for Vascular Medicine and Biology,

Society of Interventional Radiology, and the ACC/AHA Task Force on Practice Guidelines Lawrie(Writing Committee to Develop Guidelines for the Management of Patients with Peripheral Arterial Disease): endorsed by the American Association of Cardiovascular and Pulmonary Rehabilitation; National Heart, Lung, and Blood Institute; Society for Vascular Nursing; TransAtlantic Inter-Society Consensus; and Vascular Disease Foundation. Circulation. 2006;113(11):e463–654.

98. Ivanovic V, McKusick MA, Johnson CM 3rd, Sabater EA, Andrews JC, Breen JF, et al. Renal artery stent placement: complications at a single tertiary care center. J Vasc Interv Radiol. 2003;14(2 Pt 1):217–25.
99. Rocha-Singh KJ, Novack V, Pencina M, D'Agostino R, Ansel G, Rosenfield K, et al. Objective performance goals of safety and blood pressure efficacy for clinical trials of renal artery bare metal stents in hypertensive patients with atherosclerotic renal artery stenosis. Catheter Cardiovasc Interv. 2011;78(5):779–89.
100. Henry M, Amor M, Henry I, Ethevenot G, Tzvetanov K, Courvoisier A, et al. Stents in the treatment of renal artery stenosis: long-term follow-up. J Endovasc Surg. 1999;6(1):42–51.
101. Boateng FK, Greco BA. Renal artery stenosis: prevalence of, risk factors for, and management of in-stent stenosis. Am J Kidney Dis. 2013;61(1):147–60.
102. Del Conde I, Galin ID, Trost B, Kang J, Lookstein R, Woodward M, et al. Renal artery duplex ultrasound criteria for the detection of significant in-stent restenosis. Catheter Cardiovasc Interv. 2014;83(4):612–8.
103. Rocha-Singh K, Jaff MR, Lynne Kelley E, RENAISSANCE Trial Investigators. Renal artery stenting with noninvasive duplex ultrasound follow-up: 3-year results from the RENAISSANCE renal stent trial. Catheter Cardiovasc Interv. 2008;72(6):853–62.
104. Chi YW, White CJ, Thornton S, Milani RV. Ultrasound velocity criteria for renal in-stent restenosis. J Vasc Surg. 2009;50(1):119–23.
105. Duan Y, Xiang F, Li Q, Li K, Grajo JR, Samir AE. Predictive value of duplex ultrasound for significant in-stent restenosis after percutaneous transluminal renal artery stent placement: a propensity score matching analysis. Ultrasound Med Biol. 2019;45(4):913–20.
106. Rosławiecka A, Kabłak-Ziembicka A, Badacz R, Rzeźnik D, Pieniążek P, Trystuła M, et al. Long-term outcomes and determinants of stenosis recurrence after renal artery angioplasty in hypertensive patients with renovascular disease. Postepy Kardiol Interwencyjnej. 2020;16(1):65–75.
107. Holden A, Hill A, Jaff MR, Pilmore H. Renal artery stent revascularization with embolic protection in patients with ischemic nephropathy. Kidney Int. 2006;70(5):948–55.
108. Stanley JC, David M. Hume memorial lecture. Surgical treatment of renovascular hypertension. Am J Surg. 1997;174(2):102–10.
109. Novick AC. Long-term results of surgical revascularization for renal artery disease. Urol Clin North Am. 2001;28(4):827–31.
110. Weibull H, Bergqvist D, Bergentz SE, Jonsson K, Hulthén L, Manhem P. Percutaneous transluminal renal angioplasty versus surgical reconstruction of atherosclerotic renal artery stenosis: a prospective randomized study. J Vasc Surg. 1993;18(5):841–52.
111. Lawrie GM, Morris GC Jr, Glaeser DH, DeBakey ME. Renovascular reconstruction: factors affecting long-term prognosis in 919 patients followed up to 31 years. Am J Cardiol. 1989;63(15):1085–92.
112. Gornik HL, Persu A, Adlam D, Aparicio LS, Azizi M, Boulanger M, Working Group 'Hypertension and the Kidney' of the European Society of Hypertension (ESH) and the Society for Vascular Medicine (SVM), et al. First international consensus on the diagnosis and management of fibromuscular dysplasia. J Hypertens. 2019;37(2):229–52.
113. Van der Niepen P, Robberechts T, Devos H, van Tussenbroek F, Januszewicz A, Persu A. Fibromuscular dysplasia: its various phenotypes in everyday practice in 2021. Kardiol Pol. 2021;79(7–8):733–44.
114. Arnaud C, Boulanger M, Lorthioir A, Amar L, Azarine A, Boyer L, et al. Male sex is associated with cervical artery dissection in patients with fibromuscular dysplasia. J Am Heart Assoc. 2021;10(11):e018311.

115. Persu A, Dobrowolski P, Gornik HL, Olin JW, Adlam D, Azizi M, et al. Current progress in clinical, molecular, and genetic aspects of adult fibromuscular dysplasia. Cardiovasc Res. 2022;118(1):65–83.
116. Januszewicz M, Januszewicz A, Michałowska I, Klisiewicz A, Dobrowolski P, Warchoł-Celińska E, et al. Intra-renal blood flow parameters assessed by doppler sonography in hypertensive patients with fibromuscular dysplasia—relationship to renal function and target organ damage. The ARCADIA-POL study. Pol Arch Intern Med. 2019;129(4):234–41.
117. Gavalas M, Meisner R, Labropoulos N, Gasparis A, Tassiopoulos A. Renal infarction complicating fibromuscular dysplasia. Vasc Endovasc Surg. 2014;48(7–8):445–51.
118. Abi Doumet A, Bustos B, Garrell J, Salman M, Haider L. Fibromuscular dysplasia presenting as acute unilateral renal infarction: a case report and review of two diseases. Cureus. 2023;15(3):e35933.
119. Al-Hussaini A, Abdelaty AMSEK, Gulsin GS, Arnold JR, Garcia-Guimaraes M, Premawardhana D, et al. Chronic infarct size after spontaneous coronary artery dissection: implications for pathophysiology and clinical management. Eur Heart J. 2020;41(23):2197–205.
120. Warchol-Celinska E, Prejbisz A, Dobrowolski P, et al. Systematic and multidisciplinary evaluation of fibromuscular dysplasia patients reveals high prevalence of previously undetected fibromuscular dysplasia lesions and affects clinical decisions: the ARCADIA-POL study. Hypertension. 2020;75(4):1102–9.
121. Whelton PK, Carey RM, Aronow WS, et al. 2017 ACC/AHA/AAPA/ABC/ACPM/AGS/APhA/ASH/ASPC/NMA/PCNA guideline for the prevention, detection, evaluation, and management of high blood pressure in adults: a report of the American College of Cardiology/American Heart Association Task Force on Clinical Practice Guidelines. J Am Coll Cardiol. 2018;71:e127–248.
122. Dworkin LD, Cooper CJ. Clinical practice. Renal artery stenosis. N Engl J Med. 2009;361:1972–8.
123. Arnett DK, Blumenthal RS, Albert MA, Buroker AB, Goldberger ZD, Hahn EJ, et al. 2019 ACC/AHA guideline on the primary prevention of cardiovascular disease: a report of the American College of Cardiology/American Heart Association Task Force on Clinical Practice Guidelines. Circulation. 2019;140(11):e596–646.
124. Mach F, Baigent C, Catapano AL, Koskinas KC, Casula M, Badimon L, et al. ESC Scientific Document Group. 2019 ESC/EAS Guidelines for the management of dyslipidaemias: lipid modification to reduce cardiovascular risk. Eur Heart J. 2020;41(1):111–88.
125. O'Connor S, Gornik HL, Froehlich JB, Gu X, Gray BH, Mace PD, et al. Smoking and adverse outcomes in fibromuscular dysplasia: U.S. registry report. J Am Coll Cardiol. 2016;67:1750–1.
126. Pappaccogli M, Prejbisz A, Ciurică S, Bruno RM, Aniszczuk-Hybiak A, Bracalente I, European/International Fibromuscular Dysplasia Registry and Initiative (FEIRI) and the Working Group "Hypertension and the Kidney" of the ESH, et al. Pregnancy-related complications in patients with fibromuscular dysplasia: a report from the European/international fibromuscular dysplasia registry. Hypertension. 2020;76(2):545–53.
127. Khoury MH, Hershey S, LeLeiko RM. Sex and gender differences in fibromuscular dysplasia. US Cardiol. 2024;18:e08.
128. Kadian-Dodov D, Goldfinger JZ, Gustavson S, Olin JW. Natural history of cervical artery fibromuscular dysplasia and associated neurovascular events. Cerebrovasc Dis. 2018;46(1–2):33–9.
129. Schreiber MJ, Pohl MA, Novick AC. The natural history of atherosclerotic and fibrous renal artery disease. Urol Clin North Am. 1984;11(3):383–92.
130. Goncharenko V, Gerlock AJ, Shaff MI, Hollifield JW. Progression of renal artery fibromuscular dysplasia in 42 patients as seen on angiography. Radiology. 1981;139(1):45–51.
131. de Leeuw PW, Zelis P, Kleijnen B, Schutten M, Kroon A. Follow-up of vascular lesions in fibromuscular dysplasia. No evidence for progression yet. J Hypertens. 2023;41(Suppl 3):e48.

132. Bonacina S, Grassi M, Zedde M, Zini A, Bersano A, Gandolfo C, et al. Clinical features of patients with cervical artery dissection and fibromuscular dysplasia. Stroke. 2021;52(3):821–9.
133. De Bruyne B, Manoharan G, Pijls NH, Verhamme K, Madaric J, Bartunek J, et al. Assessment of renal artery stenosis severity by pressure gradient measurements. J Am Coll Cardiol. 2006;48:1851–5.
134. Kądziela J, Jóźwik-Plebanek K, Pappaccogli M, van der Niepen P, Prejbisz A, Dobrowolski P, et al. Risks and benefits of renal artery stenting in fibromuscular dysplasia: lessons from the ARCADIA-POL study. Vasc Med. 2024;29(1):50–7.
135. Lacombe M, Ricco JB. Surgical revascularization of renal artery after complicated or failed percutaneous transluminal renal angioplasty. J Vasc Surg. 2006;44:537–44.
136. Trinquart L, Mounier-Vehier C, Sapoval M, Gagnon N, Plouin P-F. Efficacy of revascularization for renal artery stenosis caused by fibromuscular dysplasia. A systematic review and metaanalysis. Hypertension. 2010;56:525–32.
137. Cadour F, Silhol F, Iline N, Giorgi R, Lorthioir A, Amar L, et al. Insights from intravascular pressure measurement of renal artery revascularization in patients with fibromuscular dysplasia: the DYSART study. J Vasc Surg. 2022;75:939–49.
138. Persu A, Canning C, Prejbisz A, Dobrowolski P, Amar L, Chrysochou C, et al. Beyond atherosclerosis and fibromuscular dysplasia: rare causes of renovascular hypertension. Hypertension. 2021;78:898–911.

Renal Denervation for Hypertension in Chronic Kidney Disease

Agnes Bosch and Roland E. Schmieder

Introduction

Hypertension can be considered both a major cause of and a predominant accelerating factor in the progressive loss of renal function [1]. A significant proportion of Chronic Kidney Disease (CKD) patients exhibit treatment-resistant hypertension. Despite advances in pharmacological treatment, innovative therapeutic approaches to controlling hypertension are needed to slow the progression of renal function decline [2].

Renal Denervation (RDN) reduces Blood Pressure (BP) by modulating efferent and afferent renal sympathetic nerve activity [3]. Whereas initial open-label studies suggested a pronounced BP-lowering effect of RDN in patients with severe, treatment-resistant hypertension [4], the Symplicity HTN-3 trial found no statistically significant difference in BP reduction between the RDN and sham group. Subsequent analysis of the Symplicity HTN-3 trial identified several confounding factors, including incomplete denervation, drug turbulence during the run-in and follow-up phase, as well as racial and socioeconomic factors [5–7], that explained these results. Over the following years, several second-generation, sham-controlled trials were successfully conducted to document the safety and efficacy of RDN in the general hypertensive population.

A most recent meta-analysis included 10 trials, only sham-controlled randomized prospective studies with 2478 patients with uncontrolled hypertension [8]. Compared with the sham procedure, RDN reduced 24-h and office systolic BP by 4.4 mmHg (95% Confidence Interval (CI), 2.7–6.1; $P < 0.00001$) and 6.6 mmHg (95% CI, 3.6–9.7; $P < 0.0001$), respectively. The 24-h and office

A. Bosch (✉) · R. E. Schmieder
Department of Nephrology and Hypertension, Friedrich-Alexander-University Erlangen-Nürnberg (FAU), Erlangen, Germany

P. Sarafidis, R. Pontremoli (eds.), *Hypertension and Chronic Kidney Disease*, Updates in Hypertension and Cardiovascular Protection,
https://doi.org/10.1007/978-3-032-29564-4_19

diastolic BP mirrored these results (−2.6 mmHg [95% CI, −3.6 to −1.5]; $P < 0.00001$; −3.5 mmHg [9% CI, −5.4 to −1.6]; $P = 0.0003$, respectively) [8].

Overall safety and efficacy data led to a Class II recommendation for RDN use in both, the 2024 European Society of Cardiology (ESC) Guidelines for the Treatment of Hypertension and the 2023 European Society of Hypertension (ESH) Guidelines [9, 10]. When focusing on patients with CKD, both guidelines state that RDN is not currently recommended for patients with an eGFR of less than 40 ml/min/1.73 m^2, unless further evidence becomes available [9, 10].

Rationale for RDN in Patients with Chronic Kidney Disease

Increased efferent Sympathetic Nervous System (SNS) activity to the kidneys contributes to CKD progression by leading to activation of the Renin-Angiotensin System (RAS), sodium retention and decreased renal perfusion [3, 11, 12]. Afferent neural signalling from the failing native kidney to the brain is also considered a key mediator in the process of increased central SNS activity. Afferent signalling affects the entire Cardiovascular (CV) system and worsens CV and renal prognosis [11]. Indeed, several clinical studies using microneurography have revealed an inverse correlation between eGFR and SNS activity in patients with CKD [13]. Increased efferent and afferent signalling have been shown to act

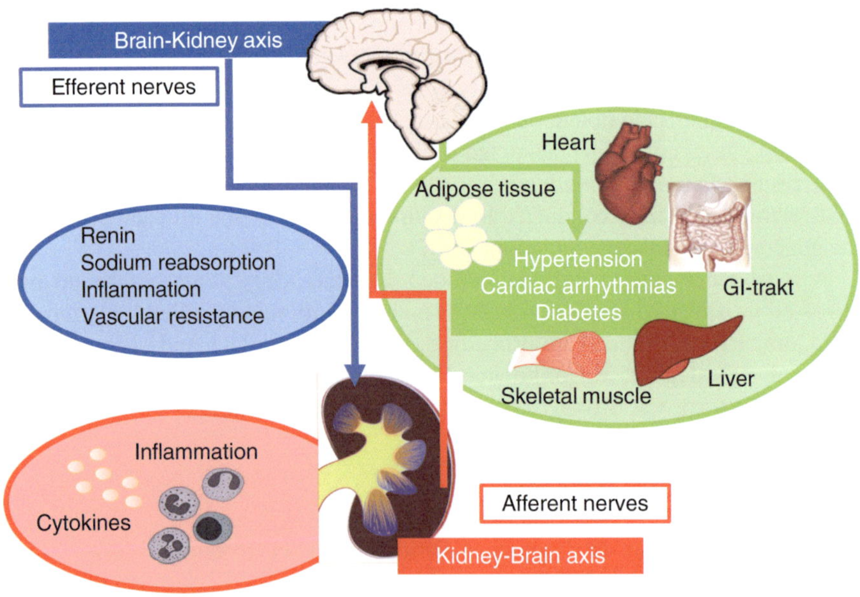

Fig. 1 Relevant efferent and afferent pathways of the bidirectional kidney-brain axis

in a vicious cycle involving increased SNS activity, CKD and hypertension (Fig. 1) [14].

While many targets are addressed in the recently recommended treatment approaches for CKD, none of the comprehensive treatment options directly address the SNS [15]. Given that both elevated BP and increased SNS activity are major progression factors of cardiorenal disease, RDN may emerge as a promising adjunctive treatment option for this patient population.

General Safety Aspects of RDN in Patients with CKD

A meta-analysis of procedure-related events in 238 patients with CKD from 11 single-centre, non-randomized, uncontrolled studies found no serious procedure-related complications (including all-cause death, major cardiovascular events, perioperative complications and hypertensive crisis) [16]. There was no incidence of electrolyte disturbances, and only a few adverse reactions were related to puncture site complications (one case of bleeding, three cases of pseudoaneurysm (1.3%) and seven cases of haematoma (2.9%)) [16]. Radiofrequency- and ultrasound-based RDN have been extensively analyzed in animal studies and found not to harm the vascular wall. In radiofrequency-based RDN, blood flow is used for cooling to protect the endothelial layer. Additionally, energy is not delivered in 360-degree plane [17]. A potential overheating of the vascular wall is directly measured, resulting in the immediate shut-off of radiofrequency delivery [18]. In ultrasound-based RDN, energy is delivered in a 360-degree plane. Ultrasound-based RDN uses a saline-filled balloon for cooling to prevent vascular injury.

Renal Artery Safety

Up to now, there is no evidence that the RDN procedure is related to the development of new renal artery stenosis. A meta-analysis of 5769 patients in 50 clinical trials showed an annular incidence of renal artery stenting after radiofrequency RDN of 0.2%, with no adverse events occurring in the distal arteries in the CKD subgroup (396 patients) [19]. A retrospective analysis of 3-year follow-up data from the Global Symplicity Registry also found rates of renal artery stenosis of less than 0.5%, with no significant difference between patients with and without CKD [20]. A recent analysis using imaging techniques also showed no association with renal artery stenosis in 557 patients after RDN (36-month follow-up) [21]. These incidence data for renal artery stenosis following RDN are comparable with the natural incidence rate of renal artery stenosis in hypertensive patients, which ranges from 0.5% to 7% [22].

Acute Kidney Injury

RDN angiography requires the use of iodinated contrast media. The potential adverse effects on renal function, such as acute kidney injury, must be discussed. Data on the short-term effects on renal function after RDN are limited. A meta-analysis of randomized controlled clinical trials involving over 2000 patients, including those with mild to moderate renal impairment, found no significant difference in the predefined safety outcomes between the RDN and sham groups, including the onset of End-Stage Kidney Disease (ESKD) [8]. However, the meta-analysis did not separately report short-term changes in renal function. A small clinical study of 30 patients with CKD stages 2–4 showed no difference in eGFR and UACR 1 month after RDN compared to baseline values [23].

The likelihood of contrast-induced acute kidney injury is thought to depend on the amount of contrast media used and the degree of renal impairment. Adequate peri-procedural patient hydration is generally recommended as a preventive strategy [18]. Alternatively, CO_2 angiography and intravascular ultrasound may be used to reduce contrast media volume [24].

The Safety and Efficacy of RDN in Patients with CKD Stages 3 and 4

Important safety and efficacy data have been obtained in the Global Symplicity Registry. Three-year follow-up data show no significant difference in eGFR decline per year between CKD and non-CKD patients 1 year after RDN [20]. A sub-analysis of only those subjects with data on both baseline and 36-month BP data confirmed these results in terms of eGFR and blood-pressure-lowering efficacy [20]. The magnitude of office and 24-h ambulatory BP reduction was similar in patients with CKD stages 3a and 3b compared to patients without CKD.seGFR remained stable and the rate of adverse renal events was low (less than 1.0%).

Data from the Erlanger Registry, a single-centre study, show similar results. With the exception of rare local adverse events, no safety signals were observed. Similar reductions in 24-h, daytime and night-time ambulatory BP, as well as office BP, have been found in patients with and without CKD at any time point up to 12 months [25].

A meta-analysis of 11 single-centre studies including 238 patients with CKD stages 2–5 showed a sustained reduction in office and 24-h ambulatory BP between baseline and 24 months after RDN [16]. The meta-analysis found a low incidence of complications: haematoma 2.9% (7/238, $p = 0.206$) and femoral pseudoaneurysm (1.3%, 3/238, $p = 0.07$) [16].

The effect of RDN on BP in patients with CKD was recently investigated in a multicentre prospective, sham-controlled, randomized, blinded, investigator-initiated trial (the RDN-CKD study, Clingov: NCT04264403) [26]. The study included 25 randomized patients with CKD stages 3a and 3b, but was stopped prematurely due to difficulties with recruitment during the pandemic. No safety

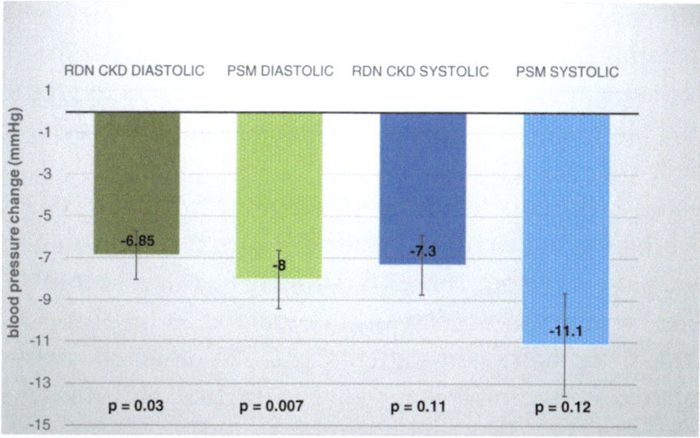

Fully coloured: Sham controlled RCT RDN-CKD. Delta Baseline to 6 months after RDN, n = 10 RDN group, n = 10 sham group
Dotted: PSM analysis of the RADIANCE Program: Delta Baseline to2 months after RDN, n = 14 RDN group, n = 12 sham group and

p-value ist given for difference of change in BP between baseline and 2 months (PSM) or 6 months (RDN-CKD) after RDN in thetreatment compared to the sham group, X+SEM are given

Fig. 2 Change in sham-corrected daytime diastolic and systolic BP after ultrasound-based renal denervation
Fully coloured: **Sham-controlled RCT RDN-CKD. Delta Baseline to 6 months after RDN, *n* = 10 RDN group, *n* = 10 sham group**
Dotted: **PSM analysis of the RADIANCE Program: Delta Baseline to 2 months after RDN, *n* = 14 RDN group, *n* = 12 sham group and *P*-value is given for difference of change in BP between baseline and 2 months (PSM) or 6 months (RDN-CKD) after RDN in the treatment compared to the sham group, X + SEM are given**

concerns were associated with ultrasound-based RDN in the study [26]. RDN was documented to reduce diastolic BP in particular under ambulatory and office BP conditions (Fig. 2).

A propensity-score-matching analysis of the RADIANCE clinical trial programme, which used ultrasound-based RDN in patients with mild CKD stage 3 (eGFR 40–60 mL/min/1.73 m^2) confirmed these results, particularly with respect to the diastolic BP reduction. Patients receiving RDN experienced a greater reduction in BP than the matched sham patients (Fig. 2).

The Safety and Efficacy of RDN in Patients with End-Stage Kidney Disease

In patients with advanced CKD, we encounter various procedural challenges. These patients often display very small or atrophic renal arteries [27], a finding that has been confirmed by a case series of RDN treatment in patients with ESKD [11]. Second-generation RDN catheters have been proven effective in sham-controlled trials and can be applied to treat renal arteries with an internal diameter of 3–8 mm [18]. In 2011, we successfully treated a patient with ESRD, without any complications, achieving excellent BP reduction [28]. Subsequently, two case series involving a total of 18 patients from different RDN sites [11, 29] confirmed the safety and efficacy of RDN in patients undergoing chronic haemodialysis. A recently published study of 14 dialysis patients (seven on haemodialysis and seven on peritoneal dialysis) showed that RDN treatment was equally safe and effective for both groups of patients [30]. RDN did not alter dialysis treatment schedules, and there were no reports of acute intradialytic hypotension [30].

In a proof-of-concept study, patients with ESKD showed no major safety issues. The study reported a reduction in office systolic BP at 3, 6 and 12 months after RDN in the nine treated patients (from 166 ± 16.0 mmHg to 148 ± 11 mmHg, 150 ± 14 mmHg and 138 ± 17 mmHg, respectively) compared to baseline. No change was observed in the three untreated patients [11]. Sympathetic nerve activity, as assessed by microneurography, was reduced in two patients who underwent repeat measurements [11]. In another study, a similar reduction in 24-h ambulatory BP 6 months after RDN was observed while all haemodialysis parameters remained constant and antihypertensive medication was unchanged [29].

A randomized controlled trial in patients with ESKD on haemodialysis and treatment-resistant hypertension also found no significant peri-procedural complication of RDN. The study compared the BP-lowering efficacy up to 1 year after RDN (12 patients) with the BP effect of medical treatment (12 patients) [31]. The average number of antihypertensive medications remained stable throughout the study [31]. Systolic and diastolic office BP and 24-h ambulatory BP showed early and sustained reductions after RDN (24-h ambulatory systolic BP: baseline: 175 ± 11 mmHg, 12 months after RDN: 149 ± 17 mmHg) [31].

Potential Nephroprotective Effects of RDN

To date, three single-centre observational studies from independent research groups have shown evidence that RDN attenuates and even halts the progressive loss of renal function in patients with CKD (Table 1).

It remains unclear whether the observed beneficial effects are purely related to the BP reduction and/or to the interruption of the sympathetic drive to the kidneys. Overall, definitive evidence that RDN attenuates the progressive decline in renal function in patients with CKD is still lacking.

Intensive research is ongoing in this area. The RDN ADPKD study (Clingov: NCT05460169) is currently investigating safety, reduction in BP and renal outcome

Table 1 Renal function after RDN: data from three single-centre observational studies

Study	Number of patients, patient characteristics	eGFR after RDN	eGFR years before RDN	Albuminuria after RDN
Hering et al. [24]	15 patients with resistant hypertension, stage 3–4 CKD	Stabilization of eGFR 12 months after RDN	Not assessed	UACR tended to gradually decrease after RDN (not significant)
Ott et al. [33]	27 patients with resistant hypertension, stage 3 CKD	Stabilization of eGFR 12 months after RDN	Less decline of eGFR compared to the eGFR decline the last 3 years prior to RDN	Reduction in albuminuria after RDN in patients with elevated UACR
Hering et al. [34]	46 patients with resistant hypertension, stage 3 CKD	eGFR increased at 3 months and remained unchanged at 6, 12 months and 24 months post procedure	Decline in eGFR from months 60 to 12 months and from 12 months to baseline prior to RDN	Not assessed
Kiuchi et al. [23]	30 patients with resistant hypertension, stage 2–4 CKD	eGFR increased from baseline after RDN, the difference remained significant at all time points through the end of follow-up at 24 months	Not assessed	UACR was lower 3 month after RDN compared to baseline, decrease was sustained until the 24th month after RDN

CKD chronic kidney disease, *eGFR* estimated glomerular filtration rate, *RDN* renal denervation, *UACR* urine albumin creatinine ratio

parameters (e.g. cyst growth by MRI and measured GFR). The study uses ultrasound-based RDN in patients with autosomal-dominant polycystic kidney disease with a follow-up period of 3 years.

Conclusion

Clinical trials and observational studies in patients with CKD have found clinically meaningful reductions in systolic and diastolic BP over 3 years after RDN, without revealing any safety concern. Consequently, RDN may represent a promising additional treatment option for patients with CKD and uncontrolled hypertension. Further randomized controlled data are needed to support these findings, particularly in patients with advanced CKD stages.

As the ESH 2023 [10] and ESC 2024 [9] guidelines do not, in general, recommend RDN for patients with an eGFR of less than 40 ml/min/1.73^2, due to lack of data and not due to any safety concerns, an individualized approach in patients with CKD and uncontrolled hypertension is advisable. Most recently, data have become available [26, 32] that support the application of RDN on an individual basis in patients with CKD and uncontrolled hypertension. As recommended by the guidelines, patient preference should be incorporated into shared decision-making, and RDN should only be performed in specialized excellence centres with extensive experience in RDN.

References

1. Ott C, Schmieder RE. Diagnosis and treatment of arterial hypertension 2021. Kidney Int. 2022;101(1):36–46.
2. Sarafidis P, Schmieder R, Burnier M, Persu A, Januszewicz A, Halimi JM, et al. A European Renal Association (ERA) synopsis for nephrology practice of the 2023 European Society of Hypertension (ESH) guidelines for the management of arterial hypertension. Nephrol Dial Transplant. 2024;39(6):929–43.
3. DiBona GF, Esler M. Translational medicine: the antihypertensive effect of renal denervation. Am J Physiol Regul Integr Comp Physiol. 2010;298(2):R245–53.
4. Esler MD, Krum H, Schlaich M, Schmieder RE, Bohm M, Sobotka PA. Renal sympathetic denervation for treatment of drug-resistant hypertension: one-year results from the Symplicity HTN-2 randomized, controlled trial. Circulation. 2012;126(25):2976–82.
5. Kandzari DE, Bhatt DL, Brar S, Devireddy CM, Esler M, Fahy M, et al. Predictors of blood pressure response in the SYMPLICITY HTN-3 trial. Eur Heart J. 2015;36(4):219–27.
6. Bhatt DL, Kandzari DE, O'Neill WW, D'Agostino R, Flack JM, Katzen BT, et al. A controlled trial of renal denervation for resistant hypertension. N Engl J Med. 2014;370(15):1393–401.
7. Schmieder RE. Renal denervation–a valid treatment option despite SYMPLICITY HTN-3. Nat Rev Cardiol. 2014;11(11):638.
8. Vukadinovic D, Lauder L, Kandzari DE, Bhatt DL, Kirtane AJ, Edelman ER, et al. Effects of catheter-based renal denervation in hypertension: a systematic review and meta-analysis. Circulation. 2024;150:1599.
9. McEvoy JW, McCarthy CP, Bruno RM, Brouwers S, Canavan MD, Ceconi C, et al. ESC guidelines for the management of elevated blood pressure and hypertension. Eur Heart J. 2024;45(38):3912–4018.
10. Mancia G, Kreutz R, Brunstrom M, Burnier M, Grassi G, Januszewicz A, et al. 2023 ESH guidelines for the management of arterial hypertension the task force for the management of arterial hypertension of the European Society of Hypertension: endorsed by the International Society of Hypertension (ISH) and the European Renal Association (ERA). J Hypertens. 2023;41(12):1874–2071.
11. Schlaich MP, Bart B, Hering D, Walton A, Marusic P, Mahfoud F, et al. Feasibility of catheter-based renal nerve ablation and effects on sympathetic nerve activity and blood pressure in patients with end-stage renal disease. Int J Cardiol. 2013;168(3):2214–20.
12. Veelken R, Schmieder RE. Renal denervation–implications for chronic kidney disease. Nat Rev Nephrol. 2014;10(6):305–13.
13. Grassi G, Biffi A, Seravalle G, Bertoli S, Airoldi F, Corrao G, et al. Sympathetic nerve traffic overactivity in chronic kidney disease: a systematic review and meta-analysis. J Hypertens. 2021;39(3):408–16.
14. Esler MD, Osborn JW, Schlaich MP. Sympathetic pathophysiology in hypertension origins: the path to renal denervation. Hypertension. 2024;81(6):1194–205.
15. Kidney Disease: Improving global outcomes CKDWG. KDIGO 2024 clinical practice guideline for the evaluation and management of chronic kidney disease. Kidney Int. 2024;105(4S):S117–314.
16. Xia M, Liu T, Chen D, Huang Y. Efficacy and safety of renal denervation for hypertension in patients with chronic kidney disease: a meta-analysis. Int J Hyperth. 2021;38(1):732–42.

17. Barbato E, Azizi M, Schmieder RE, Lauder L, Bohm M, Brouwers S, et al. Renal denervation in the management of hypertension in adults. A clinical consensus statement of the ESC Council on hypertension and the European Association of Percutaneous Cardiovascular Interventions (EAPCI). Eur Heart J. 2023;44:1313.
18. Lauder L, Kandzari DE, Luscher TF, Mahfoud F. Renal denervation in the management of hypertension. EuroIntervention. 2024;20(8):e467–e78.
19. Townsend RR, Walton A, Hettrick DA, Hickey GL, Weil J, Sharp ASP, et al. Review and meta-analysis of renal artery damage following percutaneous renal denervation with radiofrequency renal artery ablation. EuroIntervention. 2020;16(1):89–96.
20. Ott C, Mahfoud F, Mancia G, Narkiewicz K, Ruilope LM, Fahy M, et al. Renal denervation in patients with versus without chronic kidney disease: results from the global SYMPLICITY registry with follow-up data of 3 years. Nephrol Dial Transplant. 2022;37(2):304–10.
21. Mahfoud F, Kandzari DE, Townsend RR, Kario K, Weber MA, Schmieder RE, Tsioufis K, Parmari G, Uretskyj S, Gibsonk M, Liu M, McKennal P, Böhm M. Tct-481 renal artery Imaging through long-term follow-up following radiofrequency renal denervation: Results from the spyral clinical trial program. J Am Coll Cardiol. 2024;84(18 Suppl):B157.
22. Kalra PA, Guo H, Kausz AT, Gilbertson DT, Liu J, Chen SC, et al. Atherosclerotic renovascular disease in United States patients aged 67 years or older: risk factors, revascularization, and prognosis. Kidney Int. 2005;68(1):293–301.
23. Kiuchi MG, Graciano ML, Carreira MA, Kiuchi T, Chen S, Lugon JR. Long-term effects of renal sympathetic denervation on hypertensive patients with mild to moderate chronic kidney disease. J Clin Hypertens (Greenwich). 2016;18(3):190–6.
24. Hering D, Mahfoud F, Walton AS, Krum H, Lambert GW, Lambert EA, et al. Renal denervation in moderate to severe CKD. J Am Soc Nephrol. 2012;23(7):1250–7.
25. Gunes-Altan M, Schmid A, Ott C, Bosch A, Pietschner R, Schiffer M, et al. Blood pressure reduction after renal denervation in patients with or without chronic kidney disease. Clin Kidney J. 2024;17(1):sfad237.
26. Kannenkeril DS, R.E., Böhm M, Mahfoud FR, LC, Stegbauer J, der v, Giet MS, M, Veelken R, Uder M, Schmid A. Renal denervation is effective in reducing blood pressure in patients with ckd: results of a multicenter, prospective, randomized, sham- controlled, blinded, investigator-initiated trial. J Am Soc Nephrol. 2024;35(10S):10.1681. https://doi.org/10.1681/ASN.20246pzzaq23.
27. Manaktala R, Tafur-Soto JD, White CJ. Renal artery stenosis in the patient with hypertension: prevalence, impact and management. Integr Blood Press Control. 2020;13:71–82.
28. Ott C, Schmid A, Ditting T, Sobotka PA, Veelken R, Uder M, et al. Renal denervation in a hypertensive patient with end-stage renal disease and small arteries: a direction for future research. J Clin Hypertens (Greenwich). 2012;14(11):799–801.
29. Ott C, Schmid A, Ditting T, Veelken R, Uder M, Schmieder RE. Effects of renal denervation on blood pressure in hypertensive patients with end-stage renal disease: a single centre experience. Clin Exp Nephrol. 2019;23(6):749–55.
30. Gangemi CGA, Ortalda V, Tavella D, Caletti C, Fezzi S, Bianco B, De Tomi E, Gambaro G, Ribichini FL. Renal denervation in dialysis patients: long-term outcomes in a real-world setting. Clin Kidney J. 2025;18:sfaf149.
31. Scalise F, Sole A, Singh G, Sorropago A, Sorropago G, Ballabeni C, et al. Renal denervation in patients with end-stage renal disease and resistant hypertension on long-term haemodialysis. J Hypertens. 2020;38(5):936–42.
32. Schlaich M, Mahfoud F, Narkiewicz K, Ruilope L, Sharif F, Ribichini FL, Böhm M. Radiofrequency renal denervation in patients with severe CKD, including patients on dialysis: analysis from the global SYMPLICITY registry DEFINE. J Am Soc Nephrol. 2024;TH-PO1178:35(10S). https://doi.org/10.1681/ASN.2024fzrm66ak.
33. Ott C, Mahfoud F, Schmid A, Toennes SW, Ewen S, Ditting T, et al. Renal denervation preserves renal function in patients with chronic kidney disease and resistant hypertension. J Hypertens. 2015;33(6):1261–6.
34. Hering D, Marusic P, Duval J, Sata Y, Head GA, Denton KM, et al. Effect of renal denervation on kidney function in patients with chronic kidney disease. Int J Cardiol. 2017;232:93–7.

MIX
Papier aus verantwortungsvollen Quellen
Paper from responsible sources
FSC® C105338

If you have any concerns about our products,
you can contact us on
ProductSafety@springernature.com

In case Publisher is established outside the EU,
the EU authorized representative is:
Springer Nature Customer Service Center GmbH
Europaplatz 3, 69115 Heidelberg, Germany

Printed by Libri Plureos GmbH
in Hamburg, Germany